Chemical Speciation of Organic and Inorganic Components of Environmental and Biological Interest in Natural Fluids

Chemical Speciation of Organic and Inorganic Components of Environmental and Biological Interest in Natural Fluids: Behaviour, Interaction and Sequestration

Special Issue Editors

Francesco Crea
Alberto Pettignano

MDPI • Basel • Beijing • Wuhan • Barcelona • Belgrade • Manchester • Tokyo • Cluj • Tianjin

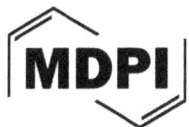

Special Issue Editors
Francesco Crea
University of Messina
Italy

Alberto Pettignano
University of Palermo
Italy

Editorial Office
MDPI
St. Alban-Anlage 66
4052 Basel, Switzerland

This is a reprint of articles from the Special Issue published online in the open access journal *Molecules* (ISSN 1420-3049) (available at: https://www.mdpi.com/journal/molecules/special_issues/chemical_speciation_natural_fluids).

For citation purposes, cite each article independently as indicated on the article page online and as indicated below:

LastName, A.A.; LastName, B.B.; LastName, C.C. Article Title. *Journal Name* **Year**, *Article Number*, Page Range.

ISBN 978-3-03928-452-8 (Pbk)
ISBN 978-3-03928-453-5 (PDF)

© 2020 by the authors. Articles in this book are Open Access and distributed under the Creative Commons Attribution (CC BY) license, which allows users to download, copy and build upon published articles, as long as the author and publisher are properly credited, which ensures maximum dissemination and a wider impact of our publications.

The book as a whole is distributed by MDPI under the terms and conditions of the Creative Commons license CC BY-NC-ND.

Contents

About the Special Issue Editors vii

Francesco Crea and Alberto Pettignano
Special Issue "Chemical Speciation of Organic and Inorganic Components of Environmental and Biological Interest in Natural Fluids:
Behaviour, Interaction and Sequestration"
Reprinted from: *Molecules* 2020, 25, 826, doi:10.3390/molecules25040826 1

Giuseppe Arena and Enrico Rizzarelli
Zn^{2+} Interaction with Amyloid-B: Affinity and Speciation
Reprinted from: *Molecules* 2019, 24, 2796, doi:10.3390/molecules24152796 5

Cezary Grochowski, Eliza Blicharska, Jacek Baj, Aleksandra Mierzwińska, Karolina Brzozowska, Alicja Forma and Ryszard Maciejewski
Serum iron, Magnesium, Copper, and Manganese Levels in Alcoholism: A Systematic Review
Reprinted from: *Molecules* 2019, 24, 1361, doi:10.3390/molecules24071361 25

Xiaoping Yu, Chenglong Liu, Yafei Guo and Tianlong Deng
Speciation Analysis of Trace Arsenic, Mercury, Selenium and Antimony in Environmental and Biological Samples Based on Hyphenated Techniques
Reprinted from: *Molecules* 2019, 24, 926, doi:10.3390/molecules24050926 39

Francesco Crea, Concetta De Stefano, Anna Irto, Gabriele Lando, Stefano Materazzi, Demetrio Milea, Alberto Pettignano and Silvio Sammartano
Understanding the Solution Behavior of Epinephrine in the Presence of Toxic Cations:
A Thermodynamic Investigation in Different Experimental Conditions
Reprinted from: *Molecules* 2020, 25, 511, doi:10.3390/molecules25030511 63

Anna Irto, Paola Cardiano, Salvatore Cataldo, Karam Chand, Rosalia Maria Cigala, Francesco Crea, Concetta De Stefano, Giuseppe Gattuso, Nicola Muratore, Alberto Pettignano, Silvio Sammartano and M. Amélia Santos
Speciation Studies of Bifunctional 3-Hydroxy-4-Pyridinone Ligands in the Presence of Zn^{2+} at Different Ionic Strengths and Temperatures
Reprinted from: *Molecules* 2019, 24, 4084, doi:10.3390/molecules24224084 89

András Ozsváth, Linda Bíró, Eszter Márta Nagy, Péter Buglyó, Daniele Sanna and Etelka Farkas
Trends and Exceptions in the Interaction of Hydroxamic Acid Derivatives of Common Di- and Tripeptides with Some 3d and 4d Metal Ions in Aqueous Solution
Reprinted from: *Molecules* 2019, 24, 3941, doi:10.3390/molecules24213941 119

Roberta Risoluti, Giuseppina Gullifa, Elena Carcassi, Francesca Buiarelli, Li W. Wo and Stefano Materazzi
Modeling Solid State Stability for Speciation: A Ten-Year Long Study
Reprinted from: *Molecules* 2019, 24, 3013, doi:10.3390/molecules24163013 145

Dorota Adamczyk-Szabela, Katarzyna Lisowska, Zdzisława Romanowska-Duda and Wojciech M. Wolf
Associated Effects of Cadmium and Copper Alter the Heavy Metals Uptake by *Melissa Officinalis*
Reprinted from: *Molecules* 2019, 24, 2458, doi:10.3390/molecules24132458 155

Cezary Grochowski, Eliza Blicharska, Jacek Bogucki, Jędrzej Proch, Aleksandra Mierzwińska, Jacek Baj, Jakub Litak, Arkadiusz Podkowiński, Jolanta Flieger, Grzegorz Teresiński, Ryszard Maciejewski, Przemysław Niedzielski and Piotr Rzymski
Increased Aluminum Content in Certain Brain Structures is Correlated with Higher Silicon Concentration in Alcoholic Use Disorder
Reprinted from: *Molecules* **2019**, *24*, 1721, doi:10.3390/molecules24091721 . . . . **167**

Katarzyna Karaś and Marcin Frankowski
Analysis of Hazardous Elements in Children Toys: Multi-Elemental Determination by Chromatography and Spectrometry Methods
Reprinted from: *Molecules* **2018**, *23*, 3017, doi:10.3390/molecules23113017 . . . . **179**

Zhou Tong, Jinsheng Duan, Yancan Wu, Qiongqiong Liu, Qibao He, Yanhong Shi, Linsheng Yu and Haiqun Cao
Evaluation of Highly Detectable Pesticides Sprayed in *Brassica napus* L.: Degradation Behavior and Risk Assessment for Honeybees
Reprinted from: *Molecules* **2018**, *23*, 2482, doi:10.3390/molecules23102482 . . . . **197**

About the Special Issue Editors

Francesco Crea (Professor) graduated in Chemistry with full honors in July 1997 at University of Messina. In November 1997, he obtained his Professional Qualification of Chemist according to Italian law. He conducted his research doctorate in Chemical Sciences as a three-year course in 1998–2001 at the University of Messina, and in 2002, was awarded his Ph.D. In September 2002, he began work as researcher in the Academic Scientific-Disciplinary Sector CHIM01 of Analytical Chemistry at the Department of Inorganic Chemistry, Analytical Chemistry, and Physical Chemistry of University of Messina. In December 2010, he was appointed Associate Professor at the same Academic Scientific-Disciplinary Sector at the Department of Chemical Science of the University of Messina. His research is mainly focused on the study of the thermodynamics of solutions with particular reference to 1. Speciation of polyelectrolytes: acid–base properties and complexing ability towards different classes of organic and inorganic ligands; 2. Modeling in HPLC: modeling of the separation of linear and branched polyamines by IC chromatography; 3. Speciation of UO_2^{2+} in different ionic media, interaction with carboxylic acids at low molecular weight and formation of hydrolytic heterometal species; 4. Determination of the solubility and activity coefficients of different classes of organic ligands in different ionic media. He is co-author of 100 scientific papers published in international journals and more than 80 contributions to national and international congresses.

Alberto Pettignano (Professor) graduated in Chemistry in July 2000 with cum laude at the University of Messina. In 11/2000, he obtained his Professional Qualification of Chemist, according to Italian law. In 2004, he was awarded his Ph.D. in Chemistry, curriculum Analytical Chemistry from the University of Messina. He was a visiting Ph.D. student during Jan/2003 to Mar/2003 in the laboratories of Professor Gregory R. Choppin (R.O. Lawton Distinguished Professor of Chemistry, emeritus), Department of Chemistry and Biochemistry, Florida State University, Tallahassee. From 2008, he has been Researcher of the Academic Scientific-Disciplinary Sector CHIM01 (Analytical Chemistry) at the Department of Physics and Chemistry of the University of Palermo. In 2018, he was Associate Professor of the Academic Scientific-Disciplinary Sector CHIM01 (Analytical Chemistry) at the Department of Physics and Chemistry of the University of Palermo. His main research topics are summarized in the following points. 1. Anionic coordination: Interaction of protonated polyamines with polycarboxylates, sulfate, fluoride, and carbonate; 2. Speciation of ligands of biological and environmental interest: acid–base equilibria of phytate and of ATP in aqueous solutions containing different ionic media and at different ionic strengths and the dependence of thermodynamic parameters on ionic strength using several models; 3. Speciation of uranyl ion in presence of ligands of biological interest: thermodynamic parameters of hydrolytic species of uranyl ion and of complex species formed with polyamine, polyaminocarboxylates, amino acids, and ATP; 4. Setting up of suitable chemical models for the study of the acid–base properties of natural and synthetic polyelectrolytes and for their complexation capability towards metal ions; 5. Speciation of organometal compounds of tin(IV) and of mercury(II); 6. Sequestration capability of organic ligands towards several transition metal ions: interaction of phytate with Pd^{2+} ion; interaction of synthetic polyelectrolytes (polyacrylates and polymethacrylates) with Cd^{2+} and Cu^{2+} ions, etc.; 7. Natural and synthetic adsorbent materials for the organic and inorganic pollutants removal from aqueous solutions. He is reviewer of several scientific journals. He is co-author of 51 articles published on International ISI journals. He has presented the results of his research at numerous national and international meetings.

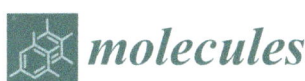

Editorial

Special Issue "Chemical Speciation of Organic and Inorganic Components of Environmental and Biological Interest in Natural Fluids: Behaviour, Interaction and Sequestration"

Francesco Crea [1],* and Alberto Pettignano [2],*

1. Dipartimento di Scienze Chimiche, Università di Messina, Viale Ferdinando Stagno d'Alcontres, 31, I-98166 Messina (Vill. S. Agata), Italy
2. Dipartimento di Fisica e Chimica, Università di Palermo, Viale delle Scienze, I-90128 Palermo, Italy
* Correspondence: fcrea@unime.it (F.C.); alberto.pettignano@unipa.it (A.P.)

Received: 11 February 2020; Accepted: 12 February 2020; Published: 13 February 2020

Several different definitions were in the past proposed to describe the term chemical speciation, and some of them were accepted from the scientific community. Some examples of such definitions are as follows: "Chemical speciation can be defined as the process of identification and quantification of the different forms or phases in which an element is present in a material" or as "the description of quantities, types of species, forms or phases present in a material" [1,2].

Many authors used the term chemical speciation to explain different reaction types: (i) the chemical reactions that transform a set of metal compounds in a sample into another set of components, (ii) the assembly of compounds containing a given component that are present in a sample, and (iii) the process of identification and quantification of the metallic species present in a sample.

The International Union of Pure and Applied Chemistry (IUPAC) sums up that "speciation" denotes to "the distribution of an element amongst defined chemical species in a system", while the process leading to the quantitative estimation of the content of different species is called speciation analysis [3], as also reported in Ref. [4].

Over the last 2–3 decades, an increase in interest from chemists, biochemists, and biologists in techniques for chemical speciation studies has been observed, since it is now established that both bioavailability and toxicity are critically dependent on the chemical form of the given element in a given environment.

The chemical speciation now involves various sectors of the sciences, from chemistry, to biology, to biochemistry, to environmental sciences, since, as it is well known, the total concentration of an inorganic or organic component (metal or ligand) in a multicomponent natural system (fresh water, sea water, biological fluids, soil, etc.) provides insufficient information to deeply understand its behavior in those contests.

Biochemical and toxicological investigation has shown that, for living organisms, the chemical form of a specific element, or the oxidation state in which that element is introduced into the environment, is crucial, as well as the quantities [5]. Therefore, to get information on the activity of specific elements in the environment, more particularly for those in contact with living organisms, it is necessary to determine not only the total content of the element but also to gain an indication of its individual chemical and physical form.

As an example, in the case of metal toxicity, it is generally accepted that the free (hydrated) metal ion is the form most toxic to aquatic life. Strongly complexed metal, or metal associated with colloidal particles, is much less toxic [6].

Chemical speciation has been presenting great relevance, leading to the development of various methods of analysis used in the areas of health, food quality control, and the environment.

Metals and metalloids are present in all compartments of our environment and the environmental pathways of these elements are of high importance in relation to their toxicity towards flora and fauna. Their concentration levels, mobility, and transformation and accumulation processes in the ecosystem depend on parameters such as pH, redox conditions, oxidation states, temperature, the presence of organic matter, and microbiological activity. All these factors strongly influence the biogeochemical cycles of elements in our environment.

For this reason, as guest editors, we thought about proposing the Special Issue: "Chemical Speciation of Organic and Inorganic Components of Environmental and Biological Interest in Natural Fluids: Behaviour, Interaction, and Sequestration" in the Molecules journal. The primary goal was to involve scientists from different sectors who could propose scientific contributions that, even with different approaches, involve the sector of chemical speciation and speciation analysis.

The Special Issue had satisfactory feedback from researchers, with contributions having cross-field character and being of interest for different industrial, pharmaceutical, chemical, and biological fields [7–17].

The Special Issue is accessible through the following link: https://www.mdpi.com/journal/molecules/special_issues/chemical_speciation_natural_fluids

As guest editors for this Special Issue, we would like to thank all the authors and co-authors for their contributions and all the reviewers for their efforts in carefully evaluating the manuscripts. Moreover, we would like to appreciate the editorial office of the Molecules journal for their kind assistance in preparing this Special Issue and, in particular, Ms. Katie Zhang, managing editor of the "Analytical Chemistry" section, for her precious help during the various stages of the organization and programming of the Special Issue.

Funding: This research received no external funding.

Conflicts of Interest: The authors declare no conflict of interest.

References

1. Ure, A.M. Trace element speciation in soils, soil extracts and solutions. *Microchim. Acta* **1991**, *104*, 49–57. [CrossRef]
2. Ure, A.M.; Davidson, C.M. *Chemical Speciation in the Environment*, 2nd ed.; University of Strathdyde: Glasgow, Scotland, 2001.
3. Templeton, D.M.; Ariese, F.; Cornelis, R.; Danielsson, L.-G.; Muntau, H.; van Leeuwen, H.P.; Lobinski, R. IUPAC guidelines for terms related to speciation of trace elements. *Pure Appl. Chem.* **2000**, *72*, 453–1470.
4. Sperling, M.; Karst, U. Advances in Speciation Techniques and Methodology. *Trends Anal. Chem.* **2018**, *104*, 1–3. [CrossRef]
5. Liu, W.X.; Li, X.D.; Shen, Z.G.; Wang, D.C.; Wai, O.W.H.; Li, Y.S. Multivariate statistical study of heavy metal enrichment in sediments of the Pearl River estuary. *Environ. Pollut.* **2003**, *121*, 377–388. [CrossRef]
6. Florence, T.M.; Batley, G.E.; Benes, P. Chemical Speciation in Natural Waters. *C. R C Crit. Rev. Anal. Chem.* **1980**, *9*, 219–296. [CrossRef]
7. Crea, F.; De Stefano, C.; Irto, A.; Lando, G.; Materazzi, S.; Milea, D.; Pettignano, A.; Sammartano, S. Understanding the Solution Behavior of Epinephrine in the Presence of Toxic Cations: A Thermodynamic Investigation in Different Experimental Conditions. *Molecules* **2020**, *25*, 511. [CrossRef] [PubMed]
8. Irto, A.; Cardiano, P.; Cataldo, S.; Chand, K.; Cigala, R.M.; Crea, F.; De Stefano, C.; Gattuso, G.; Muratore, M.; Pettignano, A.; et al. Speciation Studies of Bifunctional 3-Hydroxy-4-Pyridinone Ligands in the Presence of Zn^{2+} at Different Ionic Strengths and Temperatures. *Molecules* **2019**, *24*, 4084. [CrossRef] [PubMed]
9. Ozsváth, A.; Bíró, L.; Nagy, E.M.; Buglyó, P.; Sanna, D.; Farkas, E. Trends and Exceptions in the Interaction of Hydroxamic Acid Derivatives of Common Di- and Tripeptides with Some 3d and 4d Metal Ions in Aqueous Solution. *Molecules* **2019**, *24*, 3941. [CrossRef] [PubMed]
10. Risoluti, R.; Gullifa, G.; Carcassi, E.; Buiarelli, F.; Wo, L.W.; Materazzi, M. Modeling Solid State Stability for Speciation: A Ten-Year Long Study. *Molecules* **2019**, *24*, 3013. [CrossRef] [PubMed]

11. Adamczyk-Szabela, D.; Lisowska, K.; Romanowska-Duda, Z.; Wolf, W.M. Associated Effects of Cadmium and Copper Alter the Heavy Metals Uptake by Melissa Officinalis. *Molecules* **2019**, *24*, 2458. [CrossRef] [PubMed]
12. Grochowski, C.; Blicharska, E.; Bogucki, J.; Proch, J.; Mierzwińska, A.; Baj, J.; Litak, J.; Podkowiński, A.; Flieger, J.; Teresiński, G.; et al. Increased Aluminum Content in Certain Brain Structures is Correlated with Higher Silicon Concentration in Alcoholic Use Disorder. *Molecules* **2019**, *24*, 1721. [CrossRef] [PubMed]
13. Karaś, K.; Frankowski, M. Analysis of Hazardous Elements in Children Toys: Multi-Elemental Determination by Chromatography and Spectrometry Methods. *Molecules* **2018**, *23*, 3017. [CrossRef] [PubMed]
14. Tong, Z.; Duan, J.; Wu, Y.; Liu, Q.; He, Q.; Shi, Y.; Yu, L.; Cao, H. Evaluation of Highly Detectable Pesticides Sprayed in *Brassica napus* L.: Degradation Behavior and Risk Assessment for Honeybees. *Molecules* **2018**, *23*, 2482. [CrossRef] [PubMed]
15. Arena, G.; Rizzarelli, E. Zn^{2+} Interaction with Amyloid-B: Affinity and Speciation. *Molecules* **2019**, *24*, 2796. [CrossRef] [PubMed]
16. Grochowski, C.; Blicharska, E.; Baj, J.; Mierzwińska, A.; Brzozowska, K.; Forma, A.; Maciejewski, R. Serum iron, Magnesium, Copper, and Manganese Levels in Alcoholism: A Systematic Review. *Molecules* **2019**, *24*, 1361. [CrossRef] [PubMed]
17. Yu, X.; Liu, C.; Guo, Y.; Deng, T. Speciation Analysis of Trace Arsenic, Mercury, Selenium and Antimony in Environmental and Biological Samples Based on Hyphenated Techniques. *Molecules* **2019**, *24*, 926. [CrossRef] [PubMed]

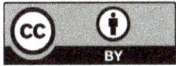

© 2020 by the authors. Licensee MDPI, Basel, Switzerland. This article is an open access article distributed under the terms and conditions of the Creative Commons Attribution (CC BY) license (http://creativecommons.org/licenses/by/4.0/).

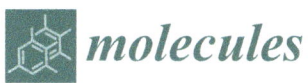

Review

Zn^{2+} Interaction with Amyloid-β: Affinity and Speciation

Giuseppe Arena [1,2,*] and Enrico Rizzarelli [1,2,3]

1. Department of Chemical Sciences, University of Catania, Viale Andrea Doria 6, 95125 Catania, Italy
2. Consorzio Interuniversitario di Ricerca in Chimica dei Metalli nei Sistemi Biologici (C.I.R.C.M.S.B.), 70125 Bari, Italy
3. Institute of Crystallography—CNR—UOS Catania, Via Paolo Gaifami 9, 95126 Catania, Italy
* Correspondence: garena@unict.it; Tel.: +39-(0)95-738-5071

Received: 10 July 2019; Accepted: 29 July 2019; Published: 31 July 2019

Abstract: Conflicting values, obtained by different techniques and often under different experimental conditions have been reported on the affinity of Zn^{2+} for amyloid-β, that is recognized as the major interaction responsible for Alzheimer's disease. Here, we compare the approaches employed so far, i.e., the evaluation of K_d and the determination of the stability constants to quantitatively express the affinity of Zn^{2+} for the amyloid-β peptide, evidencing the pros and cons of the two approaches. We also comment on the different techniques and conditions employed that may lead to divergent data. Through the analysis of the species distribution obtained for two selected examples, we show the implications that the speciation, based on stoichiometric constants rather than on K_d, may have on data interpretation. The paper also demonstrates that the problem is further complicated by the occurrence of multiple equilibria over a relatively narrow pH range.

Keywords: speciation; amyloid-β; Zn^{2+}; affinity

1. Introduction

As of 2018, there were over 50 million people worldwide with dementia, more than 50% of whom lived in low and middle-income countries. This figure is forecast to double by 2030 (82 million people) and more than triple by 2050 (152 million people). It is estimated that, around the world, there will be a new case every three seconds [1]. Much of this increase will be in rapidly developing and heavily populated regions such as China, India and Latin America. Already 58% of people with dementia live in low and middle-income countries, but by 2050 this will rise to 68% [2]. Dementia primarily affects older people. This is particularly relevant to countries like China, India, and their south Asian and western Pacific neighbors, that have the fastest growing elderly population but also this poses major problems worldwide since the world's population is ageing. Up to the age of 65, dementia develops in only about one person in 1000. The chance of having the condition rises sharply with age to one person in 20 over the age of 65. Over the age of 80, this figure increases to one person in five [3]. As to the economic burden, the total estimated worldwide cost of dementia in 2018 was 1 trillion US $, and this figure is expected to rise to 2 trillion US $ by 2030, which represents more than 1% of global GDP [2].

Noteworthily, according to a 2018 report about two thirds of the 50 million people suffering from dementia have Alzheimer's disease (AD), a progressive and devastating neurodegenerative brain disorder first described in 1906, that is also the most common cause of dementia in elderly people [1]. AD is characterized by the brain deposition of neurofibrillary tangles and senile plaques, a hallmark of this pathological disorder. Plaques consist mainly of insoluble amyloid-β (Aβ) fibril deposits [4–6]. The amyloid peptides (Aβ) are generated by the proteolytic action of α-, β- and γ- secretases on the large transmembrane amyloid precursor protein (APP) [7–12] and contain predominantly forty

(Aβ(1–40)) and forty two (Aβ(1–42)) aminoacid residues; though less abundant, Aβ(1–42) is more neurotoxic than Aβ(1–40) [13–16].

The observation that high concentrations of metal ions are co-localized in the core of Alzheimer's amyloid plaques has generated great interest in the effects of metal ions on β peptide misfolding and aggregation. Exposure to a number of metal ions is considered a risk factor for the onset of the disease; some metal ions accelerate protein aggregation, stabilize amyloid fibrils, and increase the neurotoxic effects of Aβ peptides in vitro [17]. Metal ions belonging to the *d* block like zinc, copper, and iron have been thought to be pathogenic agents in AD owing to the accumulation of these metals in amyloid deposits [18–20] and in the cortical tissues of AD patients [21]. In fact, it has been shown that these metals induce Aβ aggregation [22,23] and fibril formation [24,25].

Thus, it is not surprising that the interaction of transition metal ions with the Aβ peptides has attracted a considerable attention in recent years due to its impact on AD; in particular, a large number of reports, some of which contradicting one another, indicate that Cu and Zn have significant effects on the Aβ peptide aggregation and the stabilization of neurotoxic soluble Aβ oligomers [10]. There is still some debate on whether Aβ aggregation is the cause or only a consequence of AD and whether the oligomers are the toxic species responsible for synaptic dysfunction and neuronal cell loss in AD [26,27]. Lee et al. found that zinc ions are able to more effectively destabilize fibril structures than copper ions; according to this study, Zn^{2+} ions would promote the formation and stability of Aβ oligomers, whereas they reduce the stability of Aβ fibrils [28]. Evidence shows that the presence of Zn^{2+} can avoid [29] or delay the conversion of Aβ(1–40) into fibrils [30] but also rapidly promotes Aβ(1–40) aggregation to oligomeric species [22,31]; Mannini et al. suggest that the latter process results from the redirection of Aβ(1–40) aggregation as a result of intermediate species becoming kinetically trapped and no longer being capable of forming fibrils [32].

Previously we reviewed the affinity of Cu^{2+} to Aβ and examined the implications that a correct speciation may have on the interpretation of data obtained through different techniques [33]. In the present paper, we focus on the coordination of Zn^{2+} to Aβ and discuss the possible implications of species distribution on metal concentration-dependent effects on Aβ aggregates and their toxicities.

2. Zn^{2+} Interaction with Amyloid-β

The complexity of biological systems makes it difficult to quantitate interactions between metal ions and biomolecules directly in vivo. A viable route is to determine the affinity of a metal ion to a biomolecule in vitro and to extend the information obtained in vitro to in vivo conditions; the in vitro study should be carried out in conditions approaching the in vivo conditions as much as the specific technique permits. In our specific case, such a route is severely hampered by the poor solubility of Aβ in water. Consequently, fragments of the whole protein have to be employed which retain/model the binding characteristics of the native molecule; this becomes an even greater challenge when dealing with metal complexes, that often are much less soluble than the biomolecule itself.

2.1. Aβ(1–16)-Peg

Amyloid-β consists of a mixture of peptides containing 39–42 aminoacid residues (see Introduction). The aminoacid sequence of human Aβ(1–42) is reported in Figure 1a.

H_2N-Asp^1-Ala^2-Glu^3-Phe^4-Arg^5-His^6-Asp^7-Ser^8-Gly^9-Tyr^{10}-Glu^{11}-Val^{12}-His^{13}-His^{14}-Glm^{15}-Lys^{16}-Leu^{17}-Val^{18}-Phe^{19}-Phe^{20}-Ala^{21}-Glu^{22}-Asp^{23}-Val^{24}-Gly^{25}-Ser^{26}-Asp^{27}-Lys^{28}-Gly^{29}-Ala^{30}-Ile^{31}-Ile^{32}-Gly^{33}-Leu^{34}-Met^{35}-Val^{36}-Gly^{37}-Gly^{38}-Val^{39}-Val^{40}-Ile^{41}-Ala^{42}-COOH

(a) Human Aβ(1–42).

Figure 1. Cont.

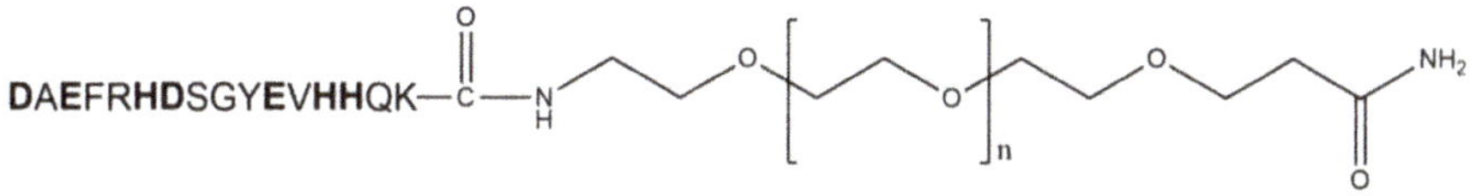

DAEFRHDSGYEVHHQK—C(=O)—NH—CH₂CH₂—O—[CH₂CH₂O]ₙ—CH₂CH₂—O—CH₂CH₂—O—CH₂CH₂—C(=O)—NH₂

(b) Aβ(1–16)-Peg.

Figure 1. Aminoacid sequence of Aβ(1–42) (a) and schematic representation of Aβ(1–16)-PEG (b)

Neither one of the amyloid-β main peptides (Aβ(1–40) and Aβ(1–42)) are soluble enough to allow for an investigation by potentiometry, the technique of choice for a reliable speciation, to see how the species concentration changes with pH or, in more general terms, with the concentration of the titrant. Thus shorter peptides that reproduce and, at least partly, retain the binding characteristics of these longer fragments have to be used. Although there are some discrepancies on the speciation/coordination mode of the most investigated metal ions (i.e., Cu^{2+} and Zn^{2+}) [26,33,34], it is now well-established that in amyloid-β, the metal binding sites are located in the N-terminal hydrophilic region encompassing the amino acid residues 1–16 (Aβ(1–16)) [35,36]. Unfortunately, neither the Cu^{2+} nor Zn^{2+} complexes with the peptide reportedly containing the metal binding sites (i.e., Aβ(1–16)) can be fully characterized in aqueous solution due the formation of precipitates that prevent scanning a wide range of metal:ligand ratios. In order to overcome such a major obstacle, Aβ(1-16) has been derivatized by attaching a polyethylene glycol (PEG) chain to the C-terminus thus rendering the peptide soluble in water. It has been shown that Aβ(1–16)-PEG (Figure 1b) forms with both Cu^{2+} and Zn^{2+} complexes soluble enough to allow for a detailed potentiometric and spectroscopic characterization of the Aβ(1–16)PEG-metal ion systems [34,37]. Donor atoms potentially involved in the coordination to the metal ion are indicated in bold in Figure 1b.

2.2. Zn^{2+} in Alzheimer's Disease

Zinc is an essential nutrient and the second most abundant trace element in the body [38,39]. It has a wide range of biologically relevant functions including the regulation of gene expression, protein synthesis, and cellular signaling [40]. The alteration of zinc homeostasis is involved in neurological diseases such as Alzheimer's disease, Parkinson's disease, and amyotrophic lateral sclerosis. According to some findings, zinc would reduce oxidative stress by binding to thiol groups, decreasing their oxidation [41,42]. Zinc dysregulation is reportedly involved in two types of neuropathology: (i) Alzheimer's disease, and (ii) the so-called 'excitotoxicity' which injures neurons after ischemia, hemorrhage, seizures, or mechanical brain traumas and also affects the rate and severity of AD pathophysiology [43]. Zinc may reach concentration values as high as 1 mM in AD plaques of patients [18]. The role of zinc in amyloid fibrils formation has also been demonstrated by experiments showing that the solubilization of Aβ from post-mortem brain tissue was significantly increased by suitable Zn^{2+} chelators [44]. Although Zn^{2+} binding to Aβ is well established, the effects of such a binding, in terms of metal-dependent aggregation and toxicity, are still controversial. High concentrations promote Aβ-induced toxicity both in vitro [45] and in vivo [46]. According to others, low levels of this metal ion reduce Aβ toxicity and thus exert a neuroprotective effect [47–50]. Thus, zinc would have concentration-dependent effects that may also be linked to the number of Zn^{2+} ions bound to Aβ [34].

3. Zn^{2+} Affinity for Aβ

The key parameter in the interaction of Zn^{2+} with Aβ is the affinity for the ligand(s) of interest. The determination of the stability constants of the complex(es) resulting from the binding of a metal ion (Zn^{2+} in this specific case) to Aβ is the indispensable bridge linking the model to the naturally occurring system. Fortunately, the interest in the formation of metal complexes in aqueous solutions has gone beyond the initial purpose of interpreting the structure and the mechanism of formation of a relatively simple complex in solution. Nowadays, studies of the metal-binding affinity of biologically relevant ligands are ubiquitous in bioinorganic chemistry [34,37,51–56] and are valuable for the information that they can provide about metal speciation.

Knowing the stability constant values allows to have the species distribution over the pH interval of interest as well as to compare Zn^{2+} affinity for Aβ with that of other ligands. This can provide valuable information on the competition of Aβ for other ligands and vice versa [57]. This is considered of particular interest, as it might be possible to create therapeutic drugs for AD that safely target the Aβ-Zn interaction [43,58]. A thorough speciation might even help explaining why Zn^{2+} inhibits the β-aggregation of both Aβ(1–40) and Aβ(1–42) in a concentration-dependent manner (*vide infra*) [29].

3.1. Stability Constant and Speciation

A still debated issue in bioinorganic chemistry is whether metal binding to a given protein site is under thermodynamic or kinetic control [59]. This is a controversial issue as some authors suggest that the metal chemistry of some compartments (e.g., the cytoplasm) is under kinetic control [60], whilst others indicate that metal binding in specific protein sites in vitro is under thermodynamic control [59]. Whatever the situation may be in nature and although the entire process cannot be assumed the summation of the individual steps determining the cascade of events, understanding the thermodynamics of some of the steps involved in the cascade may be crucial to shed light on the entire process. Thus, the thermodynamic characterization of the equilibrium (or the equilibria), eventually reached, becomes the starting point to study a binding process [61]. Unfortunately, the picture for Zn^{2+}-amyloid-β affinity is further complicated by the spread of values (and species) reported in literature for Zn^{2+}-Aβ binding (Table 1) [34,57,62–67].

Table 1. Literature values for Zn^{2+} binding to Aβ fragments.

Aβ Fragment [a]	K_d (μM)	pH	T (°C)	Conc. (μM)	Method	Buffer	Background Salt	Ref.
1–40	5/0.1	7.4	20	-	Radioact. Sat.bind.	TRIS (20mM)	0.1 M NaCl + 1mM $MnCl_2$	62
1–40	3.5	7.4	20	-	Radioact. Sat.bind.	TRIS (50mM)	1 M KCl	63
1–40	300	7.4	n.s.[b]	3	Tyr. fl.	TRIS/HEPES (10 mM)	0.1 M NaCl	64
1–42	57	7.4	n.s.[b]	3	Tyr. fl.	TRIS (10 mM)	0.1 M NaCl	64
1–28	1.1	7.2	20	10	Tyr. fl. Zn/Cu Compet.	Phosphate (10 mM)	none	65
1–40	1.2	7.2	20	50	NMR	Phosphate (10 mM)	none	65
1–28	6.6	7.2	20	10	Tyr. fl. Zn/Cu Compet.	HEPES (10 mM)	none	65
1–16	22/71 [c,d]	7.4	25	20/140 [c]	ITC	HEPES/TRIS (20 mM) [e]	0.1 M NaCl	57
1–28	10/30 [c,d]	7.4	25	20/140 [c]	ITC	HEPES/TRIS (20 mM) [e]	0.1 M NaCl	57
1–40	7/3 [c]	7.4	25	10/70 [c]	ITC	HEPES/TRIS [e] (20 mM) [e]	0.1 M NaCl	57
1–16	14	7.4	n.s.[b]	10	Fl. Zincon Compet.	HEPES (20 mM)	0.1 M NaCl	57
1–28	12	7.4	n.s.[b]	10	Fl. Zincon Compet.	HEPES (20 mM)	0.1 M NaCl	57

Table 1. Cont.

Aβ Fragment [a]	K_d (µM)	pH	T (°C)	Conc. (µM)	Method	Buffer	Background Salt	Ref.
1–40/1–42	7/7	7.4	n.s. [b]	10	Fl. Zincon Compet.	HEPES (20 mM)	0.1 M NaCl	57
1–40	65	7.4	n.s. [b]	4	Tyr. fl.	HEPES (20 mM)	0.1 M NaCl	66
1–42	91	7.4	n.s. [b]	4	Tyr. fl.	HEPES (20 mM)	0.1 M NaCl	66
1–40	60	7.4	n.s. [b]	4	Tyr. fl.	TRIS (10 mM)	0.1 M NaCl	66
1–40	184	7.4	n.s. [b]	4	Tyr. fl.	TRIS (100 mM)	0.1 M NaCl	66
1–40	11/2 [f]	7.3	n.s. [b]	12	Fl. Zincon Compet.	HEPES (50 mM)	0.1 M NaCl	66
1–16-PEG	- [g]	-	25	1–4 (×10³)	Potentiometry	No Buffer	0.2 M KCl	34
1–16	9	7.1	25	- [h]	UV-Vis Compet. [h]	HEPES (50 mM)	none	67

a. Only data for soluble fragments are shown in the table; b. not specified; c. the two values were obtained by using the 'low' and 'high' concentrations shown in the adjacent column; d. the best fit yielded a stoichiometry of about 1.5; e. experiments were also run by using cacodylate buffer; f. the two values were obtained by competition with Zincon after incubation for 3 and 30 min, respectively; g. no value is reported as the best model contains more than one Zn^{2+} complex near neutrality- ten protonation constants are reported; h. determined by UV-Vis competition experiments with a new water-soluble Zn^{2+} chelator-Aβ was added to a solution of the chelator (60 µM) and Zn^{2+} (50 µM), final Aβ/Zn^{2+} ratio was 10/1.

Although the table contains a few entries, these have all been extracted from only half a dozen papers. Compared to the interaction of Aβ fragments with Cu^{2+} [33] the data available for the analogous interaction with Zn^{2+} are relatively scarce. Perhaps the paucity of data has to do with Zn^{2+} being spectroscopically silent. Please note that the data listed in the table concern different Aβ peptides ranging from Aβ (1–16) to Aβ (1–42). This originates from the commonly accepted view that these peptides retain the binding characteristics of the amyloid-β that cannot be investigated due to its scarce solubility.

All the entries listed in the second column are concentration constants and as such must be retained valid only at or near the conditions at which they were determined [68]. Intentionally, no distinction is made between ^cK_d and ^aK_d, i.e., between conditional and apparent constants [26,66,69,70]. It is worth emphasizing, though, that according to the accepted definition the conditional dissociation constant, ^cK_d, is the apparent dissociation constant that depends on the pH value and the ionic background employed while ^aK_d is the apparent dissociation constant measured in a given buffer or in the presence of a competing ligand. ^aK_d can easily be converted to ^cK_d by taking into account the competition with other ligand(s), be it a deliberately introduced competing ligand and/or the buffer, if the buffer forms complexes with the metal ion of interest. However, for the sake of clarity, the footnote of Table 1 specifies whether the value refers to a ^cK_d or a ^aK_d according to the source reference. The reader will appreciate that the values significantly depend on the experimental conditions used.

Despite the efforts and the variety of techniques and methodologies employed for the quantification of the metal-protein dissociation constants K_d, yet there exist significant discrepancies in the literature (Table 1); these may result from the fairly different experimental conditions employed and/or, more likely, from the significantly different concentrations and Zn^{2+}/Aβ ratios explored. The values reported so far range from 1.1 to 300 µM, although there is a general consensus that K_d falls in the low micromolar range. Even the stoichiometry of the interactions of Aβ with metal ions is somewhat elusive; in fact, for Zn^{2+}-Aβ complexes, stoichiometries ranging from 1:1 to 3:1 have been reported [63,66,71]. Before commenting on the different techniques/methodologies employed to obtain speciation, it is worth delineating a number of issues that must be born in mind when presenting/discussing a K_d. When using a competing ligand (L) preliminarily evidence should be provided that no ternary (Aβ-M-L or M-Aβ-M') complex are formed that are the rule rather than the exception. In the context of the present work (Aβ binding to metal ions) this long known concept [72] has been brought up by two research groups recently [73,74].

On the other hand, when working with a high M/L it should also be explored whether binuclear complexes form. An often-overlooked issue is that values of stability constants may be compared only when they refer to species having the same stoichiometry [33,70]. For example, species having the same M/Aβ ratio but a different number of protons (e.g., MAβH and MAβ) cannot be compared; the same applies to species in which the number of protons displaced from the molecule backbone is different (e.g., MAβ and MAβH$_{-1}$) [33]. In connection with the last point, in Table 1 only reference 34 provides absolute values for the binding constants (*vide infra*). We shall briefly discuss the advantages and disadvantages inherent in the determination of absolute and dissociation constants.

To avoid confusion between Aβ and the overall stability constant (conventionally denoted as β) Aβ will be indicated as L throughout the next couple of paragraphs that specifically deal with absolute (stoichiometric) constants; please note that Aβ may denote any fragment of the amyloid-β. We shall assume that *i*. our system contains only one metal cation and one ligand; *ii*. the ligand can take up or release protons; and *iii*. the metal ion and the resulting complexes may hydrolyse. If the metal ion interacts with the ligand in a protic solvent like water, we may write the following equilibrium:

$$iM + kL + jH \rightleftharpoons M_iL_kH_j \tag{1}$$

and its associated overall stability constant, $\beta_{M_iL_kH_j}$:

$$\beta_{M_iL_kH_j} = \frac{[M_iL_kH_j]}{[M]^i[L]^k[H]^j} \tag{2}$$

where $[M_iL_kH_j]$, [M], [H] and [L] are the free concentrations of the complex, the metal ion, the ligand and the proton, respectively (charges are omitted for simplicity). Equation (2) does not represent a thermodynamic stability constant but a stoichiometric stability constant, expressed in terms of concentration quotients, and as such is valid only under the conditions (temperature, pressure, ionic strength) at which is determined whilst thermodynamic constants are dependent only upon temperature and pressure [68]. In order to replace activities, used to express a 'true' thermodynamic constant, with concentrations, an inert electrolyte is added. In the presence of relatively large concentrations of "neutral" or inert electrolytes which are assumed not to form complexes with the reacting species, the activity coefficients can be taken as constant. In $[M_iL_kH_j]$ the subscript *j* may have negative values; hence, in the simplest case a species may be represented by the formula MLH$_{-1}$. Such a formula, *per se* ambiguous, indicates that the ML complex has lost a proton, which may either have been released from a water molecule coordinated to the metal ion or from the ligand backbone (e.g., from a peptide nitrogen) if the number of protons that are released exceeds the maximum number of protons that may dissociate from the ligand in the absence of a metal ion. In both cases the species is indicated as [MLH$_{-1}$]; further details on the mathematics behind this may be found in reference [75]. The intentional ambiguity of the MLH$_{-1}$ symbolism is due to the difficulty to identify the origin of the extra-proton that is detected in solution (often by potentiometry, *vide infra*). Note also that if *i* in the expression of β_{ikj}, (2), is null, β_{ikj} refers to the overall protonation constant of the ligand. On the other hand, if *k* is null, β_{ikj} will refer to the metal ion hydrolysis; for example, β_{10-2} refers to [M(OH)$_2$].

An alternative way to quantify the binding of the metal ion to Aβ is to consider the dissociation equilibrium. In this case, the most common parameter used as a quantitative measure of the binding affinity of a species (e.g., a metal ion) to Aβ is the dissociation constant, K_d, expressed by the following equilibrium and its related constant:

$$MA\beta \rightleftharpoons M' + A\beta' \tag{3}$$

$$K_d = \frac{[M'][A\beta']}{[MA\beta]} \tag{4}$$

where [MAβ], [M'] and [Aβ'] denote the concentration of the MAβ complex, the free concentration of the metal and Aβ, respectively; in equations (3–4) charges are omitted for simplicity. K_d is not an absolute constant but is a concentration quotient derived in conditions in which the concentration of one or more reactants is fixed at a particular constant value and thus is strictly valid only for the experimental conditions used, i.e., temperature, pressure, ionic strength, competing ligand (if any) and, much more so, pH. Originally, the concept of 'apparent/conditional' stability constant was introduced by Schwartzenbach for EDTA metal complexes [76–78] and is used to determine the pH at which EDTA may be employed as a complexing agent for quantitative analysis [79]. It should be noted that [M'] and [Aβ'] are not the parameters defined in Equation (2); they are in fact the total concentrations of free metal ion and Aβ, respectively, present in all their forms at a given pH. It must be emphasized that [Aβ'] is not the concentration of the fully deprotonated ligand but it rather represents an equilibrium mixture of differently protonated ligand species, $H_nAβ$ (i.e., Aβ, HAβ, $H_2Aβ$ ... . $H_nAβ$ etc.). Analogously, [M'] denotes the total concentration of the metal ion not bound to Aβ, since the metal ion may hydrolyze and/or interact with a ligand other than Aβ. As detailed above, nowadays in the bioinorganic area a distinction is made between the apparent, ^aK_d, and the conditional, ^cK_d, constant.

In any case K_d proves useful since it allows to consider the complex dissociation as if both M' and Aβ' were present under one form only (for a more detailed description please refer to the IUBMB-IUPAC recommendations) [80]. If the system is investigated at a fixed pH, there is no need to determine the protonation constants of the ligand; obviously it holds that there must be no other competing equilibria influencing either [M'] and/or [Aβ'], which must strictly remain constant. If these conditions are not met, K_d value will also reflect the changes of [M'] and/or [Aβ'] due, for example, to competing metal hydrolysis and complexation and/or to protonation/deprotonation equilibria. In such cases, corrections should be introduced to take into account the competing equilibria between the metal ion and the ligands (e.g., a competing ligand and/or the buffer).

K_d has one undisputable advantage: it gives an idea of the binding affinity of the metal to the biomolecule. In fact, Equation (4) clearly shows that K_d= [M'] when [Aβ'] is equal to [MAβ]. This means that, when 50% of the initial Aβ is bound to the metal ion, the free metal ion concentration (usually denoted as $[M]_{50}$) is numerically equivalent to the K_d value and any procedure leading to the calculation of $[M]_{50}$ may thus provide the K_d value [33,54]. It follows that any K_d value lesser than the free metal ion concentration of a given physiological compartment implies the formation of significant amounts of MAβ. If the metal ion binds to more than one site within the same biomolecule, $[M]_{50}$ may be considered an 'average' of the dissociation constants of each single site. Perhaps it is worth mentioning again that comparisons between K_d values determined under seemingly analogous conditions should be avoided as in some cases K_d may refer to different species. The potential for error in these studies is high, however, since many competing equilibria may be present even in in vitro solution and must be taken into consideration.

3.2. Main Techniques Employed to Determine the Binding Constant

As indicated by Table 1, several techniques have been used to determine the binding affinity of Zn^{2+} to the Aβ. We shall briefly comment on the main techniques (i.e., potentiometry, calorimetry and fluorescence spectroscopy) and highlight the advantages and pitfalls that must be addressed when determining metal–ligand binding constants of biological systems.

3.2.1. Potentiometry

Potentiometry has long been regarded as the most accurate method to determine binding affinities of metal complexes as it provides universally applicable stability constants [81]. With the introduction of accurate and precise glass electrodes, pH-metry has become the technique of choice. It is the only technique that can provide pH-independent stability constants and hence a detailed description of the individual species formed over a relatively large pH interval. It is an indirect technique based on the extra-proton displacement caused by the metal ion. This implies that the protonation constants of the ligand be determined before measuring the actual complexation constant(s). This is not an easy task by itself as a biomolecule may contain several protons that can dissociate in the absence of a metal ion. For instance, ten protonation constants had to be determined for Aβ before proceeding to the investigation of the Zn^{2+}-Aβ reported in Table 1 [34,37]. Moreover, it is mandatory that protonation and complexation constants be determined under the same experimental conditions, including ionic strength; usually, the background salt should be one hundred times more concentrated than the reacting species to ensure that coefficients are constant and, thus, justify the use of stoichiometric constants. With the advent of excellent commercially available packages (PSEQUAD [82], HYPERQUAD [75]) data processing and modelling has become increasingly more objective. These packages minimize the function:

$$U = \Sigma (X_{calc} - X_{obs})^2 \qquad (5)$$

where, depending on the program, X may be the analytical concentration, the volume added or the potential; for example, the most commonly used software (HYPERQUAD) minimizes the error square sum in measured potentials. The constants obtained through this procedure express the explicit metal and proton stoichiometries of complexes. Unfortunately, this technique requires millimolar solutions. Though accurate, this methodology is time consuming since several titrations must be carried out to determine both protonation and complexation constants; in addition, compared with other techniques, it requires relatively large concentrations of biomolecule, which may pose solubility and cost problems.

3.2.2. Calorimetry

In the last decade, isothermal titration calorimetry (ITC) has been used to determine K_d [26,57,70,83]. ITC is particularly suitable for the study of the interactions of biomolecules with spectroscopically silent metal ions like Zn^{2+} that lack traditional spectroscopic signatures characteristic of other metal ions associated with d–d transitions [84]. The introduction of calorimeters, that make use of small volume cells and have fairly low detection limits by Microcal (now Malvern) and Calorimetry Science Corporation (now TA Instruments), determined the surge in popularity for the study of chemical binding phenomena and the widespread use of isothermal titration calorimetry [61,85–87]. Calorimeters belonging to this class directly produce the time derivative of the thermogram (dQ/dt vs. time) that can be integrated over time to give the heat produced or absorbed during the chosen time interval. Since ITC experiments provide a quantity, the gross heat (Q), that includes a number of additive terms, they need to be carefully designed to obtain the net heat of reaction. Suggestions/advices to avoid the pitfalls concerning the production of good quality data can be found in references [61,84–87].

The determinability and the accuracy of K, ΔH, and the stoichiometry factor n basically depend on the so-called Wiseman 'c' value:

$$c = n \, K_f C_R \qquad (6)$$

where n, K_f and C_R are the stoichiometric factor, the binding constant and the total macromolecule concentration [88]. The 'c' value should fall in the range 10 < c < 1000. A more recent treatment linking properties of the reaction (K_f and ΔH) and properties of the calorimeter (V_R and δQ) demonstrates that the following condition:

$$K_f/|\Delta H| < 4.72 \, V_R/\delta Q \qquad (7)$$

should be satisfied, where V_R and δQ are the active reaction volume of the cell and the uncertainty in the heat per data point in the titration, respectively [86]; this narrows down the Wiseman window and thus the c value should range from 50 to 500. However, the lower boundary is still a matter of debate [61,89,90]. Like in potentiometry, the function U is minimized:

$$U = \Sigma (Q_{exp,corr} - Q_{calc})^2 \qquad (8)$$

where $Q_{exp,corr}$ is the experimental value of the 'net' heat generated in a reaction step (*vide infra*). Q_{calc}, is related to the change, δn_i, in the number of moles of the *i*-th chemical species by Equation (9):

$$Q_{calc} = -\sum_{i=1}^{n} \delta n_i \Delta H_i \qquad (9)$$

δn_i values, that represent the change in the number of moles of the *i*-th reaction component, are calculated with a given set of stability constants and experimental conditions.

As ITC experiments are often conducted at constant pH they do not require prior knowledge of protonation constants. By contrast, only 'apparent' constants are produced; best fit yielding non-integer stoichiometries (e.g., 1.5), whose interpretation is rather puzzling, are sometimes reported [57]. Apparent constants can be turned into 'conditional' constants but this introduces a further degree of uncertainty due to error propagation. In any case, the 'apparent' constant thus obtained does not refer to a specific species.

Recently, a new package of the HYPERQUAD suite, HypCal, has been published that can provide stoichiometric (absolute) formation rather than 'apparent' dissociation constants [91]. Although calorimetry does not require the prior knowledge of a protein pK_a values, can provide K, ΔH and ΔS values and is in principle applicable to larger molecules than potentiometry it suffers from major drawbacks. The physical quantity measured (heat, Q_{exp}) must be corrected for all non-chemical energy terms (stirring, dilution of titrant and titrate, etc.) to obtain the 'net heat' value, $Q_{exp,corr}$, before processing the data. Secondly, the heat contribution resulting from the interaction with components of the solution other than the analyte (e.g., a competing ligand employed in a titration, the buffer, hydrolysis of the metal ion) must be precisely known in the conditions employed for the actual titration under study (i.e., temperature, ionic background).

3.2.3. Spectroscopy

Spectroscopic titrations may also be used to quantitate Zn^{2+} binding to Aβ. Despite the similarity between spectroscopic and calorimetric titrations was evidenced by Bolles et al. long ago [92], only recently has UV-Vis spectroscopy been used to determine the apparent zinc association constant to Aβ [67]. Unlike calorimetry, spectroscopy follows the change of signals directly and necessitates concentrations lower than those used in calorimetric experiments. Although spectroscopy has been used to determine stoichiometric association constants in relatively complex systems [93] has not gained much popularity in metal–biomolecule studies. This is surprising if one considers that packages that can provide stoichiometric constants like PSEQUAD [82], HYPERQUAD [75], SPECFIT [94] have been available for some time now; incidentally, these programs utilize a multi-wavelength treatment of spectral data thus minimizing the risks of creating artifacts associated with a single-wavelength treatment. Aβ has a fluorophore (tyrosine in position 10) that can be exploited to run spectrofluorometric titrations. In spectrofluorometric titrations signals may be followed directly too, with the additional advantage that very low concentrations can be explored. Titrations based on the intrinsic tyrosine fluorescence [64,66] as well as competition experiments [57,65] have been used to determine Zn^{2+} binding to Aβ. However, both types of experiments were used to determine apparent and not stoichiometric constants.

Job plots often obtained from spectroscopic experiments are only indicative as they can conceal contributions resulting from additional species that are formed in the same mixture. Garzon-Rodriguez et al., who used this method to model Zn^{2+} and Cu^{2+} complexation with Aβ(1–40), Aβ(1–42) and an Aβ(1–40) fragment having a tryptophan in position four, clearly state that the Job plots obtained via fluorescence measurements show maxima corresponding to peptide-to-metal stoichiometry between 1:1 and 1:2. Incidentally, the Job plots for Cu^{2+} ion showed the stoichiometry closer to 1:1 with some possible contribution from a 2:1 peptide-metal complex, which again highlights the limits of this methodology [64].

3.2.4. NMR

NMR may also be used to determine the association constant(s). However, this technique requires relatively large amounts of material; furthermore, the buffer (if any) must be deuterated in ^{1}H-NMR studies, and this may render the method fairly expensive. Moreover, people who have been extensively using this technique explicitly state that K_d resulting from their NMR study is not a quantitative measure of the binding of zinc by the molecule but rather a measure of which residues are most involved in the binding [65].

3.2.5. Other Techniques

In addition to those briefly illustrated above, in principle other techniques (e.g., CD, EPR and ESI-MS) might be used to determine the association constant(s). Like UV-vis and fluorescence, CD requires that the bands of each individual complex differ from each other enough to allow for the determination of the concentration of each complex species. As this is not often the case, CD as well as EPR have been used to validate the model obtained through potentiometric measurements.

ESI-MS involves a 'significant alteration of the physical environment of the reaction studied' (i.e., transition to the gas phase) and thus requires validation for the specific reaction studied or combination with other techniques [70,95]. For example, within the framework of Zn-Aβ interaction/speciation, Damante et al. have combined potentiometric, NMR, and ESI-MS investigations to demonstrate that the Aβ(1–16) is able to coordinate up to three zinc ions [34].

3.3. Use of Speciation Data

The data listed in Table 1 shows that to date there have been many inconsistencies in the literature on both the affinity of Zn^{2+} for Aβ as well as on the stoichiometry of the species resulting from Zn^{2+} interaction with Aβ peptides. Bush et al. reported on a highly specific pH-dependent high- and a low-affinity binding; they also reported different Zn^{2+}: Aβ ratios (stoichiometry) for such low and high affinity bindings [62] derived from Scatchard plots. The existence of a high- and low-affinity binding site is also reported by Danielsson et al. [65], based on NMR results, whilst Clements et al. found no evidence for the higher affinity binding site [63]. Based on Job-plots obtained via fluorescence measurements Garzon-Rodriguez et al. reported for Zn^{2+} a peptide-to-metal stoichiometry between 1:1 and 1:2 while they found no evidence for a high affinity binding [64]. Tougu et al. highlighted that the 'interaction of Zn^{2+} with the amyloid peptides cannot be characterized by a single conditional K_d value' and stressed that likely 'in the case of zinc the K_d value does not belong to a single and well-defined Zn^{2+}-Aβ complex' [66]. Clements et al. pointed out that the composition of the buffer, the different experimental conditions employed and/or, more likely the significantly different Zn/Aβ ratio explored may be responsible for some of the above discrepancies [63]. It has been reported that high concentrations of metals ions, like zinc, copper and iron, may induce Aβ aggregation [22,23] and fibril formation [24,25], while low concentrations of zinc and copper selectively lower the highly toxic Aβ oligomeric species [20,50]. Zawisza et al. underlined that the range of values of stability constants which can be determined by the different methods may be the source of significant controversies, particularly in Aβ research. They also pointed out that 'the description of the coordination process in terms of sets of pH-independent cumulative stability constants', as those expressed by Equation (2), is the only method that can describe individual components of the chemical equilibrium under given conditions [70].

Though different authors [34,57,62–67,70] have attempted to explain/reconcile the diverging data concerning Zn^{2+} affinity constants for Aβ, the correlation between zinc-binding affinity, metal coordination features, the morphology of zinc-containing aggregates and their different toxicity are all still matter of discussion.

In the examples that follow, we show that the determination of the stoichiometry of the Zn^{2+} complexes (mono-, bi-nuclear, protonated, hydroxo-complexes) as well as of their stability constants over a wide pH range, may allow to correlate a given property with a specific species that is formed in determined conditions (pH, buffer, competing ligand, etc.); this may avoid, for example, to correlate results obtained through different techniques (and experimental conditions) with 'high-' and/or 'low-affinity', which very likely reflect a mixture of Zn^{2+}-Aβ species. Perhaps it is worthy stressing that the methods and the procedures used for evaluation of binding constant values for the Zn^{2+}-Aβ peptides actually measure average parameters of the mixture of complexes with the exception of potentiometric studies. Moreover, the most common techniques briefly reviewed above make use of sizably different concentrations which implies the formation of different chemical species and may account, at least in part, for the spread of the values listed in Table 1.

In the first example that reproduces two ITC titrations run with different Zn^{2+} and Aβ concentrations we highlight the problems associated with the use of apparent binding constant instead of stoichiometric constants (Figure 2). For the sake of simplicity, reactant concentrations (and conditions) were taken from reference [57], although the discussion that follows might be extended to similar experiments, whose conclusions are based on K_d. For the sake of visual clarity, species forming below ten percent are not plotted in the figures. The computation of the species distribution has been carried out by using the only set of stoichiometric constants available in the literature [34].

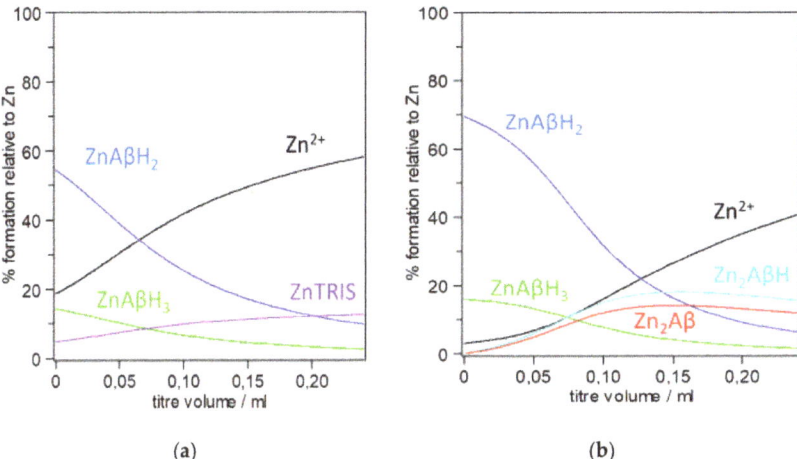

Figure 2. Computed species distribution reproducing the addition of Zn^{2+} to Aβ(1–16)PEG in 20 mM TRIS buffer, 100 mM NaCl, pH 7.4, t = 25 °C; (a) C_{Zn} = 5 × 10^{-4}, $C_{Aβ}$ = 20 μM; Zn^{2+} (black line), ZnAβH$_3$ (green line), ZnAβH$_2$ (blue line), ZnTRIS (fuchsia line); (b) C_{Zn} = 3 × 10^{-3} M, $C_{Aβ}$ = 140 μM; free Zn^{2+} (black line), ZnAβH$_3$ (green line), ZnAβH$_2$ (blue line), Zn$_2$AβH (turquoise line), Zn$_2$Aβ (red line). Aβ(1–16)PEG protonation constants from [37]; TRIS protonation and Zinc-TRIS formation constants and Zn^{2+} hydrolysis constants from [96]. Species percentage was computed by using HYSS [97].

Figure 2 prompts a few considerations that are crucial to the correlation of results with the species actually existing in solution. Figure 2a,b show that multiple species are formed in both cases. This strongly supports the assertion by Togu et al. that in the case of 'zinc ^aK_d value likely does not belong to a single and well-defined Zn^{2+}-Aβ complex' [66]; this view is shared by Damante et al. who, based on a multi-technique investigation, have also highlighted that the data obtained just below pH 7 cannot be attributed to a single complex species [34]. A second consideration focuses on the significant difference between the two titrations depicted in Figure 2a,b. Only mononuclear zinc complexes ([Zn(Aβ)H$_3$] and [Zn(Aβ)H$_2$]) are formed in Aβ more dilute solutions (Figure 2a), while binuclear Zn^{2+} species also form in more concentrated Aβ solutions (Figure 2b). Furthermore, although both the mononuclear species of Figure 2a have the same Zn/Aβ ratio (1:1) their contribution to the total measured heat is unlikely to be the same since they have a different number of protons. Moreover, a complex with the buffer tends to form in the final region of the titration (~12%), which will contribute to the total heat (Figure 2a). The nature of the buffer, its concentration as well as the peptide/buffer ratio opens a new chapter since the buffer may act as a competitive metal-binding agent and as such often has an appreciable effect on the metal speciation in solution. In the effective words of Magyar et al., buffers are 'non-innocent' components of the solution investigated in vitro [59]. Togu et al. have highlighted that ^aK_d for Zn^{2+}-Aβ complex is higher at higher concentrations of TRIS, while there is no difference between the ^aK_d values in 20 mmol/L HEPES, and in 10 mmol/L TRIS [66]. Johnson et al. have pointed out that buffers can significantly affect the interpretation of thermodynamic data; they have also provided a good example illustrating how complexes with and proton transfer to a buffer may be accounted for [84]. Taking into account the contribution of the complex formed with the buffer to the measured physical quantity (Q_{exp}) might help at least in part unravelling some of the discrepancies reported in the literature. The presence of a buffer, while particularly relevant for some techniques (e.g., ITC), may also affect the interpretation of results obtained through spectroscopic experiments (e.g., NMR). For example, commenting on their NMR data, Danielson et al. have underlined that 'quantitative results may be somewhat biased, due to metal–phosphate complex', i.e., the buffer used in their experiments [65]. In more concentrated solutions (Figure 2b), binuclear species ([Zn_2(Aβ)] and [Zn_2(Aβ)H]) are also formed which together total ca. 30% of total zinc at the end of the titration while in the same region the zinc complex with the buffer is just below 10% (~8%, not shown in the figure). The formation of multiple coexisting species probably accounts for the non-integer stoichiometries obtained when fitting the ITC data obtained for the titration represented in Figure 2b as well as for the different number of protons transferred to the buffer when zinc is added to a peptide solution or when the peptide is added to a zinc solution [57]. Noteworthily, even in regions where the total Zn^{2+} over the total Aβ concentration is approximately equal to 1.5 (i.e., titre = 0.12), the percentage of Zn^{2+} binuclear species that are formed roughly matches that of the mononuclear species. Thus, assumptions on the Zn/Aβ ratio, often referred to as stoichiometry, of the species resulting from the binding of the metal ion to Aβ fragments should be made with extreme caution as the interaction is more complex than it might seem at first sight. Perhaps, the relevance of binuclear species is even more evident if we consider that the synapse is the main arena of molecular events that lead to neurodegenerative disorders involving Aβ peptides and that Zn^{2+}, as well as other metal ions, is released into the synaptic cleft in the process of Glu-mediated neurotransmission. Zawisza et al. have figured out that the metal ion concentrations in the glutamatergic cleft is of the order of 0.1 mM and, locally and temporarily, might be even higher at the site of release [70]. It has to be evidenced that at the end of the run represented in Figure 2a,b, the Zn/Aβ ratio is about 4.5 and 3, respectively. The amount of 'free' Zn^{2+} calculated for the in vitro experiments depicted in Figure 2 should not lead to the conclusion that free Zn^{2+} exists in vivo since in human zinc metabolism, several ligands (e.g., low molecular weight ligands, proteins) participate in cellular uptake, extrusion, and re-distribution [98]. The potential for misinterpretation in metal ion-peptide studies is high since many competing equilibria are present in solution and this further stresses the necessity to have stoichiometric constants as they can provide valuable information about metal speciation and exchange in biological systems [33,59].

Incidentally, a ubiquitous ligand, OH^-, is often overlooked. The hydroxo ion may be of paramount importance since all measurements in vitro tend to reproduce naturally occurring conditions and are thus carried out at or around physiological pH values; at these pH values, even if in the presence of a strongly coordinating ligand OH^- does not cause the formation of metal ion hydroxide, more often than not comes in as a 'third' ligand thereby leading to the formation of hydroxo species of the type $M_iL_k(OH)_j$. In cases where stoichiometric constants cannot be obtained, due the complexity of biological systems, we as well as other authors emphasize that the characteristics of complexes should never be compared unless it can be proved that they have the same stoichiometries [33,70].

In the second example, we deal with an interesting result, reported by Yoshiike et al., who in an effort to see whether some metal ions (viz. Zn^{2+} and Cu^{2+}) promote or inhibit the formation of aggregates, performed a series of experiments on Aβ(1–40) and Aβ(1–42) by using different techniques and methods [29]. Based on fluorescence, UV, CD, cell culture experiments, they reported that 'Zn(II) and, to a lesser extent, Cu(II) prevent Aβ from forming β-sheet conformations in an as-yet-undetermined manner', evidencing that 'with concentrations greater than 10 µM, both Zn(II) and Cu(II) effectively suppressed β-aggregation, resulting in an increase in cell viability'. Indeed, conflicting views on whether Zn^{2+} has beneficial or detrimental effects have been reported [22,26–32]. A speciation based on the use of absolute (stoichiometric) stability constants might help explaining why in the experiments reported in [29], Zn^{2+} inhibits the β-aggregation of both Aβ(1–40) and Aβ(1–42) in a concentration-dependent manner. To this end, we computed the species distribution with a view to modelling the intriguing effect of Zn^{2+} on the inhibition of aggregates reported by Yoshiike et al. [29]. These authors explored *inter alia* Zn^{2+} concentrations ranging from zero up to 100 µM in a medium containing 5 µM Aβ(1–40) in order to understand why low Zn^{2+} concentrations decrease the formation of toxic fibrils whilst concentrations greater than 10 µM inhibit the formation of β-aggregates and increase cell viability; interestingly it was also reported that the effect of Zn^{2+} concentration tends to level off above 40 µM.

Similarly to what we did to obtain the species distribution for the examples shown in Figure 2, we used the set of data reported in literature for the representative Aβ(1–16) PEG peptide and investigated Zn^{2+} concentrations ranging from 0.05 to 70 µM (0,05, 2, 5, 10, 20, 30, 40, 50, 60 and 70 µM) while keeping Aβ concentration constant (5 µM) as done by Yoshiike et al. in their experiment on Aβ(1–40) [29]. Figure 3a–c and d show selected species distribution obtained at 2, 5, 10 and 70 µM, respectively.

Species whose formation is less than five percent are not shown. Figure 3a–d show neither 'free' Zn^{2+} (not bound to Aβ) nor ZnTRIS; the latter species is just above thirty percent (relative to total zinc) in the conditions depicted in Figure 3d. Figure 3a,b show that sizable amounts of Zn^{2+}-Aβ complex species are formed as the Zn/Aβ ratio reaches the 1:1 value (i.e., 5 µM, Figure 3b). As pointed out for the experiments reproduced in Figure 2a,b, the picture is more complex that one may think. The species distribution strengthens the view that in the case of zinc the K_d value does not belong to a single and well-defined Zn^{2+}-Aβ complex [66] but is rather represented by a complex mixture that above a certain Zn^{2+}/Aβ ratio involves both mono- and bi-nuclear species [34]. Noteworthy, significant percentages of zinc species are formed 'with concentrations greater than 10 µM' and Zn/Aβ ratios equal to or greater than two, i.e., at the concentration where zinc effectively suppressed β-aggregation (ThT results in [29]), and increased cell viability (MTT results in [29]).

Moreover, the species distribution shown in Figure 3 helps explain why zinc-promoted non-β-sheet aggregates are destabilized when pH lowers slightly as found around the site of inflammation [29]. In fact, at pH = 6.8 the percentage of Zn^{2+}-Aβ species is sizably smaller than that detected at pH 7.4 and this supports the hypothesis that an 'aberrant increase in β-aggregation in the presence of zinc may represent the pathological mechanism by which acidosis induces the liberation of Aβ from Zn(II)' [29].

In order to have an overview of both the mono- and bi-nuclear species formed over the range explored and to find a possible link between the species and the effect observed, we have reported the sum of the percentages of mono-, bi-nuclear zinc species and Zn-TRIS versus the concentration of Zn^{2+} added (Figure 4).

For the sake of visual clarity, Figure 4 does not show the percentage of the species resulting from the interaction of Zn^{2+} with the buffer (relative to zinc concentration) calculated for each Zn^{2+} concentration (0.05, 2, 5 µM etc.). As anticipated, such a percentage is just above 20% at 0.05 µM increases to about 30% at 70 µM, and may be retained constant over the entire interval, considering the wide range of zinc concentrations and Zn/Aβ ratios investigated. Figure 4 would indicate that the effective suppression of β-aggregation and the consequent increase in cell viability does not depend on zinc concentration as much as on the amount of Zn-Aβ species formed. The trend represented by the sum of zinc mono-and binuclear species (green bars) levels off and mirrors that observed by Yoshiike et al. in their experiments. Although a more confident statement about the physiological significance of the link between speciation and effect would require a more detailed study, it might be speculated that the main species that are formed in in the presence of excess Zn^{2+} might be responsible for both the inhibition of the formation of β-aggregates as well as the increase of cellular viability. Overall, our data support the idea that Zn^{2+} and much more so Zn^{2+}-Aβ species have a protective role against β-amyloid toxicity [26,29].

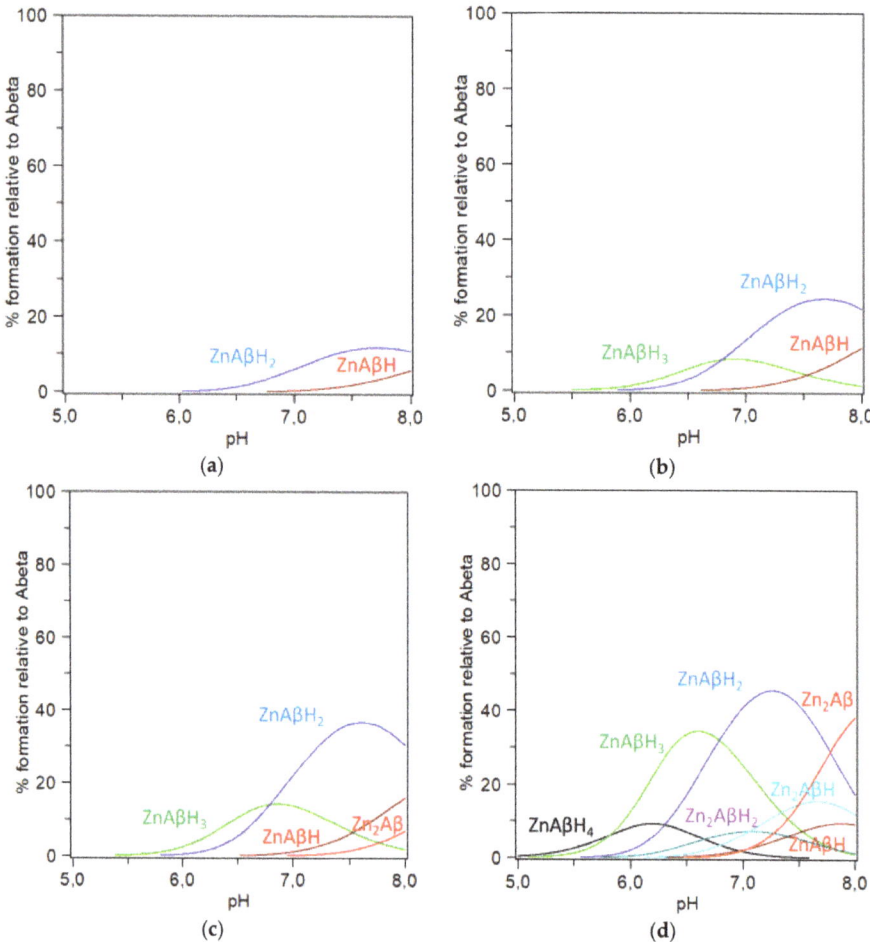

Figure 3. Computed species distribution mimicking the assays by Yoshiike et al. [29] who investigated the concentration dependent inhibition of β-aggregates (ThT test) and the increase of cell (MTT test). Figure 3a–d reproduce the addition of Zn^{2+} to Aβ(1–16)PEG in 20 mM TRIS buffer at pH 7.4, t = 25 °C; $C_{Aβ}$ = 5 μM in all diagrams; (a) C_{Zn} = 2 μM; ZnAβH$_2$ (blue line), ZnAβH (amaranth line); (b) C_{Zn} = 5 μM, ZnAβH$_3$ (green line), ZnAβH$_2$ (blue line), ZnAβH (amaranth line); (c) C_{Zn} = 10 μM, ZnAβH$_3$ (green line), ZnAβH$_2$ (blue line), ZnAβH (amaranth line), Zn$_2$Aβ (red line); (d) C_{Zn} = 70 μM, ZnAβH$_4$ (black line), ZnAβH$_3$ (green line), ZnAβH$_2$ (blue line), ZnAβH (amaranth line), Zn$_2$AβH$_2$ (fuchsia line), Zn$_2$AβH (turquoise line), Zn$_2$Aβ (red line). Aβ(1–16) PEG protonation constants from reference [37]; TRIS protonation, Zinc-TRIS formation and Zn^{2+} hydrolysis constant from reference [96]. Species percentage was computed by using HYSS [97].

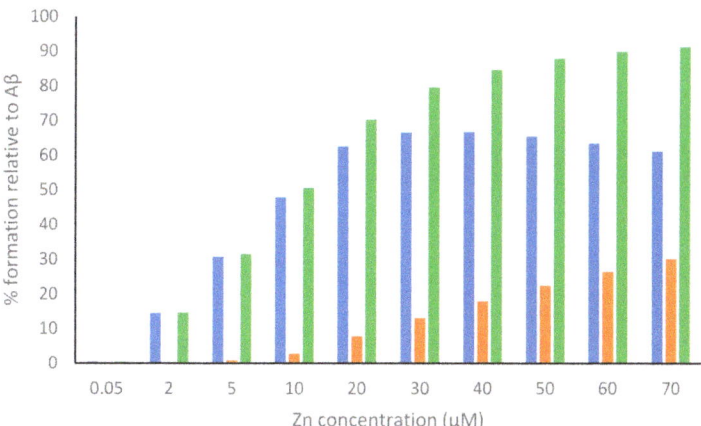

Figure 4. Total percentage of mono-, bi-nuclear species computed at pH = 7.4 for the experiments reported in Figure 6 of [29]. Blue, red and green represent the total percentage of all mono-nuclear, bi-nuclear and mono- plus bi-nuclear species, respectively.

4. Concluding Remarks

It must be underlined that there is nothing wrong with the determination of an apparent (K_d) constant and often this is the only stability constant that may be accessed experimentally at a given pH value when for instance, neither the protonation constants nor the speciation of the metal ion with the protein (or fragments of the protein) are available. However, we emphasize that using an apparent Kd to draw conclusions on the structure of the complex species formed may be misleading since, as underlined when commenting the terms (M' and Aβ') that appear in the equation expressing K_d (Eq. 4), M' and Aβ'are in fact the total concentrations of free metal ion and free Aβ, respectively, present in all their forms at a given pH. As a consequence, the apparent ^aK_d should be used only to compare values measured under the same conditions and in particular the same buffer and the same concentration of the buffer [26,66].

The determination of stoichiometric constants (where feasible) can be a time-consuming and tedious procedure, since numerous titrations under various conditions (different concentrations as well as different metal/Aβ ratios) must be carried out to avoid bias and to ensure that the calculated stoichiometric constants provide, in fact, the best descriptions of the system. However, these efforts may be rewarding; as emphasized by Magyar et al. as the binding interactions of the peptide(s) with metal ions are described on a truly quantitative basis we will gain a much greater understanding of the roles and relationships of metals in biology and biological processes [59].

If the experiment to measure the binding constant is well planned and all the parameters (pH, ionic strength, buffer etc.) influencing this thermodynamic quantity are duly taken into account, Einstein's statement that reads

'A theory is the more impressive the greater the simplicity of its premise is, the more different kinds of things it relates, and the more extended is its area of applicability. It [thermodynamics] is the only physical theory of universal content concerning which I am convinced that, within the framework of applicability of its basic concepts it will never be overthrown' will be more appropriate than ever [99].

Funding: This research was in part funded by MIUR under Grant PRIN 2015 (2015MP34H3 and PRA 2016-2018, University of Catania).

Conflicts of Interest: The authors declare no conflict of interest.

References

1. World Alzheimer Report 2018. Available online: https://www.alz.co.uk/research/WorldAlzheimerReport2018.pdf (accessed on 13 May 2019).
2. Dementia statistics. Available online: https://www.alz.co.uk/research/statistics (accessed on 13 May 2019).
3. Frequently Asked Questions. Available online: https://www.alz.co.uk/info/faq (accessed on 13 May 2019).
4. Masters, C.L.; Simms, G.; Weinman, N.A.; Multhaup, G.; McDonald, R.L.; Beyreuther, K. Amyloid plaque core protein in Alzheimer disease and Down syndrome. *Proc. Natl. Acad. Sci. USA* **1985**, *82*, 4245–4249. [CrossRef] [PubMed]
5. Glenner, G.G.; Wong, C.W. Alzheimer's disease: Initial report of the purification and characterization of a novel cerebrovascular amyloid protein. *Biochem. Biophys. Res. Commun.* **1984**, *120*, 885–890. [CrossRef]
6. Mucke, L. *Neuroscience*: Alzheimer's disease. *Nature* **2009**, *461*, 895–897. [CrossRef] [PubMed]
7. Kuo, Y.M.; Emmerling, M.R.; Vigo-Pelfrey, C.; Kasunic, T.C.; Kirkpatric, J.B.; Murdoch, G.H.; Ball, M.J.; Rother, A.E. Water-soluble Aβ (N-40, N-42) Oligomers in Normal and Alzheimer Disease Brains. *J. Biol. Chem.* **1996**, *271*, 4077–4081. [CrossRef] [PubMed]
8. Checler, F. Processing of the beta-amyloid precursor protein and its regulation in Alzheimer's disease. *J. Neurochem.* **1995**, *65*, 1431–1444. [CrossRef] [PubMed]
9. Selkoe, D.J. Alzheimer's disease: Genes, proteins, and therapy. *J. Physiol. Rev.* **2001**, *81*, 741–766. [CrossRef]
10. Rana, M.; Sharma, A.K.M. Cu and Zn interactions with Aβ peptides: Consequence of coordination on aggregation and formation of neurotoxic soluble Aβ oligomers. *Metallomics* **2019**, *11*, 64–84. [CrossRef] [PubMed]
11. Jarrett, J.T.; Berger, E.P.; Lansbury, P.T. The C-Terminus of the β Protein is Critical in Amyloidogenesis. *Ann. N. Y. Acad. Sci.* **1993**, *695*, 144–148. [CrossRef]
12. Hartmann, T.; Bieger, S.C.; Brühl, B.; Tienari, P.J.; Ida, N.; Allsop, D.G.; Roberts, W.C.; Masters, L.; Dotti, C.G.; Unsicker, K.; et al. Distinct sites of intracellular production for Alzheimer's disease Aβ 40/42 amyloid peptides. *Nat. Med.* **1997**, *3*, 1016–1020. [CrossRef]
13. Bibl, M.; Esselmann, H.; Mollenhauer, B.; Weniger, G.; Welge, V.; Liess, M.; Lewczuk, P.; Otto, M.; Schulz, J.B.; Trenkwalder, C.; et al. Wiltfang, J. Blood-based neurochemical diagnosis of vascular dementia: A pilot study. *J. Neurochem.* **2007**, *103*, 467–474. [CrossRef]
14. Schoonenboom, N.S.; Mulder, C.; Van Kamp, G.J.; Mehta, S.P.; Scheltens, P.; Blankenstein, M.A.; Mehta, P.D. Amyloid beta 38, 40, and 42 species in cerebrospinal fluid: More of the same? *Ann. Neurol.* **2005**, *58*, 139–142. [CrossRef] [PubMed]
15. Burdick, D.; Soreghan, B.; Kwon, M.; Kosmoski, J.; Knauer, M.; Henschen, A.; Yates, J.; Cotman, C.; Glabe, C. Assembly and aggregation properties of synthetic Alzheimer's A4/beta amyloid peptide analogs. *J. Biol. Chem.* **1992**, *267*, 546–554. [PubMed]
16. Jarrett, J.T.; Berger, E.P.; Lansbury, P.T., Jr. The carboxy terminus of the beta. amyloid protein is critical for the seeding of amyloid formation: Implications for the pathogenesis of Alzheimer's disease. *Biochemistry* **1993**, *32*, 4693–4697. [CrossRef] [PubMed]
17. Ricchelli, F.; Drago, D.; Filippi, B.; Tognona, G.; Zatta, P. Aluminum-triggered structural modifications and aggregation of β-amyloids. *Cell. Mol. Life Sci.* **2005**, *62*, 1724–1733. [CrossRef] [PubMed]
18. Lovell, M.A.; Robertson, J.D.; Teesdale, W.J.; Campbell, J.L.; Markesbery, W.R. Copper, iron and zinc in Alzheimer's disease senile plaques. *J. Neurol. Sci.* **1998**, *158*, 47–52. [CrossRef]
19. Maynard, C.J.; Bush, A.I.; Masters, C.L.; Cappai, R.; Li, Q.X. Metals and amyloid-beta in Alzheimer's disease. *Int. J. Exp. Path.* **2005**, *86*, 147–159. [CrossRef] [PubMed]
20. Gaggelli, E.; Janicka-Klos, A.; Jankowska, E.; Kozlowski, H.; Migliorini, C.; Molteni, E.; Valensin, D.; Valensin, G.; Wieczerzak, E. NMR Studies of the Zn^{2+} Interactions with Rat and Human β-Amyloid (1–28) Peptides in Water-Micelle Environment. *J. Phys. Chem. B.* **2008**, *112*, 100–109. [CrossRef]
21. Religa, D.; Strozik, D.; Cherny, R.A.; Volitakis, I.; Haroutunian, V.; Winblad, B.; Naslund, J.; Bush, A.I. Elevated cortical zinc in Alzheimer disease. *Neurology* **2006**, *67*, 69–75. [CrossRef]
22. Bush, A.I.; Pettingell, W.H.; Multhaup, G.; Paradis, M.D.; Vonsattel, J.P.; Gusella, J.F.; Beyreuther, K.; Masters, C.L.; Tanzi, R.E. Rapid induction of Alzheimer A beta amyloid formation by zinc. *Science* **1994**, *265*, 1464–1467. [CrossRef]

23. Huang, X.; Atwood, C.S.; Moir, R.D.; Hartshorn, M.A.; Vonsatell, J.P.; Tanzi, R.E.; Bush, A.I. Zinc-induced Alzheimer's Aβ1–40 Aggregation Is Mediated by Conformational Factors. *J. Biol. Chem.* **1997**, *272*, 26464–26470. [CrossRef]
24. Morgan, D.M.; Dong, J.; Jacob, J.; Lu, K.; Apkarian, R.P.; Thiyagarajan, P.; Lynn, D.G. Metal switch for amyloid formation: Insight into the structure of the nucleus. *J. Am. Chem. Soc.* **2002**, *124*, 12644–12645. [CrossRef] [PubMed]
25. Syme, C.D.; Nadal, R.C.; Rigby, S.E.J.; Viles, J.H. Copper Binding to the Amyloid-(A) Peptide Associated with Alzheimer's Disease. *J. Biol. Chem.* **2004**, *279*, 18169–18177. [CrossRef] [PubMed]
26. Faller, P.; Hureau, C. Bioinorganic chemistry of copper and zinc ions coordinated to amyloid-b peptide. *Dalton Trans.* **2009**, 1080–1094. [CrossRef] [PubMed]
27. Haass, C.; Selkoe, D.J. Soluble protein oligomers in neurodegeneration: Lessons from the Alzheimer's amyloid beta-peptide. *Nat. Rev. Mol. Cell Biol.* **2007**, *8*, 101–112. [CrossRef] [PubMed]
28. Lee, M.; Kim, J.I.; Na, S.; Eom, K. Metal ions affect the formation and stability of amyloid β aggregates at multiple length scales. *Phys.Chem.Chem.Phys.* **2018**, *20*, 8951–8961. [CrossRef] [PubMed]
29. Yoshiike, Y.; Tanemura, K.; Murayama, O.; Akagi, T.; Murayama, M.; Sato, S.; Sun, X.; Tanaka, N.; Takashima, A. New Insights on How Metals Disrupt Amyloid β-Aggregation and Their Effects on Amyloid-β Cytotoxicity. *J. Biol. Chem.* **2001**, *276*, 32293–32299. [CrossRef] [PubMed]
30. Abelein, A.; Graslund, A.; Danielsson, J. Zinc as chaperone-mimicking agent for retardation of amyloid β peptide fibril formation. *Proc. Natl. Acad. Sci. USA* **2015**, *112*, 5407–5412. [CrossRef] [PubMed]
31. Lim, K.H.; Kim, Y.K.; Chang, Y.-T. Investigations of the Molecular Mechanism of Metal-Induced Aβ (1–40) Amyloidogenesis. *Biochemistry* **2007**, *46*, 13523–13532. [CrossRef]
32. Mannini, B.; Habchi, J.; Chia, S.K.R.; Ruggeri, F.S.; Perni, M.; Knowles, T.P.J.; Dobson, C.M.; Vendruscolo, M. Stabilization and characterization of cytotoxic $Aβ_{40}$ oligomers isolated from an aggregation reaction in the presence of zinc ions. *ACS Chem Neurosci.* **2018**, *9*, 2959–2971. [CrossRef]
33. Arena, G.; Pappalardo, G.; Sovago, I.; Rizzarelli, E. Copper(II) interaction with amyloid-β: Affinity and speciation. *Coord. Chem. Rev.* **2012**, *256*, 3–12. [CrossRef]
34. Damante, C.A.; Osz, K.; Nagy, Z.; Pappalardo, G.; Grasso, G.; Impellizzeri, G.; Rizzarelli, E.; Sóvágó, I. Metal Loading Capacity of Aβ N-Terminus: A Combined Potentiometric and Spectroscopic Study of Zinc(II) Complexes with Aβ(1–16), Its Short or Mutated Peptide Fragments and Its Polyethylene Glycol-ylated Analogue. *Inorg. Chem.* **2009**, *48*, 10405–10415. [CrossRef]
35. Kozin, S.A.; Zirah, S.; Rebuffat, S.; Hoa, G.H.B.; Debey, P. Zinc Binding to Alzheimer's Aβ(1–16) Peptide Results in Stable Soluble Complex. *Biochem. Biophys. Res. Commun.* **2001**, *285*, 959–964. [CrossRef] [PubMed]
36. Mekmouche, Y.; Coppel, Y.; Hochgrafe, K.; Guiloreau, L.; Talmard, C.; Mazarguil, H.; Faller, P. Characterization of the Zn^{II} Binding to the Peptide Amyloid-$β^{1-16}$ linked to Alzheimer's Disease. *ChemBioChem* **2005**, *6*, 1663–1671. [CrossRef] [PubMed]
37. Damante, C.A.; Osz, K.; Nagy, Z.; Pappalardo, G.; Grasso, G.; Impellizzeri, G.; Rizzarelli, E.; Sóvágó, I. The Metal Loading Ability of β-Amyloid N-Terminus: A Combined Potentiometric and Spectroscopic Study of Copper(II) Complexes with β-Amyloid(1–16), Its Short or Mutated Peptide Fragments and Its Polyethylene Glycol (PEG)-ylated Analogue. *Inorg. Chem.* **2008**, *47*, 9669–9683. [CrossRef] [PubMed]
38. Vallee, B.L.; Falchuk, K.H. Zinc and gene expression. *Philos. Trans. R. Soc. Lond. B. Biol. Sci.* **1981**, *294*, 185–197. [CrossRef] [PubMed]
39. Coleman, J.E. Zinc proteins: Enzymes, storage proteins, transcription factors, and replication proteins. *Annu Rev. Biochem.* **1992**, *61*, 897–946. [CrossRef] [PubMed]
40. Foster, M.; Samman, S. Zinc and redox signaling: Perturbations associated with cardiovascular disease and diabetes mellitus. *Antioxid. Redox Signal.* **2010**, *13*, 1549–1573. [CrossRef]
41. Takeda, A. Zinc homeostasis and functions of zinc in the brain. *BioMetals* **2001**, *14*, 343–351. [CrossRef]
42. Cuajungco, M.P.; Lees, G.J. Zinc and Alzheimer's disease: Is there a direct link? *Brain. Res. Rev.* **1997**, *23*, 219–236. [CrossRef]
43. Frederickson, C.J.; Bush, A.I. Synaptically released zinc: Physiological functions and pathological effects. *BioMetals* **2001**, *14*, 353–366. [CrossRef]

44. Cherny, R.A.; Legg, J.T.; McLean, C.A.; Fairlie, D.P.; Huang, X.; Atwood, C.S.; Beyreuther, K.; Tanzi, R.E.; Masters, C.L.; Bush, A.I. Aqueous dissolution of Alzheimer's disease Abeta amyloid deposits by biometal depletion. *J. Biol Chem.* **1999**, *274*, 23223–23228. [CrossRef] [PubMed]
45. Lovell, M.A.; Xie, C.; Markeshery, W.R. Protection against amyloid beta peptide toxicity by zinc. *Brain Res.* **1999**, *823*, 88–95. [CrossRef]
46. Bishop, G.M.; Robinson, S.R. The amyloid paradox: Amyloid-beta-metal complexes can be neurotoxic and neuroprotective. *Brain Pathol.* **2004**, *14*, 448–452. [CrossRef] [PubMed]
47. Moreira, P.; Pereira, C.; Santos, M.S.; Oliveira, C. Effect of zinc ions on the cytotoxicity induced by the amyloid beta-peptide. *Antioxid. Redox Signaling* **2000**, *2*, 317–325. [CrossRef] [PubMed]
48. Zhu, Y.J.; Lin, H.; Lal, R. Fresh and nonfibrillar amyloid beta protein(1–40) induces rapid cellular degeneration in aged human fibroblasts: Evidence for AbetaP-channel-mediated cellular toxicity. *FASEB J.* **2000**, *14*, 1244–1254. [CrossRef] [PubMed]
49. Cuajungco, M.P.; Goldstein, L.E.; Nunomura, A.; Smith, M.A.; Lim, J.T.; Atwood, C.S.; Huang, X.; Farrag, Y.W.; Perry, G.; Bush, A.I. Evidence that the β-Amyloid Plaques of Alzheimer's Disease Represent the Redox-silencing and Entombment of Aβ by Zinc. *J. Biol. Chem.* **2000**, *275*, 19439–19442. [CrossRef]
50. Garai, K.; Sahoo, B.; Kaushalya, S.K.; Desai, R.; Maiti, S. Zinc Lowers Amyloid-β Toxicity by Selectively Precipitating Aggregation Intermediates. *Biochemistry* **2007**, *46*, 10655–10663. [CrossRef]
51. Gaggelli, E.; Kozlowski, H.; Valensin, D.; Valensin, G. Copper homeostasis and neurodegenerative disorders (Alzheimer's, prion, and Parkinson's diseases and amyotrophic lateral sclerosis). *Chem. Rev.* **2006**, *106*, 1995–2044. [CrossRef]
52. Kowalik-Jankowska, T.; Ruta, M.; Wisniewska, K.; Lankiewicz, L. Coordination abilities of the 1-16 and 1-28 fragments of beta-amyloid peptide towards copper(II) ions: A combined potentiometric and spectroscopic study. *J. Inorg. Biochem.* **2003**, *95*, 270–282. [CrossRef]
53. Arena, G.; Bindoni, M.; Cardile, V.; Maccarrone, G.; Riello, M.C.; Rizzarelli, E.; Sciuto, S.J. Cytotoxic and cytostatic activity of copper(II) complexes. Importance of the speciation for the correct interpretation of the in vitro biological results. *Inorg. Biochem.* **1993**, *50*, 31–45. [CrossRef]
54. Kozlowski, H.; Łuczkowski, M.; Remelli, M. Prion proteins and copper ions. Biological and chemical controversies. *Dalton Trans.* **2010**, *39*, 6371–6385. [CrossRef] [PubMed]
55. Copper complex species within a fragment of the N-terminal repeat region in opossum PrP protein. *Dalton Trans.* **2010**, *40*, 2441–2450.
56. Travaglia, A.; Arena, G.; Fattorusso, R.; Isernia, C.; La Mendola, D.; Malgieri, G.; Nicoletti, V.G.; Rizzarelli, E. The inorganic perspective of nerve growth factor: Interactions of Cu^{2+} and Zn^{2+} with the N-terminus fragment of nerve growth factor encompassing the recognition domain of the TrkA receptor. *Chem. Eur. J.* **2011**, *17*, 3726–3738. [CrossRef] [PubMed]
57. Talmard, C.; Bouzan, A.; Faller, P. Zinc Binding to Amyloid-â: Isothermal Titration Calorimetry and Zn Competition Experiments with Zn Sensors. *Biochemistry* **2007**, *46*, 13658–13666. [CrossRef] [PubMed]
58. Ayton, S.; Belaidi, A.A.; Lei, P.; Bush, A.I. Targeting Transition Metals for Neuroprotection in Alzheimer's Disease. In *Neuroprotection in Alzheimer's Disease*; Gozes, I., Ed.; Elsevier Inc.: Amsterdam, The Netherlands, 2017; Chapter 10; pp. 193–215. [CrossRef]
59. Magyar, J.S.; Godwin, H.A. Spectropotentiometric analysis of metal binding to structural zinc-binding sites: Accounting quantitatively for pH and metal ion buffering effects. *Anal. Biochem.* **2003**, *320*, 39–54. [CrossRef]
60. Outten, C.E.; O'Halloran, T.V. Femtomolar sensitivity of metalloregulatory proteins controlling zinc homeostasis. *Science* **2001**, *292*, 2488–2492. [CrossRef] [PubMed]
61. Arena, G.; Sgarlata, C. Modern Calorimetry: An Invaluable Tool in Supramolecular Chemistry. In *Comprehensive Supramolecular Chemistry II*; Atwood, J.L., Gokel, G.W., Barbour, L.J., Eds.; Elsevier: Amsterdam, The Netherlands, 2016; Volume 2. [CrossRef]
62. Bush, A.I.; Pettingell, W.H.D.; Paradis, M.; Tanzi, R.E. Modulation of A beta adhesiveness and secretase site cleavage by zinc. *J. Biol. Chem.* **1994**, *269*, 12152–12158. [PubMed]
63. Clements, A.; Allsop, D.; Walsh, D.M.; Williams, C.H. Aggregation and metal-binding properties of mutant forms of the amyloid A beta peptide of Alzheimer's disease. *J. Neurochem.* **1996**, *66*, 740–747. [CrossRef]
64. Garzon-Rodriguez, W.; Yatsimirsky, A.K.; Glabe, C.G. Binding of Zn(II), Cu(II), and Fe(II) ions to Alzheimer's A beta peptide studied by fluorescence. *Bioorg. Med. Chem. Lett.* **1999**, *9*, 2243–2248. [CrossRef]

65. Danielsson, J.; Pierattelli, R.; Banci, L.; Graslund, A. High-resolution NMR studies of the zinc-binding site of the Alzheimer's amyloid b-peptide. *FEBS J.* **2007**, *274*, 46–59. [CrossRef]
66. Tõugu, V.; Karafin, A.; Palumaa, P. Binding of zinc(II) and copper(II) to the full-length Alzheimer's amyloid-b peptide. *J. Neurochem.* **2008**, *104*, 1249–1259. [CrossRef] [PubMed]
67. Noel, S.; Bustos Rodriguez, S.; Sayen, S.; Guillon, E.; Faller, P.; Hureau, C. Use of a new water-soluble Zn sensor to determine Zn affinity for the amyloid-β peptide and relevant mutants. *Metallomics* **2014**, *6*, 1220–1222. [CrossRef] [PubMed]
68. Nancollas, G.H.; Tomson, M.B. Guidelines for the determination of stability constants. *Pure Appl. Chem.* **1982**, *54*, 2675–2692. [CrossRef]
69. Sokolowska, M.; Bal, W. Cu(II) complexation by 'non-coordinating' N-2-hydroxyethylpiperazine-N'-2-ethanesulfonic acid (HEPES buffer). *J. Inorg. Biochem.* **2005**, *99*, 1653–1660. [CrossRef] [PubMed]
70. Zawisza, I.; Rozga, M.; Bal, W. Affinity of copper and zinc ions to proteins and peptides related to neurodegenerative conditions (Aβ, APP, α-synuclein, PrP). *Coord. Chem. Rev.* **2012**, *256*, 2297–2307. [CrossRef]
71. Atwood, C.S.; Scarpa, R.C.; Huang, X.; Moir, R.D.; Jones, W.D.; Fairlie, D.P.; Tanzi, R.E.; Bush, A.I. Characterization of copper interactions with alzheimer amyloid beta peptides: Identification of an attomolar-affinity copper binding site on amyloid beta1-42. *J. Neurochem.* **2000**, *75*, 1219–1233. [CrossRef] [PubMed]
72. Margerum, D.W.; Dukes, G.R. Kinetics and mechanisms of metal-ion and proton-transfer reactions. In *Metal Ions in Biological Systems*; Sigel, H., Ed.; Dekker: New York, NY, USA, 1974; Volume 1, pp. 158–207.
73. Arena, G.; La Mendola, D.; Pappalardo, G.; Sovago, I.; Rizzarelli, E. Interactions of Cu2+ with prion family peptide fragments: Considerations on affinity, speciation and coordination. *Coord. Chem. Rev.* **2012**, *256*, 2202–2218. [CrossRef]
74. Santoro, A.; Wezynfeld, N.E.; Stefaniak, E.; Pomorski, A.; Płonka, D.; Krezel, A.; Bal, W.; Faller, P. Cu transfer from amyloid-β4–16 to metallothionein-3: the role of the neurotransmitter glutamate and metallothionein-3 Zn(II)-load states. *Chem. Commun.* **2018**, *54*, 12634–12637. [CrossRef]
75. Gans, P.; Sabatini, A.; Vacca, A. Investigation of equilibria in solution. Determination of equilibrium constants with the HYPERQUAD suite of programs. *Talanta* **1996**, *43*, 1739–1753. [CrossRef]
76. Schwarzenbach, G. *Die Komplexometrische Titration*, 2nd ed.Oberostendorf, Germany, 1956.
77. Irving, H. *Complexometric Titration*; Methuen & Co.: London, UK, 1957.
78. Flaschka, H.A. *EDTA Titrations*; Pergamon Press: London, UK, 1959.
79. Harris, D. *Quantitative Chemical Analysis*, 6th ed.; W.H. Freeman & Co.: New York, NY, USA, 2003.
80. Alberty, A.R. Recommendations for nomenclature and tables in biochemical thermodynamics (IUPAC Recommendations 1994). *Pure Appl. Chem.* **1994**, *66*, 1641–1666. [CrossRef]
81. Pettit, L.D.; Hefford, R.J. Stereoselectivity in the metal complexes of aminoacids and dipeptides. In *Metal Ions in Biological Systems*; Sigel, H., Ed.; Marcel Dekker: New York, NY, USA, 1979; Volume 9, pp. 174–209.
82. Zékány, L.; Nagypál, I. *Computational Methods for the Determination of Formation Constants*; Leggett, D.J., Ed.; Plenum Press: New York, NY, USA, 1985; pp. 291–355.
83. Faller, P.; Hureau, C.; Dorlet, P.; Hellwige, P.; Coppel, Y.; Collin, F.; Alies, B. Methods and techniques to study the bioinorganic chemistry of metal–peptide complexes linked to neurodegenerative diseases. *Coord. Chem. Rev.* **2012**, *256*, 2381–2396.
84. Johnson, R.A.; Manley, O.; Spuches, A.M.; Grossoehme, N.E. Dissecting ITC data of metal ions binding to ligands and proteins. *Biochim. et Biophysica. Acta.* **2016**, *1860*, 892–901. [CrossRef] [PubMed]
85. Velazquez Campoy, A.; Freire, E. ITC in the post-genomic era . . . ? Priceless. *Biophys. Chem.* **2005**, *115*, 115–124. [CrossRef] [PubMed]
86. Hansen, L.D.; Fellingham, G.W.; Russell, D.J. Simultaneous determination of equilibrium constants and enthalpy changes by titration calorimetry: Methods, instruments, and uncertainties. *Anal. Biochem.* **2011**, *409*, 220–229. [CrossRef]
87. Demarse, N.A.; Quinn, C.F.; Eggett, D.L.; Russell, D.J.; Hansen, L.D. Calibration of nanowatt isothermal titration calorimeters with overflow reaction vessels. *Anal. Biochem.* **2011**, *417*, 247–255. [CrossRef]
88. Wiseman, T.; Williston, S.; Brandts, J.F.; Lint, L.N. Rapid measurement of binding constants and heats of binding using a new titration calorimeter. *Anal. Biochem.* **1989**, *179*, 131–137. [CrossRef]

89. Turnbull, W.B.; Daranas, A.H. On the value of c: Can low affinity systems be studied by isothermal titration calorimetry? *J. Am. Chem. Soc.* **2003**, *125*, 14859–14866. [CrossRef] [PubMed]
90. Tellinghuisen, J. Isothermal titration calorimetry at very low c. *Anal. Biochem.* **2008**, *373*, 395–397. [CrossRef] [PubMed]
91. Arena, G.; Gans, P.; Sgarlata, C. HypCal, a general-purpose computer program for the determination of standard reaction enthalpy and binding constant values by means of calorimetry. *Anal. Bioanal. Chem.* **2016**, *408*, 6413–6422. [CrossRef] [PubMed]
92. Bolles, T.F.; Drago, R.S. A Calorimetric Procedure for Determining Free Energies, Enthalpies, and Entropies for the Formation of Acid-Base Adducts. *J. Am. Chem. Soc.* **1965**, *87*, 5015–5019. [CrossRef]
93. Sgarlata, C.; Arena, G.; Longo, E.; Zhang, D.; Yang, Y.; Bartsch, R.A. Heavy metal separation with polymer inclusion membranes. *J. Membr. Sci.* **2008**, *323*, 444–451. [CrossRef]
94. Specfit, Spectrum Software Associates, Chapel Hill, NC. Available online: http://www.kingkongsci.co.uk/specfitglobalanalysis.htm (accessed on 13 May 2019).
95. Smirnova, J.; Zhukova, L.; Witkiewicz-Kucharczyk, A.; Kopera, E.; Olędzki, J.; Wysłouch-Cieszyńska, A.; Palumaa, P.; Hartwig, A.; Bal, W. Quantitative electrospray ionization mass spectrometry of zinc finger oxidation: The reaction of XPA zinc finger with H_2O_2. *Anal. Biochem.* **2007**, *369*, 226–231. [CrossRef] [PubMed]
96. Martell, A.E.; Smith, R.M. *Critical Stability Constants*; Volume 6 (Second Supplement); Plenum Press: New York, NY, USA, 1989.
97. Protonic Software. Available online: http://www.hyperquad.co.uk/hyss.htm (accessed on 13 May 2019).
98. Maret, W. Analyzing free zinc(II) ion concentrations in cell biology with fluorescent chelating molecules. *Metallomics* **2015**, *7*, 202–211. [CrossRef] [PubMed]
99. Brecher, K. A guide for the perplexed. *Nature* **1979**, *278*, 215–218. [CrossRef]

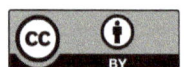

© 2019 by the authors. Licensee MDPI, Basel, Switzerland. This article is an open access article distributed under the terms and conditions of the Creative Commons Attribution (CC BY) license (http://creativecommons.org/licenses/by/4.0/).

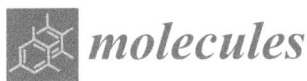

Review

Serum iron, Magnesium, Copper, and Manganese Levels in Alcoholism: A Systematic Review

Cezary Grochowski [1,2,*], Eliza Blicharska [3], Jacek Baj [1], Aleksandra Mierzwińska [4], Karolina Brzozowska [4], Alicja Forma [4] and Ryszard Maciejewski [1]

1. Chair and Department of Anatomy, Medical University of Lublin, 20-090 Lublin, Poland; jacek.baj@me.com (J.B.); maciejewski.r@gmail.com (R.M.)
2. Department of Neurosurgery and Pediatric Neurosurgery, Medical University of Lublin, 20-090 Lublin, Poland
3. Department of Analytical Chemistry, Medical University of Lublin, 20-090 Lublin, Poland; bayrena@o2.pl
4. Department of Forensic Medicine, Medical University of Lublin, 20-090 Lublin, Poland; mierzwinska.aa@gmail.com (A.M.); brzozowskak@gmail.com (K.B.); aforma@o2pl (A.F.)
* Correspondence: cezary.grochowski@o2.pl

Academic Editors: Francesco Crea and Alberto Pettignano
Received: 22 March 2019; Accepted: 6 April 2019; Published: 7 April 2019

Abstract: The aim of this paper was to review recent literature (from 2000 onwards) and summarize the newest findings on fluctuations in the concentration of some essential macro- and microelements in those patients with a history of chronic alcohol abuse. The focus was mainly on four elements which the authors found of particular interest: Iron, magnesium, copper, and manganese. After independently reviewing over 50 articles, the results were consistent with regard to iron and magnesium. On the other hand, data were limited, and in some cases contradictory, as far as copper and manganese were concerned. Iron overload and magnesium deficiency are two common results of an excessive and prolonged consumption of alcohol. An increase in the levels of iron can be seen both in the serum and within the cells, hepatocytes in particular. This is due to a number of factors: Increased ferritin levels, lower hepcidin levels, as well as some fluctuations in the concentration of the TfR receptor for transferrin, among others. Hypomagnesemia is universally observed among those suffering from alcoholism. Again, the causes for this are numerous and include malnutrition, drug abuse, respiratory alkalosis, and gastrointestinal problems, apart from the direct influence of excessive alcohol intake. Unfortunately, studies regarding the levels of both copper and manganese in the case of (alcoholic) liver disease are scarce and often contradictory. Still, the authors have attempted to summarize and give a thorough insight into the literature available, bearing in mind the difficulties involved in the studies. Frequent comorbidities and mutual relationships between the elements in question are just some of the complications in the study of this topic.

Keywords: alcoholism; alcoholic liver disease; iron; magnesium; copper; manganese; deficiency

1. Introduction

Fluctuations in the concentration of minerals, vitamins, and ions in the human body are common among those patients who consume excessively high amounts of alcohol. Changes in these amounts are observed mainly due to an inappropriate nutritional status, alcohol-induced vomiting, diarrhea or excessive urination. Deficiency or excessive amounts of particular ions may induce more or less severe dysfunctions, including impairments in the proper functioning of the cardiovascular, nervous, and skeletal systems. In the following review paper, mainly iron, magnesium, manganese, and copper levels among alcohol-dependent people have been investigated. The main aim was to investigate potential changes in the concentration of these ions under the condition of chronic increased alcohol consumption. Over fifty articles have been reviewed by four independent authors, dating from the year 2000 onwards. The results were mostly conclusive with regard to the levels of iron and magnesium in those patients who suffer from alcohol dependence. All reviewed papers indicate an increase in the levels of serum iron and hepatic iron overload [1]. Iron is an essential element in a number of biochemical reactions. It forms complexes with oxygen, mainly in hemoglobin and myoglobin. Iron is also found in the active sites of enzymes responsible for oxidation and reduction reactions. The accumulation of iron in the liver is associated with increased ferritin synthesis and a reduced amount of hepcidin produced. Due to an increased synthesis of ferritin, more iron can be stored in the body [2]. Additionally, pathologically decreased amounts of hepcidin lead to an accumulation of iron. This is because of an increased efflux of these ions to the outside of the cell via ferroportin, thus increasing the level of iron in the bloodstream. Magnesium is an essential element responsible for the proper function of a number of enzymes in the organism [3]. Magnesium ions, for instance, are needed for the enzymes active in the production of ATP. Additionally, an ATP molecule itself is found in the form of a chelate with magnesium ion. Copper is an essential transition metal that acts as a cofactor for a number of enzymes, thus ensuring proper metabolism and homeostasis. It participates in the metabolism of lipids, as well as redox balance and iron mobilization—with the latter being an interesting relationship to be further explored in the context of (alcoholic) liver disease and iron overload. Finally, the role of manganese in the body's metabolism is mostly thanks to its function as a coenzyme: It is a structural part of arginase (essential in the proper metabolism of urea), among others. Manganese also acts as an activator of numerous enzymes in the Krebs cycle, particularly in the decarboxylation process. It is essential for proper bone growth. In higher concentrations, manganese can act as a neurotoxin which is then deposited in the brain, in particular the basal ganglia, affecting proper function [4]. Chronic alcohol consumption leads to structural changes in the brain [5–7]. Unfortunately, studies regarding the levels of both copper and manganese in the case of (alcoholic) liver disease are scarce and often contradictory. Still, the authors have attempted to summarize and draw conclusions, as well as propose potential future directions for research from the literature currently available.

Healthy Ranges

Iron levels differ between individuals and can indicate a number of metabolic disorders [8]. A healthy adult should have about 1700–2000 mg of iron in the form of heme iron, about 130–150 mg as a cofactor of a number of enzymes, as well as up to 1000 mg of stored iron held in reserves. An increase in iron stores is commonly seen in hemochromatosis as well as in non-alcoholic fatty liver disease (NAFLD), as a manifestation of the metabolic syndrome [9]. On the other hand, iron stores deficiency is common among patients suffering from anemia [10]. Ferritin is the most sensitive and specific indicator of iron deficiency [11,12]. Ferritin levels below 30 µg/L are an indicator of iron deficiency. Other serum markers of iron stores include transferrin–iron saturation [TS] and serum iron levels themselves [13–15]. All of the abovementioned markers are higher in people who consume mild or moderate amounts of alcohol compared to those in nondrinkers [16].

The total magnesium body content of a healthy individual should oscillate at around 20 mmol/kg of fat-free tissue. That is, an average healthy adult individual weighing 70 kg will have around 25 g of total body magnesium. Ninety-nine percent of the body's magnesium is in the form of intracellular magnesium and hence, magnesium serum levels cannot be used to diagnose magnesium deficiency or overload.

In physiological conditions, a healthy adult body contains 80 mg of copper with the concentration being highest in the eye, the heart, the liver, and the brain. The serum copper levels should fall at around 109 µg/100 mL, with 90% bound in the form of ceruloplasmin and the remaining copper loosely associated with serum albumins. Increased copper levels are associated with Alzheimer's disease.

Healthy ranges of manganese levels are 4–15 µg/L in the blood, 1–8 µg/L in urine, and 0.4–0.85 µg/L in serum. Excess manganese tends to accumulate in the basal ganglia of the brain. Normal manganese levels in the brain average 1–2 µg/g dry weight and vary depending on the region of the brain. An increase in the brain's manganese levels is associated with neurological disorders, Parkinson's disease in particular.

2. Iron Levels in Alcoholism

2.1. Concentration of Iron in the Liver

Pathologically high amounts of ferritin are usually diagnosed accidentally through screening tests or typical check-ups. The most common causes for high concentration of iron in the organism are alcoholism, inflammation, cytolysis, and metabolic syndrome. Patients with chronic hematologic diseases (either acquired or congenital), or those whose iron supplementation is excessively high, like alkalized patients or sportsmen, are particularly exposed to the risk of hyperphosphatemia. If ferritin concentration is excessively high, congenital hemochromatosis must initially be taken into account and excluded as the causative factor. Magnetic resonance imaging (MRI) of the liver is a useful tool in the diagnosis and treatment of hemochromatosis [17]. The majority of the serum ferritin is in a glycosylated form (60–90%), and macrophages are the source of it. The nonglycosylated fraction constitutes approximately 20–40%, with cytolysis being the major source. Appropriate levels of ferritin in the organism are 30–300 mg/L and 15–200 mg/L for men and women, respectively. Hyperphosphatemia occurs frequently in the case of chronic alcoholism. The prevalence varies from 40% even up to 70%. Interestingly, iron levels in the organism are not proportional to the amount of consumed alcohol. This can be explained because of the direct effects of alcohol. Ethanol induces synthesis of ferritin and decreases the amount of produced hepcidin in the body. Normally, ferritin concentration remains at <1000 mg/L, and the concentration of transferrin remains at a regular level as well. Among alcoholics, the concentration of ferritin exceeds 1000 mg/L, and the saturation of transferrin exceeds 60%. Excessively high levels of both transferrin and ferritin can be observed for up to 6 weeks after alcohol withdrawal. Additionally, other clinical consequences associated with excessive alcohol consumption, including acute or chronic hepatitis, might cause an increase in the levels of ferritin even up to >10.000 mg/L. During inflammation, a number of proinflammatory cytokines are released, including IL-1, IL-6, and TNF-alfa [18]. Particularly IL-6 stimulates the synthesis of ferritin and hepcidin. Increased amounts of hepcidin stimulate the uptake of iron by the enterocytes and macrophages, which is associated with increased synthesis of ferritin [19].

2.2. Iron Accumulation and the Role of Hepcidin

An excessive consumption of alcohol is responsible for a disturbance in iron metabolism in the organism. Accumulation of iron can damage a number of different organs—mainly the liver. Moreover, deficiency of iron due to macrocytic anemia or accumulation of iron in the liver among people who consume excessive amounts of alcohol can lead to hematologic disorders. One of the functions of hepatocytes is the synthesis of hepcidin, which is associated with control of iron accumulation and the location of iron in the organism. Hepcidin inhibits the transport of iron from enterocytes to the blood. It was observed that increased alcohol consumption lowers the expression of the gene coding hepcidin. Moreover, alcohol is proven to cause intracellular oxidative stress [20]. This is enhanced due to iron accumulation in the liver leading to hepatic steatosis, fibrosis, and eventually cirrhosis.

2.3. sTfR Receptor as a Marker in Alcoholism

Distortions of the iron metabolism among alcoholics are associated with deficiency or excessive amounts of iron in the organism, which may lead to hematologic disorders. Transferrin receptor TfR is a glycoprotein localized in the cell membrane of immature erythrocytes, which are found in the bone marrow. Its function is the transport of iron to the inside of the cells, previously binding to transferrin. Synthesis of the TfR receptor and transferrin depends on the activity of erythrocytes and the need for iron in the organism. Recently, sTfR was observed to be a beneficial marker in the diagnosis of iron deficiency, while other markers like hemoglobin levels or mean corpuscular volume (MCV) are at an appropriate level. Research has shown that average percentages of carbohydrate-deficient transferrin (CTD), alanine aminotransferase (ALT), gamma-glutamylotransferase (GGT), and MCV were significantly increased in the group of alcoholic patients in comparison to the control group. It was also observed that transferrin levels were not changed between the studied groups. However, transferrin iron saturation was much higher in the group of alcohol-dependent people. The level of sTfR is a beneficial method for the identification of iron deficiency in the organism. However, some conditions must first be followed, which are that other markers remain undisturbed and that sTfR is not strictly associated with acute phase reactions. There is a correlation between sTfR level and erythropoiesis and iron demand in the organism. Among healthy people, approximately 80% of this receptor is found in the bone marrow. The level of sTfR is therefore strictly associated with the activity of erythropoiesis in the bone marrow. This means that in case of anemia due to iron deficiency, the level of this receptor increases in the serum. Nevertheless, information is lacking when it comes to sTfR concentration in the conditions of excessive iron concentration in the body. This explains why the normal concentration of sTfR among alcoholic patients may inform about proliferation in the course of erythropoiesis. Since this level remains unchanged, iron absorption through transferrin receptor remains intact as well. A likely explanation for this is that the sTfR level depends on the suppression of hepcidin expression induced by ethanol. In the case of excessive absorption of iron in the intestinal tract (and thus, higher iron concentration in the blood), the ability of iron transport to the enterocytes and the speed of erythropoiesis remain intact. The concentration of sTfR in the serum does not depend on the metabolic status of the hepatocytes, age, and duration of alcohol addiction or alcohol withdrawal. As such, it can be concluded that neither alcohol consumption nor alcohol abstinence change the amount of transferrin receptors found in the serum.

2.4. Concentration of Iron in the Brain

Chronic alcohol abuse can lead to abnormally high amounts of iron in the organism, including in the brain [9]. An overload of iron can lead to neurotoxicity in the brain [21]. However, it is important to note that iron concentration is normally rather high due to its high metabolic rate and the need for iron as an enzymatic cofactor for myelination or catecholamine synthesis.

One of the methods that enable the monitoring of iron concentration in the brain is an MRI technique called quantitative susceptibility mapping [22,23]. The results of this research paper have shown an increase of iron concentration in all regions of the brain, with some differences in the deposited amounts depending on the specific region in the brain. The increase in iron concentration varied from 7% to 15%. Most significant differences were observed mainly in the caudate nucleus, the putamen, and the globus pallidus, as well as in the dentate nucleus. Such high concentrations of iron in deep grey matter are comparable to those in the liver in some cases [24].

Some evidence suggests that brain function restoration is possible following a period of abstinence from alcohol [25].

3. Magnesium Levels in Alcoholism

3.1. Alcohol as a Reason of Hypomagnesemia

Hypomagnesemia is a frequently occurring electrolyte disorder due to a number of possible causes. These include drug abuse, malnutrition, respiratory alkalosis, excessive alcohol intake or gastrointestinal problems. According to a recent report published by the Mayo Clinic, the risk of developing hypomagnesemia among people who excessively consume alcohol varies from 30% even up to 80% [26]. This condition is observed when the serum magnesium concentration is below 0.66 mmol/L. However, clinical symptoms are observed when it falls further still, below 0.5 mmol/L.

Severe deficiency of magnesium ions can lead to a severe imbalance in the body's homeostasis [27,28]. Magnesium is essential for protein synthesis and a number of enzymatic reactions [29]. Furthermore, there is a correlation between the amount of magnesium ions and a number of other elements, including phosphorus, calcium or potassium [30]. As such, any imbalance in one of these may eventually induce other consequences similar to those caused by magnesium deficiency. Magnesium deficiency, for instance, leads to hypocalcemia, since it affects the magnesium-dependent adenyl cyclase generation of cyclic adenosine monophosphate. As a consequence, this decreases the amount of parathormone in the body. Therefore, it leads to changes in the functioning of the cell membranes and causes disorders of the nervous and cardiac systems, as well as inappropriate functioning of the muscles [31]. The pathogenic mechanisms of hypomagnesemia also include magnesuria, which may be related to hypophosphatemia, metabolic acidosis, or direct effect of the alcohol on the amount of the ions in the organism [32].

3.2. Concentration of Ionized Magnesium in the Erythrocytes and Blood Plasma

A disturbed pattern of magnesium levels in the organism is commonly observed among those patients with a history of chronic alcohol abuse. Ionized magnesium constitutes approximately 67% of the total pool of the magnesium in the body, but only 1% of this amount is found in the blood serum. As such, the relationship between extracellular and intracellular ion concentration can be studied, which may present more clearly the effect of the intake of the alcohol on these amounts. Hypomagnesemia of alcohol-dependent patients is mainly due to alcohol-induced vomiting and diarrhea, excessive urination, and an inappropriate diet lacking in a proper vitamin and microelements supplementation. The research so far is consistent in reporting that alcohol consumption only affects the amount of the ionized magnesium, with little or no effect on the total magnesium concentration [33].

In the study performed by Ordak et al. [34], the amount of ionized magnesium in the erythrocytes and blood plasma of both alcohol-dependent people and the control group was investigated. The results indicated that the amount of magnesium in the erythrocytes in the alcohol-dependent group was almost twice as low compared to that in the control group. However, the amount of ionized magnesium in the blood plasma in both groups remained unchanged. Interestingly, the total amount of magnesium in the blood plasma and the erythrocytes differed between the two groups. A significant decrease was observed in the alcohol-dependent group compared to the control group. Additionally, SF-36 questionnaires performed in both groups showed that individuals with lower total magnesium concentration tend to have a lower quality of life. They were more impulsive and susceptible to mental disturbances, as well as suffered from sleeping disorders. Furthermore, a correlation was found between the amount of ionized magnesium and physiological changes as analyzed by the Bried symptom inventory, the Barratt impulsiveness scale, and the sleep disorder questionnaire.

3.3. Hypomagnesemia and Cardiovascular System

Alcohol consumption may also lead to changes of the cardiac conduction system. The cardiovascular system is usually affected when ethanol consumption exceeds 80g daily for approximately 10 years. However, lower daily doses for a longer period of time or greater doses for shorter than ten years may also lead to similar clinical consequences [35,36].

One of the dysfunctions associated with this observation may be prolongation of the QT interval. In the study performed by Moulin et al. (2015) [37], groups of both active and abstinent alcoholics were studied. The results showed that active alcoholics exhibited a higher heart rate. Furthermore, 12 out of 166 individuals, among whom 10 were active alcoholics, were observed with prolonged QT interval. Hypomagnesemia has been shown in 50% of those individuals with a prolonged QT interval. The study showed that active alcoholics were three times more likely to develop hypomagnesemia, and at least nine times more likely to exhibit a prolonged QT interval. This suggests that hypomagnesemia caused by alcoholism may be a relevant factor in the prolongation of the QT interval. In a case study performed by Hiroki Nakasone et al. (2001), a patient suffering from alcoholic liver cirrhosis was observed to have critical arrhythmia (torsade de pointes, TdP). The laboratory data showed hypomagnesemia, which could potentially lead to the development of TdP. Therapy included a supplementation of magnesium sulfate to restore appropriate magnesium levels. It can be concluded that patients with an alcoholic liver disease, along with hypomagnesemia and hypocalcemia and a prolonged QT interval, are at higher risk of developing torsade de pointes.

Other studies, including research by Paulo Borini et al. (2001), presented similar results of prolonged QT intervals in female alcoholics alike [38].

3.4. Effects of the Hypomagnesemia on the Digestive System

Considerable magnesium deficiency has also been observed among alcoholics with pancreatitis caused by excessive alcohol intake. Magnesium deficiency was higher among alcoholics with pancreatitis than among those where this condition was not present [39,40]. The research concludes that continuous intake of alcohol may lead to the greater magnesium deficiency over time.

In the study performed by Turecky in 2006, a group of 44 patients with liver steatosis (either alcoholic or non-alcoholic) and a control group were investigated [41]. The study explored whether alcohol consumption is responsible for magnesium deficiency and whether liver disorders may also play a significant role. The results showed hypomagnesemia in both groups. Patients suffering from hepatic steatosis showed distortions in the secretion of bile acids as well. This consequently lowers the amount of endogenous magnesium concentration, as the increased amounts of fatty acids in the intestinal lumen form insoluble soaps with magnesium.

Since hypomagnesemia was also observed in the group of non-alcoholic patients, it must be considered that alcoholism is not the only cause of hypomagnesemia among patients with hepatic steatosis.

3.5. Alcohol Intake and Paralysis

One severe consequence of excessive alcohol intake is paralysis associated with both hypokalemia and hypomagnesemia. The continual excretion of minerals and vitamins from the body may induce muscle weakness due to inappropriate amounts of ions, mainly in the intracellular environment. The treatment in the form of infusion of thiamine, glucose, potassium, and magnesium results in quick improvement of hypomagnesemia [42]. On the other hand, hypokalemia might not be improved that quickly. Nevertheless, muscle performance appears to be improved, and symptoms of the paralysis are significantly lowered [32]. Since hypomagnesemia-induced kaliuresis eventually leads to hypokalemia, potassium replacement may play a role in the treatment of paralysis.

3.6. Hypomagnesemia and Neural Dysfunctions

Since hypomagnesemia is a common electrolyte disorder associated with excessive alcohol intake, it has a great impact on every system of the organism. It includes more or less severe implications on the nervous system. One of such dysfunctions may be childhood seizures with non-neurological etiology but as a cause of hypomagnesemia [43]. In all of the cases concerning childhood seizures with no neurological background, a decreased level of magnesium has been observed. Additionally, when magnesium supplementation has been provided, the intensity of seizures was lowered. The exact mechanism of decline of magnesium and seizures has not been proposed. Nevertheless, it was studied on a rat model which showed that a decreased level of extracellular magnesium leads to lack of antagonism at the N-methyl-D-aspartate-type glutamate receptors, thus resulting in epileptiform discharges.

Even though it may be not that common, hypomagnesemia can lead to such implications as posterior reversible encephalopathy syndrome (PRES). This condition is also induced by various factors like high blood pressure, autoimmune disorders, renal failure or immunosuppressive therapy. However, there are cases of PRES induced by hypomagnesemia noted in the literature. This was confirmed by the chemical analysis of serum magnesium levels in patients with PRES. In this case, the parenteral replacement of magnesium induced rapid clinical improvement.

3.7. Hypomagnesemia and Level of Other Ions

A two-year-long hospital study was performed in 2012 by George Liamis et al. [44]. Patients chosen for the following study were a group of 107 nonselected, consecutive, adult patients (over 18 years of age) who were observed with hypomagnesemia. Among the examined group, 13 patients (12.1%) developed hypomagnesemia due to the excessive alcohol consumption. The study also showed a link between magnesium deficiency and other elements, including potassium and calcium. Additionally, the study indicated a higher incidence of hypomagnesemia in patients over the age of 65. Thus, it should be considered that hypomagnesemia induced by alcohol consumption may be more or less severe when other factors are taken into consideration. This includes the presence of other disorders like diabetes mellitus or pancreatitis, the intake of medicines such as loop and thiazide diuretics or proton pump inhibitors, age or nutritional status.

4. Copper levels in Alcoholism

4.1. Copper in the Case of Alcoholism: Deficiency or Increased Levels?

While there are a number of consistent reports on selenium and zinc deficiency and excessive alcohol consumption, reports on copper are scarcer and often inconclusive, or indeed lead to contradictory results [45]. On the one hand, copper deficiency has been reported in a number of studies on alcoholic liver disease (ALD), as well as malnutrition linked to alcoholism [46,47]. However, some studies (Rahelic et al., 2006) have also reported an increase in copper levels of patients suffering from alcoholism, as linked to zinc deficiency [48]. This goes to show just how intricate the relationship between copper levels and other metabolic conditions is [49]. Since the liver is a central organ for copper metabolism, copper deficiency has been reported in diseases where the metabolism of lipids has been disrupted, including non-alcoholic liver disease (Eigner at al., 2008), as well as liver cirrhosis in the course of alcoholism [50]. Other common diseases linked to insufficient copper concentration are obesity, metabolic syndrome, hematological disorders, and ischemic heart disease [51,52]. However, none of the above relationships have been extensively studied, and reports from 2000 onwards are lacking.

4.2. The Relationship Between Copper and Zinc

Serum copper levels remain in a close relationship with the levels of zinc in an inversely proportional relationship. The mechanism of this interaction is yet to be fully understood, but it is certain that high zinc consumption inhibits copper absorption. A difficulty in reporting and comparing copper levels is the fact that copper is mostly an extracellular element (90%), while the contents of zinc in blood serum are low at 1%, and zinc is mostly found in the intracellular environment. This has been accounted for in the study by Ordak et al., 2017, where the relationship between the concentrations of zinc in erythrocytes/copper in blood plasma in alcohol-dependent patients and the clinical parameters was explored [53]. It was concluded that copper deficiency in alcohol-dependent patients often correlates to reduced and impaired function of the central nervous system, thus affecting patients' mental and physical state. Indeed, since any increase in zinc absorption can lead to a significant copper deficiency, maintenance of the proper copper to zinc ratios is essential to the body's homeostasis. Both the levels of zinc and copper are affected in the case of alcoholism, consequently impairing day-to-day functioning.

An imbalance in the levels of copper and zinc has been linked to Alzheimer's disease (AD) (Mital et al., 2018; Sensi et al., 2018) [54,55]. Pathogenesis of Alzheimer's disease involves accumulation of the β-amyloid (Aβ) peptide in the brain. The activity of the Zn^{2+}-dependent endopeptidase neprilysin (NEP) remains in an inverse relationship with brain Aβ levels during aging and in AD—as such, zinc acts as a protective agent. An increase in the levels of copper, on the other hand, will have a negative effect both through the modulation of zinc concentration, as well as directly, since copper ions inhibit the proper function of NEP. With regard to cognitive function, copper is also linked to certain psychiatric disorders, including depression [56]. Moreover, copper deficiency can be a cause of idiopathic myelopathy in adults [57–59].

4.3. The Relationship Between Copper and Iron

Copper availability contributes to iron metabolism and homeostasis, as described by Eigner et al. 2008 [50]. However, the relationship between copper serum and liver content was explored here only in the context of patients suffering from non-alcoholic fatty liver disease (NAFLD). No similar studies have been performed with regard to hepatic iron concentrations and alcoholic liver disease (ALD). Still, it may be worthy to note that the low bioavailability of copper observed in NAFLD causes increased hepatic iron stores. This is due to a decrease in the expression of ferroportin-1 as well as the activity of ceruloplasmin ferroxidase, both of which lead to a block in the export of iron from the liver. As both copper deficiency and iron overload are commonly observed in patients with ALD, a corresponding relationship may be worth exploring in future studies. The same study also reported low liver copper concentrations in the context of increased insulin resistance and metabolic syndrome.

4.4. Copper Deficiency and Lipid Metabolism

Another notice of copper insufficiency linked to lipid synthesis and fatty liver disease was made in the paper by Morrell et al., 2017 [51]. Inadequate levels of copper may further promote the damaging effects of excessive alcohol consumption. Copper deficiency promotes dyslipidemia and increases oxidative stress, since copper is an essential cofactor of a number of antioxidant enzymes. Similarly, the study by Ordak et al. found decreased serum copper concentration among 20.4% of the examined patients with alcohol abuse history [53]. This also corresponded to worsening of the symptoms related to the central nervous system, including depressive symptoms and sleep deficiency.

4.5. Serum Copper Levels and Hepatitis C Virus (HCV) Infection

In addition to alcohol consumption, the relationship between serum copper levels (as well as zinc and selenium) and HCV infection was investigated in a paper by Gonzalez-Reimers et al. (2009) [60]. In this research paper, no interaction was found between serum copper levels and alcohol consumption, but a direct relationship was confirmed between serum Cu levels and HCV infection. Serum copper levels were significantly lower in those patients who tested positive for HCV. Moreover, the relationship between copper and serum malonaldehyde (MDA), as well as a number of cytokines, was explored, but no conclusive relationship was confirmed.

4.6. Copper Muscle Content

Finally, an interesting study by Duran Castellon et al. (2005) looked at muscle content of several elements in order to explore the pathogenesis of muscle myopathy as a common occurrence in patients with alcoholism [61]. This seems to be a combined effect of alcoholism and protein malnutrition. Increased protein catabolism, as well as protein deficiency stemming from malnutrition is commonly seen in alcoholism and may be linked to copper depletion. This leads to muscle myopathy. However, in this study, ethanol was found to have no effect on muscle copper. Rather, the decreased copper content in the muscles was due to malnutrition and, in particular, lack of protein in the diet.

5. Manganese in Alcoholism

5.1. Manganese in the Case of Alcoholism: Always Overload?

Similarly to the case of copper discussed in the above paragraph, the role of manganese in the pathogenesis of liver cirrhosis and other complications in the course of alcoholism is not yet fully understood. However, studies seem to be consistent in reporting elevated levels of manganese in the course of alcoholic liver disease. In particular, the role of manganese as a neurotoxin plays a significant role in the course of development of brain disorders related to alcohol abuse, including hepatic encephalopathy and acquired hepatocerebral degeneration [48]. In contrast to the above findings, a study was performed by Gonzalez-Perez et al. (2011), which explored the relationship between ethanol consumption and manganese levels in the bones [62]. Significant decrease of bone manganese levels was found in those patients with a history of alcohol abuse.

5.2. Manganese and Liver Cirrhosis

The study by Rahelić et al. (2006) explored the levels of a number or trace elements in patients with liver cirrhosis, including manganese [48]. No significant difference was found in the levels of manganese between the control group and the male and female patients with cirrhosis. However, there was a significant increase in the levels of magnesium in the case of patients suffering from Child-Pugh type C liver cirrhosis compared to patients with Child-Pugh A and B liver cirrhosis. The same study further investigated the relationship between manganese levels in cirrhotic patients with or without encephalopathy and ascites. No differences were found in the case of encephalopathy, which is contradictory to some studies performed in the past, which indeed found increased manganese levels as a relation to hepatic encephalopathy. Significantly higher levels of manganese were reported in the serum of those cirrhotic patients simultaneously suffering from ascites. The study goes on to discuss manganese bile secretion and its disruption in the course of cholestatic liver disease as one possible cause for increased manganese levels. Still, it is apparent that the levels of manganese as explored simply in a relationship to liver cirrhosis can vary significantly between different research studies.

5.3. Manganese as a Neurotoxin

Studies are consistent in reporting an increased deposition of manganese in the brain of patients suffering from hepatic encephalopathy (HE) [63–69]. This is depicted in the form of hyperintense MRI signals, in particular in the region of the brain called the globus pallidus [70]. Some studies have reported manganese levels that were up to seven times higher in patients with alcoholic liver disease as shown on the MRI. Again, the previously mentioned bile secretion of manganese plays a significant role in manganese crossing the blood–brain barrier in those patients suffering from cholestasis. Compromised liver function does not allow for proper detoxification, and one of the results is a free passage of neurotoxins entering the brain. As increased amounts of manganese are deposited in the brain, and in particular in the astrocytes, this causes Alzheimer type II changes, as well as selective neuronal loss in the basal ganglia [66–68]. Similar effects are seen in ammonia deposition in the brain [69]. Apart from the globus pallidus, substantia nigra reticulata is another region particularly affected [63]. Both the structure and the proper function of the brain are affected.

Another brain disorder linked to alcohol abuse and increased magnesium concentration is acquired hepatocerebral degeneration (AHE). This condition needs to be made distinct from hepatic encephalopathy, and it affects approximately 1% of patients suffering from liver cirrhosis. It exhibits itself in the form of symptoms similar to those of Wilson disease, but without the increased copper deposition. Instead, high intracerebral manganese concentration can be seen in T1-weighted MRI images, in particular in the basal ganglia, as well as some other brain areas (pituitary gland, quadrigeminal plate, caudate nucleus, subthalamic region, and red nucleus) [70].

Finally, cirrhosis-related parkinsonism commonly affects patients with a history of chronic alcohol abuse. Again, this is due to manganese deposition in the brain and is characterized by the usual symptoms of Parkinson's disease but without affecting the nigrostriatal system [71,72]. Instead, elevated levels of manganese can be found in the serum, as well as depicted in an MRI scan.

5.4. Bone Manganese Levels and Alcohol Abuse

An interesting relationship was explored in the study by Gonzalez-Perez et al. (2011) [62]. This study reported significantly lower levels of manganese in the bone tissue of patients suffering from alcoholic disease. Since appropriate levels of manganese are required for normal bone growth, as it is a cofactor of a number of essential enzymes, both the bone mass and bone synthesis were affected.

This, together with malnutrition and the deficiency of other essential elements, can be linked to the loss of bone mass and osteoporosis in patients with a history of alcohol abuse.

6. Conclusions

Chronic alcohol consumption leads to a number of metabolic disorders associated with deficiency or overloading of elements in the human body. The article is a review paper concerning, inter alia, correlation of Fe, Mg, Cu, and Mn content in people who drink alcohol. The accumulation of iron in the liver is associated with increased ferritin synthesis and a reduced amount of hepcidin produced. This results in alcohol damage of the liver, which can consequently lead to liver cirrhosis.

Excessive alcohol consumption leads to hypomagnesemia in almost all cases, differing in the severity of the deficiency. It is mainly due to malnutrition, excessive urination, diarrhea, and alcohol-induced vomiting. Interestingly, according to the research mentioned in this work, it is mainly ionized magnesium concentration which is changed. Thence, it has a significant impact on many functions and systems of the organism, including the nervous or cardiovascular system. Nicotine-dependent patients with alcoholism are at a particularly higher risk of cardiovascular disease [73]. The appropriate treatment of such a condition, like infusion of magnesium, glucose, and potassium, may give quick improvement for the patients, also lowering the harmful effects of hypomagnesemia on the organism. However, it also must be taken into consideration that deficiency of magnesium ions is strictly associated with changed concentrations of other ions like calcium, iron, manganese or copper. Therefore, there is a relationship between these values and overall effects on the organism. Moreover, other factors like age, additional diseases, and usage of medicine may have an impact on the overall concentration of the magnesium among alcohol-dependent people.

With regard to copper levels in patients suffering from alcoholism, the few studies that have been performed so far are inconsistent. Several authors investigated serum copper levels in patients both in the case of alcoholism, as well as during periods of withdrawal and after the relief of withdrawal symptoms, and observed copper deficiency. Still, a number of similar studies reported no difference in the levels of copper between alcohol-dependent individuals and control groups. In fact, higher levels of copper were reported in the case of the former in some research studies. Certainly, the close relationship between copper and zinc, and indeed the intricate relations between the metabolic pathways of various other elements add to the complexity of research on the topic.

The few studies which have been found by the authors seem to be consistent in reporting increased magnesium levels in the patients characterized by chronic alcohol abuse. In particular, the role of manganese as a neurotoxin is discussed. Alcohol abuse induces brain atrophy and neuronal loss, as well as myelin sheath degeneration, all of which seem to be reversible to some extent following periods of alcohol abstinence [74,75]. One study explored the reduction in the levels of manganese in the bones as a result of alcohol abuse.

Funding: This research received no external funding.

Conflicts of Interest: The authors declare no conflict of interest.

References

1. Lieb, M.; Palm, U.; Hock, B.; Schwarz, M.; Domke, I.; Soyka, M. Effects of alcohol consumption on iron metabolism. *Amer. J. Drug Alcoh. Abuse* **2010**, *37*, 68–73. [CrossRef]
2. Lorcerie, B.; Audia, S.; Samson, M.; Millière, A.; Falvo, N.; Leguy-Seguin, V.; Bonnotte, B. Diagnosis of hyperferritinemia in routine clinical practice. *La Presse Médicale* **2017**, *46*. [CrossRef]
3. Konrad, M.; Schlingmann, K.P.; Gudermann, T. Insights into the molecular nature of magnesium homeostasis. *Amer. J. Physiol. Renal Physiol.* **2004**, *286*. [CrossRef]
4. Saito, M.; Sawayama, T. Visualised manganese ion within the basal ganglia and long axonal tracts. *J. Neurol. Neuros. Psych.* **2009**, *80*, 695. [CrossRef]

5. Chanraud, S.; Martelli, C.; Delain, F.; Kostogianni, N.; Douaud, G.; Aubin, H.; Martinot, J. Brain Morphometry and Cognitive Performance in Detoxified Alcohol-Dependents with Preserved Psychosocial Functioning. *Neuropsychopharmacology* **2006**, *32*, 429–438. [CrossRef]
6. Mann, K.; Agartz, I.; Harper, C.; Shoaf, S.; Rawlings, R.R.; Momenan, R.; Heinz, A. Neuroimaging in Alcoholism: Ethanol and Brain Damage. *Alcohol. Clin. Exp. Res.* **2001**, *25*. [CrossRef]
7. Sutherland, G.T.; Sheedy, D.; Kril, J.J. Neuropathology of alcoholism. *Handb. Clin. Neurol.* **2014**, *125*, 603–615. [CrossRef]
8. Deugnier, Y.; Bardou-Jacquet, É.; Lainé, F. Dysmetabolic iron overload syndrome (DIOS). *La Presse Médicale* **2017**, *46*. [CrossRef]
9. Whitfield, J.B.; Zhu, G.; Madden, P.A.; Montgomery, G.W.; Heath, A.C.; Martin, N.G. Biomarker and Genomic Risk Factors for Liver Function Test Abnormality in Hazardous Drinkers. *Alcohol. Clin. Exp. Res* **2019**, *43*, 473–482. [CrossRef]
10. Bermejo, F.; García-López, S. A guide to diagnosis of iron deficiency and iron deficiency anemia in digestive diseases. *World J. Gastroenterol.* **2009**, *15*, 4638–4643. [CrossRef]
11. Soppi, E.T. Iron deficiency without anemia-a clinical challenge. *Clin. Case Rep.* **2018**, *6*, 1082–1086. [CrossRef]
12. Matos, L.C.; Batista, P.; Monteiro, N.; Ribeiro, J.; Cipriano, M.A.; Henriques, P.; Carvalho, A. Iron stores assessment in alcoholic liver disease. *Scand. J. Gastroenterol.* **2013**, *48*, 712–718. [CrossRef] [PubMed]
13. Radicheva, M.P.; Andonova, A.N.; Milcheva, H.T.; Ivanova, N.G.; Kyuchukova, S.G.; Nikolova, M.S.; Platikanova, M.S. Serum Markers of Iron Metabolism in Chronic Liver Diseases. *J. Med. Sci.* **2018**, *6*. [CrossRef]
14. Buyukasik, N.S.; Nadir, I.; Akin, F.E.; Cakal, B.; Kav, T.; Ersoy, O.; Buyukasik, Y. Serum iron parameters in cirrhosis and chronic hepatitis: Detailed description. *Turk. J. Gastroenterol.* **2011**, *22*, 606–611. [CrossRef]
15. Evangelista, A.S.; Nakhle, M.C.; Araújo, T.F.; Abrantes-Lemos, C.P.; Deguti, M.M.; Carrilho, F.J.; Cançado, E.L. HFE Genotyping in Patients with Elevated Serum Iron Indices and Liver Diseases. *BioMed. Res. Int* **2015**, 1–8. [CrossRef] [PubMed]
16. Ioannou, G.N.; Dominitz, J.A.; Weiss, N.S.; Heagerty, P.J.; Kowdley, K.V. The effect of alcohol consumption on the prevalence of iron overload, iron deficiency, and iron deficiency anemia. *Gastroenterology* **2004**, *126*, 1293–1301. [CrossRef] [PubMed]
17. Purohit, V.; Russo, D.; Salin, M. Role of iron in alcoholic liver disease: Introduction and summary of the symposium. *Alcohol* **2003**, *30*, 93–97. [CrossRef]
18. Wang, H.J. Alcohol, inflammation, and gut-liver-brain interactions in tissue damage and disease development. *World J. Gastroenterol.* **2010**, *16*, 1304. [CrossRef]
19. García-Valdecasas-Campelo, E.; González-Reimers, E.; Santolaria-Fernández, F.; Vega-Prieto, M.J.; Milena-Abril, A.; Sánchez-Pérez, M.J.; Rodríguez-Rodríguez, E. Brain atrophy in alcoholics: Relationship with alcohol intake; liver disease; nutritional status, and inflammation. *Alcohol Alcohol.* **2007**, *42*, 533–538. [CrossRef]
20. Hoek, J.B.; Cahill, A.; Pastorino, J.G. Alcohol and mitochondria: A dysfunctional relationship. *Gastroenterology* **2002**, *122*, 2049–2063. [CrossRef] [PubMed]
21. Singh, N.; Haldar, S.; Tripathi, A.K.; Horback, K.; Wong, J.; Sharma, D.; Singh, A. Brain Iron Homeostasis: From Molecular Mechanisms To Clinical Significance and Therapeutic Opportunities. *Ant. Redox Signaling* **2014**, *20*, 1324–1363. [CrossRef] [PubMed]
22. Xia, S.; Zheng, G.; Shen, W.; Liu, S.; Zhang, L.J.; Haacke, E.M.; Lu, G.M. Quantitative measurements of brain iron deposition in cirrhotic patients using susceptibility mapping. *Acta Radiologica* **2015**, *56*, 339–346. [CrossRef] [PubMed]
23. Sun, H.; Walsh, A.J.; Lebel, R.M.; Blevins, G.; Catz, I.; Lu, J.; Wilman, A.H. Validation of quantitative susceptibility mapping with Perls iron staining for subcortical gray matter. *NeuroImage* **2015**, *105*, 486–492. [CrossRef] [PubMed]
24. Juhás, M.; Sun, H.; Brown, M.R.; Mackay, M.B.; Mann, K.F.; Sommer, W.H.; Greenshaw, A.J. Deep grey matter iron accumulation in alcohol use disorder. *NeuroImage* **2017**, *148*, 115–122. [CrossRef] [PubMed]
25. Crews, F.T.; Nixon, K. Mechanisms of Neurodegeneration and Regeneration in Alcoholism. *Alcohol Alcoholism* **2009**, *44*, 115–127. [CrossRef]
26. Cheungpasitporn, W.; Thongprayoon, C.; Qian, Q. Dysmagnesemia in Hospitalized Patients: Prevalence and Prognostic Importance. *Mayo Clinic Proc.* **2015**, *90*, 1001–1010. [CrossRef]

27. Martin, K.J.; Gonzalez, E.A.; Slatopolsky, E. Clinical Consequences and Management of Hypomagnesemia. *J. Amer. Soc. Nephrol.* **2008**, *20*, 2291–2295. [CrossRef]
28. Noronha, L.J.; Matuschak, G.M. Magnesium in critical illness: Metabolism, assessment, and treatment. *Applied Physiol. Int. Care Med.* **2012**, *2*, 71–83.
29. Jahnen-Dechent, W.; Ketteler, M. Magnesium basics. *Clin. Kidney J.* **2012**, *5*, i3–i14. [CrossRef]
30. Huang, C.; Kuo, E. Mechanism of Hypokalemia in Magnesium Deficiency. *J. Amer. Soc. Nephrol.* **2007**, *18*, 2649–2652. [CrossRef]
31. Avoaroglu, D.; Inal, T.C.; Demir, M.; Attila, G.; Acartürk, E.; Evlice, Y.E.; Kayrin, L. Biochemical Indicators and Cardiac Function Tests in Chronic Alcohol Abusers. *Croat. Med. J.* **2005**, *46*, 233–237.
32. Yanagawa, Y.; Suzuki, C.; Imamura, T. Recovery of paralysis in association with an improvement of hypomagnesemia due to alcoholism. *Amer. J. Emer. Med.* **2011**, *29*. [CrossRef] [PubMed]
33. Rylander, R.; Mégevand, Y.; Lasserre, B.; Amstutz, W.; Granbom, S. Moderate alcohol consumption and urinary excretion of magnesium and calcium. *Scand. J. Clin. Labo. Invest.* **2001**, *61*, 401–405. [CrossRef]
34. Ordak, M.; Maj-Zurawska, M.; Matsumoto, H.; Bujalska-Zadrozny, M.; Kieres-Salomonski, I.; Nasierowski, T.; Wojnar, M. Ionized magnesium in plasma and erythrocytes for the assessment of low magnesium status in alcohol dependent patients. *Drug Alcohol. Dep.* **2017**, *178*, 271–276. [CrossRef]
35. DiNicolantonio, J.J.; O'Keefe, J.H.; Wilson, W. Subclinical magnesium deficiency: A principal driver of cardiovascular disease and a public health crisis. *Open Heart* **2018**, *5*, e000668. [CrossRef]
36. Schwalfenberg, G.K.; Genuis, S.J. The Importance of Magnesium in Clinical Healthcare. *Scientifica* **2017**, 4179326. [CrossRef]
37. Moulin, S.R.; Mill, J.G.; Rosa, W.C.; Hermisdorf, S.R.; Caldeira, L.D.; Zago-Gomes, E.M. QT interval prolongation associated with low magnesium in chronic alcoholics. *Drug Alcohol Dep.* **2015**, *155*, 195–201. [CrossRef]
38. Borini, P.; Terrazas, J.H.; Júnior, A.F.; Guimarães, R.C.; Borini, S.B. Female alcoholics: Electrocardiographic changes and associated metabolic and electrolytic disorders. *Arquivos Brasileiros De Cardiologia* **2003**, *81*. [CrossRef]
39. Sobral-Oliveira, M.B.; Faintuch, J.; Guarita, D.R.; Oliveira, C.P.; Carrilho, F.J. Nutritional profile of asymptomatic alcoholic patients. *Arquivos De Gastroenterologia* **2001**, *48*, 112–118. [CrossRef]
40. Papazachariou, I.M.; Martinez-Isla, A.; Efthimiou, E.; Williamson, R.C.; Girgis, S.I. Magnesium deficiency in patients with chronic pancreatitis identified by an intravenous loading test. *Clin. Chim. Acta* **2000**, *302*, 145–154. [CrossRef]
41. Turecky, L.; Kupcova, V.; Szantova, M.; Uhlikova, E.; Viktorinova, A.; Czirfusz, A. Serum magnesium levels in patients with alcoholic and non-alcoholic fatty liver. *Bratislavské lekárske listy* **2006**, *107*, 58.
42. Voma, C.; Romani, A.M. Role of Magnesium in the Regulation of Hepatic Glucose Homeostasis. *Glucose Homeost.* **2014**, *25*. [CrossRef]
43. Chen, B.B.; Prasad, C.; Kobrzynski, M.; Campbell, C.; Filler, G. Seizures Related to Hypomagnesemia. *Child. Neurol. Open* **2016**, *3*. [CrossRef]
44. Elisaf, M.; Liamis, G.; Liberopoulos, E.; Siamopoulos, K.C. Mechanisms of Hypocalcemia in Alcoholic Patients. *Nephron* **2001**, *89*, 459–460. [CrossRef]
45. Bergheim, I.; Parlesak, A.; Dierks, C.; Bode, J.C.; Bode, C. Nutritional deficiencies in German middle-class male alcohol consumers: Relation to dietary intake and severity of liver disease. *Eur. J. Clin. Nutr.* **2003**, *57*, 431–438. [CrossRef]
46. Halsted, C.H. Nutrition and Alcoholic Liver Disease. *Semin. Liv. Dis.* **2004**, *24*, 289–304. [CrossRef]
47. Shibazaki, S.; Uchiyama, S.; Tsuda, K.; Taniuchi, N. Copper deficiency caused by excessive alcohol consumption. *BMJ Case Rep.* **2017**. [CrossRef]
48. Rahelic, D.; Kujundzic, M.; Bozikov, V. Zinc, Copper, Manganese and Magnesium in Liver Cirrhosis. *Micronutr. Health Res.* **2008**, 227.
49. Collins, J.F.; Prohaska, J.R.; Knutson, M.D. Metabolic crossroads of iron and copper. *Nutr. Rev.* **2010**, *68*, 133–147. [CrossRef]
50. Aigner, E.; Theurl, I.; Haufe, H.; Seifert, M.; Hohla, F.; Scharinger, L.; Datz, C. Copper Availability Contributes to Iron Perturbations in Human Nonalcoholic Fatty Liver Disease. *Gastroenterology* **2008**, *135*, 680–688. [CrossRef]

51. Morrell, A.; Tallino, S.; Yu, L.; Burkhead, J.L. The role of insufficient copper in lipid synthesis and fatty-liver disease. *IUBMB Life* **2017**, *69*, 263–270. [CrossRef]
52. Halfdanarson, T.R.; Kumar, N.; Li, C.; Phyliky, R.L.; Hogan, W.J. Hematological manifestations of copper deficiency: A retrospective review. *Eur. J. Haematol.* **2008**, *80*, 523–531. [CrossRef]
53. Ordak, M.; Bulska, E.; Jablonka-Salach, K.; Luciuk, A.; Maj-Żurawska, M.; Matsumoto, H.; Bujalska-Zadrozny, M. Effect of Disturbances of Zinc and Copper on the Physical and Mental Health Status of Patients with Alcohol Dependence. *Biol. Trace Element Res.* **2017**, *183*, 9–15. [CrossRef]
54. Mital, M.; Bal, W.; Frączyk, T.; Drew, S.C. Interplay between Copper, Neprilysin, and N-Truncation of β-Amyloid. *Inorg. Chem.* **2018**, *57*, 6193–6197. [CrossRef]
55. Sensi, S.L.; Granzotto, A.; Siotto, M.; Squitti, R. Copper and Zinc Dysregulation in Alzheimer's Disease. *Trends Pharmacol. Sci.* **2018**, *39*, 1049–1063. [CrossRef]
56. Słupski, J.; Cubała, W.J.; Górska, N. Role of copper in depression. Relationship with ketamine treatment. *Med. Hypotheses* **2018**, *119*, 14–17. [CrossRef] [PubMed]
57. Gregg, X.T. Copper deficiency masquerading as myelodysplastic syndrome. *Blood* **2002**, *100*, 1493–1495. [CrossRef] [PubMed]
58. Kumar, N.; Gross, J.B.; Ahlskog, J.E. Copper deficiency myelopathy produces a clinical picture like subacute combined degeneration. *Neurology* **2004**, *63*, 33–39. [CrossRef] [PubMed]
59. Kumar, N. Copper Deficiency Myelopathy (Human Swayback). *Mayo Clin. Proc.* **2006**, *81*, 1371–1384. [CrossRef] [PubMed]
60. González-Reimers, E.; Martín-González, M.C.; Alemán-Valls, M.R.; De la Vega-Prieto, M.J.; Galindo-Martín, L.; Abreu-González, P.; Santolaria-Fernández, F. Relative and Combined Effects of Chronic Alcohol Consumption and HCV Infection on Serum Zinc, Copper, and Selenium. *Biol. Trace Element Res.* **2009**, *132*, 75–84. [CrossRef]
61. Durán Castellón, M.; González-Reimers, E.; López-Lirola, A.; Martín Olivera, R.; Santolaria-Fernández, F.; Galindo-Martín, L.; González-Hernández, T. Alcoholic myopathy: Lack of effect of zinc supplementation. *Food Chem. Toxicol.* **2005**, *43*, 1333–1343. [CrossRef]
62. González-Pérez, J.M.; González-Reimers, E.; DeLaVega-Prieto, M.J.; Del Carmen Durán-Castellón, M.; Viña-Rodríguez, J.; Galindo-Martín, L.; Santolaria-Fernández, F. Relative and Combined Effects of Ethanol and Protein Deficiency on Bone Manganese and Copper. *Biol. Trace Element Res.* **2011**, *147*, 226–232. [CrossRef]
63. Sureka, B.; Bansal, K.; Patidar, Y.; Rajesh, S.; Mukund, A.; Arora, A. Neurologic Manifestations of Chronic Liver Disease and Liver Cirrhosis. *Curr. Probl. Diagn. Radiol.* **2015**, *44*, 449–461. [CrossRef]
64. Pasternak, K.; Kiełczykowska, M. Alcoholism, drug addiction and macro- and microelements in experimental and clinical studies. *Alkoholizm i Narkomania* **2003**, *16*, 25–37.
65. Hartleb, M. Hepatic encephalopathy in patients with liver cirrhosis. *Gastroenterol. Klin.* **2013**, *5*, 106–122.
66. Du, K.; Liu, M.; Pan, Y.; Zhong, X.; Wei, M. Association of Serum Manganese Levels with Alzheimer's Disease and Mild Cognitive Impairment: A Systematic Review and Meta-Analysis. *Nutrients* **2017**, *9*, 231. [CrossRef] [PubMed]
67. Bowman, A.B.; Kwakye, G.F.; Herrero Hernández, E.; Aschner, M. Role of manganese in neurodegenerative diseases. *J. Trace Elements Med. Biol.* **2011**, *25*, 191–203. [CrossRef]
68. Chen, P.; Totten, M.; Zhang, Z.; Bucinca, H. Iron and manganese-related CNS toxicity: Mechanisms, diagnosis and treatment. *Expert Rev. Neur.* **2019**. (accepted). [CrossRef]
69. Butterworth, R.F. Pathophysiology of hepatic encephalopathy: A new look at ammonia. *Metabolic Brain Disease* **2002**, *17*, 221–227. [CrossRef]
70. Zuccoli, G.; Siddiqui, N.; Cravo, I.; Bailey, A.; Gallucci, M.; Harper, C.G. Neuroimaging Findings in Alcohol-Related Encephalopathies. *Amer. J. Roentgenol.* **2010**, *195*, 1378–1384. [CrossRef] [PubMed]
71. Kim, Y. Neuroimaging in Manganese-Induced Parkinsonism. *Diagn. Rehabil. Parkinsons Dis.* **2011**. [CrossRef]
72. Rivera-Mancía, S.; Ríos, C.; Montes, S. Manganese accumulation in the CNS and associated pathologies. *BioMetals* **2011**, *24*, 811–825. [CrossRef]
73. Jarvis, C.M.; Hayman, L.L.; Braun, L.T.; Schwertz, D.W.; Ferrans, C.E.; Piano, M.R. Cardiovascular Risk Factors and Metabolic Syndrome in Alcohol- and Nicotine-Dependent Men and Women. *J. Cardiovascular Nurs.* **2007**, *22*, 429–435. [CrossRef]

74. Welzel, H.; Ende, G.; Walter, S.; Diehl, A.; Demirakca, T.; Flor, H.; Mann, K. Clinical and Neuropsychological Data in Chronic Alcoholic Patients: Correlation with MR Spectroscopy and Imaging. *Alcohol. Clin. Exper. Res.* **2004**, *28*. [CrossRef]
75. Sassine, M.; Mergler, D.; Bowler, R.; Hudnell, H. Manganese accentuates adverse mental health effects associated with alcohol use disorders. *Biol. Psychiat.* **2002**, *51*, 909–921. [CrossRef]

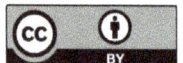

© 2019 by the authors. Licensee MDPI, Basel, Switzerland. This article is an open access article distributed under the terms and conditions of the Creative Commons Attribution (CC BY) license (http://creativecommons.org/licenses/by/4.0/).

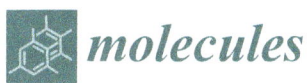

Review

Speciation Analysis of Trace Arsenic, Mercury, Selenium and Antimony in Environmental and Biological Samples Based on Hyphenated Techniques

Xiaoping Yu *, Chenglong Liu, Yafei Guo and Tianlong Deng *

Tianjin Key Laboratory of Marine Resources and Chemistry, College of Chemical Engineering and Materials Science, Tianjin University of Science & Technology, Tianjin 300457, China; 17302297916@163.com (C.L.); guoyafei@tust.edu.cn (Y.G.)
* Correspondence: yuxiaoping@tust.edu.cn (X.Y.); tldeng@tust.edu.cn (T.D.); Tel.: +86-022-60601156 (X.Y.)

Academic Editors: Francesco Crea and Alberto Pettignano
Received: 1 February 2019; Accepted: 28 February 2019; Published: 7 March 2019

Abstract: In order to obtain a well understanding of the toxicity and ecological effects of trace elements in the environment, it is necessary to determine not only the total amount, but also their existing species. Speciation analysis has become increasingly important in making risk assessments of toxic elements since the toxicity and bioavailability strongly depend on their chemical forms. Effective separation of different species in combination with highly sensitive detectors to quantify these particular species is indispensable to meet this requirement. In this paper, we present the recent progresses on the speciation analysis of trace arsenic, mercury, selenium and antimony in environmental and biological samples with an emphasis on the separation and detection techniques, especially the recent applications of high performance liquid chromatography (HPLC) hyphenated to atomic spectrometry or mass spectrometry.

Keywords: arsenic; mercury; selenium; antimony; speciation analysis; hyphenated technique

1. Introduction

Trace elements, as important components of the environment, play crucial roles in the functioning of life. Some elements such as arsenic (As), mercury (Hg) and antimony (Sb) can be highly toxic to various life forms, while some others are probably considered to be essential, but they can become toxic at higher doses. For example, selenium (Se) is widely recognized as an essential dietary component with numerous beneficial effects on health, but at levels higher than 5 µg/L will cause toxic effects [1,2]. It is generally recognized that the mobility, toxicity and bioavailability of trace elements depend strongly on their particular existing forms, and the determination of species rather than the total amount of an element is more important [3]. Usually, the ecological and healthy risk assessments of trace elements in the environment based on the species data will seem to be more reasonable and accurate than the total amount data.

"Chemical species" refers to the specific form of an element defined as to isotopic composition, electronic or oxidation state, and/or complex or molecular structure [4]. Usually, compounds that differ in isotopic composition, conformation, oxidation or electronic state, or in the nature of their complexed or covalently bound substituents, can be regarded as distinct chemical species [5]. The division suggested by Tessier et al. [6] is usually recommended in the research relevant to the species of heavy metals in soil or sediment. They distinguished and defined five fractions, i.e., exchangeable, carbonate-bound, iron and manganese oxides-bound, organic matter-bound, and the other mineral-bound metals. In addition, the BCR or modified BCR sequential extraction method [7,8] and the modified Tessier method [9] are also used to study the bound species of heavy metals in soil or sediment [10]. Nonetheless, these methods do not allow the differentiation between oxidation states of elements in aqueous phase, of which may be of great importance when considering their toxicity. As, Hg, Sb and Se probably exist in many forms in environmental and biological samples as shown in Table 1.

However, the main species existing in aquatic environments are inorganic forms, i.e., As(III), As(V); Hg(II); Sb(III), Sb(V); and Se(IV), Se(VI) [11–13], but methylation may occur in sediment environments due to the actions of microorganisms [14,15]. Selenosugars have been confirmed to be important urinary selenium metabolites, while selenohomolanthionine (SeHLan) is mainly detected in some Se-accumulating plants and yeasts [16–18]. Lipid-soluble arsenic compounds (arsenolipids) are mainly found in fish oils, fish liver, sashimi tuna, algae, et al. [19–21]. Of course, some unusual chemical species in biosamples or other complex samples probably exist. For example, tetramethylarsonium ion (TETRA), glyceryl phosphorylarsenocholine (GPAsC), and dimethylarsinothioic acid (DMAS) were found and identified in marine foods [22]; 4-aminophenylarsonic acid (4-APAA) and N-acetyl-4-hydroxyphenylarsonic acid (N-AHPAA) were found in chicken liver [23].

Table 1. Main species of As, Hg, Se and Sb commonly detected in environmental and biological samples.

Element	Species	Abbreviation	Chemical Formula
As	Arsenite (arsenous acid)	As(III)	$As(OH)_3$
	Arsenate (arsenic acid)	As(V)	$AsO(OH)_3$
	Monomethylarsenate (Monomethylarsonic acid)	MMA	$CH_3AsO(OH)_2$
	Dimethylarsonate (Dimethylarsinic acid)	DMA	$(CH_3)_2AsO(OH)$
	Trimethylarsinic oxide	TMAO	$(CH_3)_3AsO$
	Arsenocholine	AsC	$H_3C-As^--CH_2-CH_2-OH$ with CH_3 groups
	Arsenobetaine	AsB	$H_3C-As^+-CH_2-C(=O)O^-$ with CH_3 groups
	Arsenosugars	AsS	$H_3C-As^V(=O)-CH_2-R$ ribose derivative
	Roxarsone	Rox	$HO-C_6H_3(NO_2)-AsO_3H_2$
	Arsenolipids [a]		(lipid structures with $O=As(CH_3)_2$)
Hg	Inorganic bivalent mercury	Hg(II)	Hg^{2+}
	Methylmercury	MeHg	CH_3Hg^+
	Dimethylmercury	DMeHg	$(CH_3)_2Hg$
	Ethylmercury	EtHg	$CH_3CH_2Hg^+$
	Diethylmercury	DEtHg	$(CH_3CH_2)_2Hg$
	Methylethylmercury	MEtHg	$(CH_3CH_2)(CH_3)Hg$
	Phenylmercury	PhHg	$C_6H_5Hg^+$
Sb	Antimonite (Antimonous acid)	Sb(III)	$Sb(OH)_3$
	Antimonate (Antimonic acid)	Sb(V)	$SbO(OH)_3$
	Methylantimate (Methylantimonic acid)	MMSb	$CH_3SbO(OH)_2$
	Dimethylantimate (Dimethylantimonic acid)	DMSb	$(CH_3)_2SbO(OH)$
	Trimethylantimony dichloride	$TMSbCl_2$	$(CH_3)_3SbCl_2$

Table 1. Cont.

Element	Species	Abbreviation	Chemical Formula
Se	Selenite	Se(IV)	H_2SeO_3
	Selenate	Se(VI)	H_2SeO_4
	Selenomethionine	SeMet	$CH_3SeCH_2CH_2CH(NH_2)COOH$
	Selenocysteine	SeCys	$HSeCH_2CH(NH_2)COOH$
	Se-methylselenocysteine	SeMeCys	$CH_3SeCH_2CH(NH_2)COOH$
	Selenoethionine	SeEt	$CH_3CH_2SeCH_2CH_2CH(NH_2)COOH$
	Selenocystine	SeCys$_2$	$HOOCCH(NH_2)CH_2Se\text{-}SeCH_2CH(NH_2)COOH$
	Selenohomolanthionine	SeHLan	$HOOCCH(NH_2)CH_2CH_2SeCH_2CH_2CH(NH_2)COOH$
	Trimethylselenonium ion	TMSe$^+$	$(CH_3)_3Se^+$
	Selenocyanate	SeCN$^-$	$N\equiv C\text{—}Se^-$
	Selenosugar 1	SeSug 1	(structure)
	Selenosugar 2	SeSug 2	(structure)
	Selenosugar 3	SeSug 3	(structure)

[a] Some identified arsenic-containing fatty acids in cod-liver oil [21].

The lack of accurate speciation information is the major limitation for us to understand the environmental biogeochemical cycles of trace elements in the aquatic environments. In view of this, speciation analysis has become one of the fastest developed areas of analytical chemistry over the last two decades. "Speciation analysis" is defined by the IUPAC as analytical activities of identifying and/or measuring the quantities of one or more individual chemical species in a sample. It plays a unique role in the studies of biogeochemical cycles of compounds, determination of toxicity and eco-toxicity of selected elements, quality control of food products, control of medicines and pharmaceutical products, examination of occupational exposure and clinical analysis, etc. [24]. Generally, two complementary techniques are necessary for the speciation analysis of trace elements, i.e., separation and detection. The former provides an efficient and reliable separation of the species, and the latter provides adequate detection and quantification. Progresses in analytical instruments and methodology allow us to identify and measure the species presented in a particular system. Especially, the coupling of chromatographic techniques, such as gas chromatography (GC) and high performance liquid chromatography (HPLC), with a highly sensitive and selective detector, such as mass spectrometry (MS) or atomic spectrometry including atomic fluorescence spectrometry (AFS), atomic absorption spectrometry (AAS), and atomic emission spectrometry (AES) or optical emission spectrometry (OES) has been widely exploited and accepted for the speciation analysis of trace elements. Even though several reviews have been dedicated to the speciation analysis of As, Hg, Se, and Sb [25–32], this presented work reviews and discusses the different separation and detection methods for the speciation analysis of trace As, Hg, Se and Sb in environmental and biological samples with an emphasis on the hyphenated techniques.

2. Separation Techniques for Speciation Analysis

2.1. Non-Chromatographic Methods

The chemical form and quantitative information of a given element can be acquired by the application of basic chemistry methods. In other word, non-chromatographic procedures can provide simple methods to obtain sufficient information on the elemental species. Many review papers are available for the non-chromatographic speciation analysis methods [33–35], and the commonly used for As, Hg, Se and Sb include extraction and selective reduction.

2.1.1. Extraction

Extraction is usually used to separate one or a group of species from complex matrices, especially for environmental and biological samples [36,37]. Liquid-liquid extraction (LLE) is the oldest pre-concentration and isolation method for speciation analysis, and can be directly applied for the non-filtered samples with complex matrices [38]. Sequential extraction procedures using aqueous solutions, such as the Tessier or BCR method, are usually used to characterize the mobility, bioavailability, and potential toxicity of trace elements in soil and sediment. LLE may perform best for the redox labile elements such as As, Sb and Se, for which more discrete biogeochemical species may be generated due to the variations in oxidation number. At present, LLE is rarely applied for elemental species in water samples except for the extraction of different bounded species in sediment or soil. Some modified LLE methods are also used for speciation analysis. For example, ultrasonic assisted dispersive liquid-liquid microextraction (LLME) was used by Panhwar et al. [39] to analyze Se(IV) and Se(VI) in water and food samples. A vortex assisted dispersive liquid-liquid microextraction method based on the freezing of deep eutectic solvent was developed by Akramipour et al. [40] for the determination of organic and inorganic mercury in blood samples. Based on the principles of extraction, some other extracting methods have been developed including liquid phase microextraction (LPME) [41,42], solid phase extraction (SPE) [43,44], solid phase microextraction (SPME) [45–48], etc.

LPME is introduced to reduce the consumption of solvent, in which a drop of organic solvent is suspended at the tip of a microsyringe and exposed to the analytical sample. Subsequently, the drop is retracted and transferred to a particular analytical instrument after extraction. For example, speciation analysis of As(III) and As(V) based on Triton X-100 hollow fiber LPME coupled with flame atomic absorption spectrometry (FAAS) was developed by Zeng et al. [42], during which the Triton X-100 was used as an extractant and an acceptor solution; Fan [49] determined Sb(III) and total Sb in natural water by electrothermal atomic absorption spectrometry (ET-AAS) prior to separate and preconcentrate using *N*-benzoyl-*N*-phenylhydroxylamine-chloroform single drop; Single-drop gold nanoparticles for headspace microextraction and colorimetric assay of Hg(II) in environmental waters was developed by Tolessa et al. [50], and the recovery for a 10 nM spiked level was in the range of 86.8~99.8%.

SPE is popular for sample preparation in organic analysis, but it is also found to be used for speciation analysis of inorganic elements. The analytes are extracted by selective sorption and subsequently derivatized or directly detected after eluted with a small amount of organic solvent [51,52]. Sorbents with an immobilized chelating reagent such as ammonium pyrrolidine dithiocarbamate (APDC) are widely used in SPE. For example, a new magnetic SPE using octyl-immobilized silica-coated magnetic Fe_3O_4 (C_8-Fe_3O_4@SiO_2) nanoparticles was proposed by Li et al. [53] for the determination of trace Sb(III) and Sb(V) in water, during which Sb(III) forms a hydrophobic complex with APDC at pH 5.0 and is retained on C_8-Fe_3O_4@SiO_2 nanoparticles, whereas Sb(V) remains as free species in aqueous solution. A method for multi-element inorganic speciation analysis of As(III, V), Se(IV, VI) and Sb(III, V) in natural water using SPE technology was developed by Zhang et al. [54], during which TiO_2 was used to adsorb total inorganic As, Se and Sb, while As(III), Se(IV) and Sb(III) were coprecipitated with Pb-PDC. The concentration of As(V), Se(VI) and Sb(V) was subsequently calculated by the differences. Recently, Peng et al. [55] synthesized and employed functionalized multi-wall carbon nanotubes as the adsorbent for simultaneous speciation analysis of inorganic As, Se and chromium (Cr) in environmental waters by microcolumn SPE. The detection limits of 15, 38 and 16 ng/L were obtained for As(V), Cr(VI) and Se(VI), respectively.

SPME offers a fast way for species separation by collecting target analytes from the sample headspace or liquid phase directly or after derivatization. It offers the possibility to eliminate the interferences from matrices without the use of organic solvents [44,56,57]. For example, headspace

SPME coupled to miniaturized microplasma OES was developed by Zheng et al. [57] for the detection of mercury and lead in water samples. It is noted that SPME is also often used as a pretreatment method to separate or preconcentrate analytes prior to chromatographic separation [58,59]. Of course, direct coupling of SPME with particular detectors is also developed. For example, SPME was used by Panhwar et al. [45] for the determination of inorganic Sb speciation. Sb(III) forms hydrophobic complex with diethyl dithiocarbamate at pH 5.5 and subsequently adsorbed on polystyrene oleic acid imidazole polymer. A screening method was developed by Mester [60] to determine volatile metallic compounds (As, Se, Sn and Sb) in solid samples by examining the vapor phase above the sample with a SPME probe. The total analysis time was less than three minutes depending on the concentration of the target compounds.

Some assistant extracting techniques such as microwave-assisted extraction (MWAE) and ultrasound-assisted extraction (USAE) [39,61–64] have also been applied for speciation analysis so as to improve the speed of extraction. It is noted that although extraction methods can realize the determination of elemental speciation, they are usually used as pretreatment procedures for elemental speciation in complex samples followed by the chromatographic hyphenated techniques for species separation and detection [65–67]. For example, in order to determine As speciation in guano and ornithogenic sediments, MWAE was used by Lou et al. [65] to extract As(III), DMA, MMA, and As(V) in these sediments followed by the detection of HPLC-HG-AFS.

2.1.2. Selective Reduction

Selective reduction is used based on the differences of reduction potential between different species. The reduction potential can be controlled by the concentration of reductants, pH, as well as by the presence of catalysts or chelating agents. Selective reduction is generally related to the chemical vapor generation (CVG) methods, by which the volatile derivatives are produced during reduction [68,69].

It is noted that some organic Se and Hg species are not easily reduced by BH_4^-, which is the most frequently used reductant during CVG. In view of this, photochemical reduction by exposure to ultraviolet (UV) irradiation or ultrasound (US) is often used. For example, when Hg(II) and MeHg were determined by Hu et al. [70] using hydride generation ultraviolet atomization-AFS, the Hg(II) can be directly measured under the non-ultraviolet radiation mode after reducing using 0.1% (m/v) KBH_4, while the MeHg needs to be transformed into elemental mercury vapor under the ultraviolet atomization. when total Hg and MeHg in biological samples were detected by Vieira et al. [71], total Hg was measured after the tissues were digested in either formic acid or tetramethylammonium hydroxide (TMAH) following the reduction of both species by exposure the solution to UV irradiation, during which MeHg was selectively quantitated by adding of 10% v/v acetic acid into TMAH solution. Mendez et al. [72] assessed the UV and US induced redox reactions for the determination of Se(IV), Se(VI), SeMet, and SeCys in model water, enriched natural water, and soil/fly ash extracts using HG-AAS and AFS. Furthermore, Chen et al. [73] systematically studied the photochemical behaviors of selenium and some of its organic compounds in various aqueous matrices under UV irradiation at 300 nm. It was observed that the photochemical oxidation rate of Se(IV) to Se(VI) was greatly enhanced in the presence of HNO_3 at concentration larger than 1×10^{-3} M. Subsequently, the same authors [74] developed a method for the speciation analysis of Se in natural waters based on the photochemical reactions of Se(IV) and organic selenium in different aqueous solutions.

2.1.3. Miscellaneous Methods

Due to the different volatility of Hg and its compounds, thermal desorption is also used to distinguish their different species. For example, thermal release analysis in combination with AAS was developed and applied by Shuvaeva et al. [75] to determine Hg(II), MeHg, and mercury sulfide in lake sediment and plankton. Similar technique was also used by Kaercher et al. [76] for the determination of inorganic and total Hg in biological samples based on the temperature control of the measurement cell. Masking with relevant masking agents is sometimes used for speciation analysis. For example, 8-hydroxyquinoline was used as an effective masking agent by Liao and Deng [77] for As speciation analysis in porewater and sediment. In addition, in order to realize redox speciation analysis of Sb in water, Xi et al. [78] systematically tested several compounds as masking agents to inhibit the generation of stibine from Sb(V), and the results indicated that citric acid and NaF can successfully suppress this process.

It is noted that any pretreatment processes during speciation analysis even the routine processes such as the changes of pH, temperature and pressure can bring about irreversible transformation of the analyzed species. Non-chromatographic speciation analysis methods often employ multi-step procedures resulting in a high risk for the loss of analytes or species conversion. In this sense, these characteristics make such methods very difficult to automate and integrate into modern systems. Therefore, high selective and sensitive analytical methods without or with few pretreatment steps are more competent for speciation analysis.

2.2. Chromatographic Hyphenated Techniques

The most detailed information in relation to speciation analysis is no doubt derived from hyphenated techniques, in particular those involving separation by HPLC, GC or CE with ICP-MS or atomic spectrometry detectors. The main advantages of those techniques include extremely low detection limit, insignificant interference, high precision and repeatability, etc. The selection of a proper separation technique depends on the physico-chemical properties such as volatility, charge or polarity of the different species, and sometimes combination of two or more separation methods is also adopted.

2.2.1. Gas Chromatography

GC is mainly used for Hg species separation when compared with that used for As, Se and Sb, during which volatile Hg species are stripped from the sample solution after derivatization, and subsequently pre-concentrated mainly through sorptive, extraction, etc [79–81]. The trapped Hg derivatives are then released thermally and transferred quantitatively to the GC for species separation.

Because the packed columns will lead to poor reproducibility, thus capillary or multi-capillary GC is usually used to provide superior separation power and better detection limits [82]. Usually, the Hg derivatives need to be quantitatively transferred to a suitable detection system after the GC separation. A comparative study of GC coupled with AFS, AES and MS for MeHg and EtHg analysis following aqueous derivatization was conducted by Cai et al. [83], and found that both GC-AFS and GC-AES shown to be excellent techniques with detection limits in the range of sub-picogram levels. Nevado et al. [84] also evaluated the advantages and disadvantages of three hyphenated techniques including GC-MS, GC-ICP-MS and GC-pyrolysis-AFS for Hg speciation analysis in different sample matrices after aqueous ethylation with sodium tetraethylborate. Absolute detection and quantification limits were in the range of 1~4 pg for GC-MS, 0.05~0.21 pg for GC-ICP-MS, and 2~6 pg for GC-pyro-AFS.

Of course, there are also some applications of GC on the speciation analysis of As, Se and Sb [85–89]. For example, volatile organic Se compounds of dimethylselenide (DMSe) and dimethyldiselenide (DMDSe) in environmental and biological samples were determined by Ghasemi et al. [88] using a headspace hollow fiber protected LPME combined with capillary GC-MS. It is noted that although GC attracts particular attention due to its high efficiency and simplicity of coupling, however, in contrast to GC, HPLC has the ability of dealing with non-volatile compounds without any derivatization in some cases, and thus extending the range of application.

2.2.2. Liquid Chromatography

Among the most popular hyphenated techniques used for the determination of As, Hg, Se and Sb species, the coupling of various liquid chromatographies (LC) including ion-exchange chromatography

(IEC) and reverse-phase chromatography (RPC) with particular detectors has obtained the fastest development [90]. Table 2 shows the recent applications of hyphenated techniques based on LC separation for the speciation analysis of As, Hg, Sb and Se in environmental and biological samples.

Table 2. Some publications of hyphenated techniques based on LC for the speciation analysis of As, Hg, Sb and Se in environmental and biological samples in recent three years.

Element	Species	Column	Detector	Matrix	Ref.
As	As(III), As(V), DMA, MMA	Hamilton PRP-X100	ICP-MS	Rice	[91]
	As(III), As(V), DMA, MMA	Agilent ZORBAX SB-Aq	ICP-MS	Cynomolgus macaques	[92]
	As(III), As(V), DMA, MMA, AsB, AsC	Dionex IonPac AS19	ICP-MS	Ophiocordyceps sinensis	[93]
	As(III), As(V), DMA, MMA, AsB	Hamilton PRP-X100	MS	Marine samples	[94]
	As(III), As(V)	Hamilton PRP-X100	ICP-MS	Spring, well, and tap water	[95]
	As(III), As(V), DMA, MMA, AsB, AsC	Dionex IonPac AS7	ICP-MS	Bones	[96]
	As(III), As(V), DMA, MMA, AsB, AsC	Dionex IonPac AS7	ICP-MS	Fish	[97]
	As(III), As(V), DMA, MMA	Homemade capillary columns	ICP-MS	Human urine	[98]
	As(III), As(V), DMA, MMA, AsB	Hamilton PRP-X10	ICP-MS/MS	Seafood	[99]
	As(III), As(V)	Hamilton PRP-X100	ICP-MS	Mexican maize tortillas	[100]
	As(III), As(V), DMA, MMA, AsB, AsC	Dionex IonPac AS19	ICP-MS	Edible Mushrooms	[101]
	As(III), As(V), DMA, MMA, AsB	Hamilton PRP-X100	HG-AFS	Seafood	[102]
	As(III), As(V), DMA, MMA, AsB	Hamilton PRP-X10	ICP-MS/MS	Seafood	[103]
	As(III), As(V), AsB	Dionex IonPac AS9-HC	ICP-MS	Water and biota samples	[104]
	As(III), As(V)	Hamilton PRP-X100	ICP-MS	Natural water	[105]
	DMA, AsB	Spheris S5SCX	ICP-MS	Fish	[106]
	As(V), As(III), DMA, MMA	Hamilton PRP-X100	ICP-MS	Environmental waters	[107]
Hg	Hg(II), MeHg, EtHg	ZORBAX SB-C18	ICP-MS	Surface water, seawater	[51]
	Hg(II), MeHg, EtHg	Athena-C18	HG-AFS	Environmental and biological samples	[108]
	Hg(II), MeHg, EtHg	ZORBAX SB-C18	ICP-MS	Sea Cucumber	[109]
	Hg(II), MeHg, EtHg	Venusil MP-C18	CV-AFS	Natural water	[110]
	Hg(II), MeHg, EtHg	PerkinElmer C8	ICP-MS	Fish oils	[111]
	Hg(II), MeHg, PhHg	Hypersil ODS2 C18	ICP-MS	Water and fish samples	[112]
	Hg(II), MeHg	CLC-ODS C18	ICP-MS	Water	[113]
	Hg(II), MeHg	CLC-ODS C18	ICP-MS	Water	[114]
	Hg(II), MeHg, EtHg	Agilent Eclipse plus C18	ICP-MS	Rice	[115]
	Hg(II), MeHg, EtHg	Synergi Hydro-RP C18	ICP-MS	Polluted sediments	[116]
Se	Se(IV), Se(VI), SeMet, SeCys	Spheris S5 SAX	ICP-MS	Chicken breast	[117]
	Se(IV), Se(VI), SeMet, SeCys	Hamilton PRP-X100	HG-AFS	Cordyceps militaris	[118]
	Se(IV), Se(VI), SeMet, SeCys, SeMeCys	StableBond C18	ICP-MS	Rice	[119]
	Se(IV), Se(VI)	ODS-3	UV-Vis	Water and biological samples	[120]
Sb	Sb(III), Sb(V)	Hamilton PRP-X100	ICP-MS	Bottled flavored drinking water	[121]
	Sb(III), Sb(V)	Hamilton PRP-X100	ICP-MS	Matrix-rich mineral water	[122]
	Sb(III), Sb(V), TMSbCl$_2$	Hamilton PRP-X100	ICP-MS	Waters, juices	[123]
	Sb(III), Sb(V)	Hamilton PRP-X100	ICP-MS	Drinking water	[124]
	Sb(III), Sb(V)	Hamilton PRP-X100	HG-AFS	Soils, sediments, volcanic ashes	[125]
	Sb(III), Sb(V)	Hamilton PRP-X100	ICP-MS	Sediments, water	[126]

The separation of species in IEC is based on the interactions between the positively or negatively charged species and the stationary phase that contains a cationic functional group (anion exchange) or an anionic functional group (cation exchange). IEC is an ideal technique for the separation of inorganic As, Sb, Se and many charged organometallic ions such as organoselenium and organoarsenic. Buffer solutions are commonly used as eluents for IEC with concentration usually not exceeding 25 mM. RPC is used based on the partition of the analytes between a non-polar stationary phase, in which it usually contains a covalently bound C_8 or C_{18} linear hydrocarbon, and a relatively polar mobile phase. RPC is usually superior to IEC for the separation of organometallic species. Figure 1 shows the representative chromatograms of As [127], Hg [128], Se [129], and Sb [123] species in aqueous solutions separated by IEC or RPC.

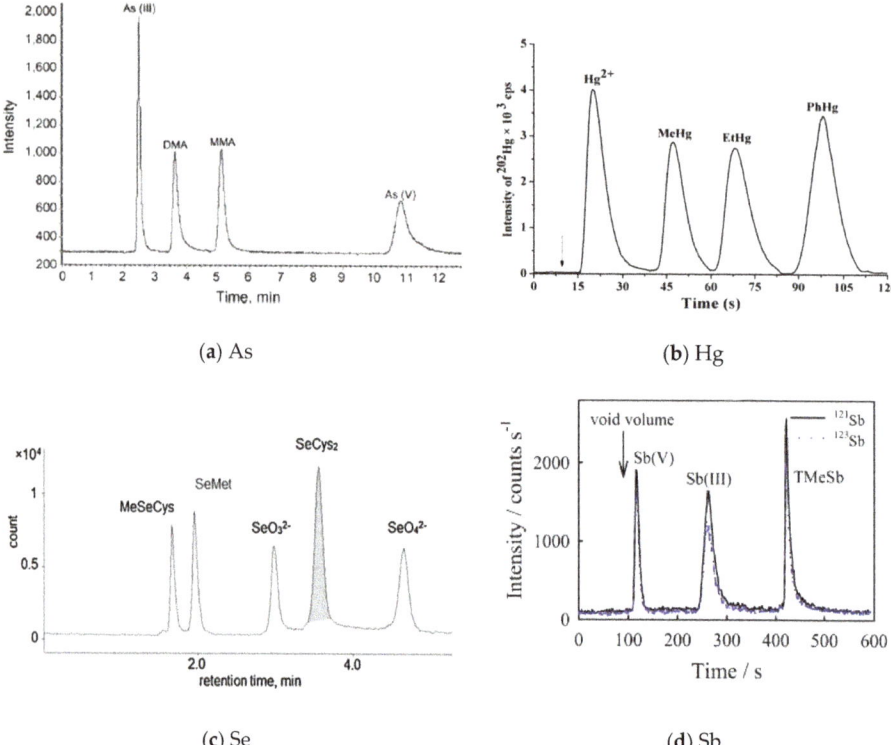

Figure 1. Representative chromatograms of As, Hg, Se, and Sb species. (**a**) As: each at 100 µg/L. Detected by HG-AFS after separated by a Hamilton PRP-X100 column (250 mm × 4.1 mm i.d., 10 µm) and eluted using 15 mM $(NH_4)_2HPO_4$ (pH 6.0) at 1.0 mL/min flow rate [127]; (**b**) Hg: each at 5.0 µg/L. Detected by ICP-MS after separated by two consecutive Zorbax SCX columns (12.5 mm × 4.6 mm i.d., 5 µm) and eluted by 2.0 mM thiourea (pH 2.0) at 1.5 mL/min flow rate [128]; (**c**) Se: Detected by ICP-MS after separated by a Dinoex IonPac AS11 anion exchange column (4 mm i.d. × 250 mm) and eluted using 10 mM $NaHCO_3$ with 2% acetonitrile (pH 11 adjusted with 20% NH_3) at 0.6 mL/min flow rate [129]; (**d**) Sb: 1 µg/L Sb(V), 2 µg/L Sb(III) and TMeSb. Detected by ICP-MS after separated by a Hamilton PRP-X100 column (250 × 4.1 mm i.d., 10 µm) and eluted using A: 20 mM EDTA + 2 mM KHP (pH 5.5), B: 20 mM + 2 mM KHP + 40 mM $(NH_4)_2CO_3$ + 1% (v/v) CH_3OH (pH 9.0) at 1.2 mL/min flow rate [123].

IEC is the most extensively used method for As, Sb and Se speciation separation, followed closely by the use of ion-pair reversed-phase chromatography (IP-RPC). Many factors, such as the pH, ionic strength, concentration and flow rate of mobile phase, the concentration and species of organic modifiers, will all influence the separation and retention of analytes in IEC and IP-RPC. For example, arsenic species are neutral, anionic or cationic depending on the pH. As a result, their retention will strongly depend on the pH of mobile phase. Therefore, anion-exchange chromatography is often used to separate As(III), As(V), MMA and DMA, while cation-exchange chromatography is used to separate AsB, AsC, TMAO, Me_4As^+ for such compounds at cationic or neutral states cannot be retained by an anion-exchange mechanism. Of course, both anion and cation exchange columns are sometimes used in a complementary fashion [130]. Based on the requirement of pH, phosphate [131], carbonate [132], nitrate [133], acetate [134] or miscellaneous [122,135] are commonly used as buffers. The anion-exchange mode with phosphate buffer elution is classically used for the separation of As(III), As(V), MMA and DMA. Sodium salt buffer leaves carbon residue upon the sampler and skimmer cones of ICP-MS resulting in the instability of plasma and the shift of retention time. Therefore, mobile phases based on ammonium salts are often used. For example, the use of NH_4NO_3 as mobile phase was shown to produce good signal stability on the ICP-MS with minimal salt deposit on the sample and skimmer cones [136].

When IP-RPC is used for species separation, a counterion is added to the mobile phase, and a secondary chemical equilibrium of the ion-pair is used to control the retention and selectivity [115,119,137]. The resolutions of species depend on the concentration and kind of ion-pair reagents, organic modifiers (e.g., methanol or acetonitrile), ionic strength, and pH of the mobile phase, etc [138]. The most used ion-pair reagent is tetrabutylammonium (TBA, including hydroxide, phosphate and bromide). Le et al. [139] investigated a series of ion pair reagents having different strength such as methanesulfonate, ethanesulfonate, propanesulfonate for the simultaneous analysis of Se and As species in a reversed phase C18 column, and found that all seven As species investigated were well separated within 16 min using hexanesulfonate as ion pair reagent. Choosing a suitable pH of eluent is also critical for species separation by IP-RPC. For example, As(III) is a neutral species, and will be eluted in the void volume at a low pH of mobile phase. But it becomes a negatively charged species when the pH of mobile phase is increased above its pK_a value of 9.2. Chromatographic column also plays an important role in the separation of species. Usually, different chromatographic columns of the same separation mechanism have different separation effects. For example, Ammann [140] investigated two different polymeric anion-exchangers: a low capacity, weakly hydrophobic material (AS11, Dionex) and a more frequently used higher capacity, higher hydrophobicmaterial (AS7, Dionex), and found that AS11 provided better retention for MMA, AsB, As(III) than AS7, whereas DMA and Cl^- were more retained on AG7. Gao et al. [119] compared the separation effects of five selenium species by two anion-exchange columns (Hamilton PRP X-100 and Dionex AS19) and three typical reversed C18 columns (Agilent Eclipse Plus C18, Waters Xselect HSS T3 and StableBond C18), and found that the StableBond C18 is more robust or has a better resolution.

When LC is employed for Hg species separation, a RP column is commonly used. However, the organic solvent concentration in the mobile phase must be as low as possible in order to reduce carbon deposit on the ICP-MS instrument interface. In order to overcome the drawback caused by organic solvent, vapor generation (VG) technique can be employed after the LC separation, by which only the volatile Hg species are introduced into the plasma. Of course, Hg(II), MeHg, EtHg and PhHg can be separated in a cation-exchange chromatographic column due to they present in positively charged ions. For example, the four species were separated and determined by Chen et al. [128] by the coupling of cation-exchange chromatographic separation with ICP-MS detection.

Both isocratic and gradient ion-exchange chromatographic systems are used for species separation. Gradient separation generally has better resolution among different species, and is often used to reduce analytical time of strong retention species. However, gradient IP-RPC is not commonly adopted when ICP-MS is used as detector due to the signal drift is likely when substantially changing the organic content of the mobile phase. In addition, as the differences in structure and charge of different species, a single chromatographic mechanism is probably not sufficient for simultaneous study of organic and inorganic species. Combination of different chromatographic modes has therefore been applied by using columns in series or column-switching systems. For example, Milstein et al. [141] successfully separated and determined As(III), As(V), MMA, DMA, AsB, and AsC by connecting cation- and anion-exchange columns in series and eluting by $(NH_4)_2CO_3$ buffer. Of course, it is noted that the mobile phase used in multidimensional chromatography should be compatible with both chromatographic mechanisms.

2.2.3. Capillary Electrophoresis

Capillary electrophoresis (CE) is discussed as a complementary technique to GC and HPLC, and is a powerful tool in element speciation with high separation capability and environmentally friendly nature due to the use of aqueous buffer solutions with moderate pH and its extremely low reagent and sample consumption [142]. For example, ten As compounds including As(III), As(V), MMA, DMA, AsB, AsC, Rox, *o*-arsanilic acid, *p*-ureidophenylarsonic acid, and 4-nitrophenylarsonic acid were simultaneously determined by Liu et al. [143] by CE coupled with ICP-MS. Of course, for the analysis of elements in complex matrices, some pretreatment steps such as microextraction techniques are often necessary prior to CE separation [144–146].

Separation by CE is usually faster than that by LC, and therefore is potentially a rapid and highly efficient separation technique. However, some problems are presented when CE is coupled to ICP-OES or ICP-MS due to liquid flow incompatibility, i.e., the liquid flow is one order of magnitude lower in CE than in ICP sample introduction system. The detection limit is often insufficient resulting from the very small sample volumes used in CE, and therefore some interface techniques were developed. For example, a novel system for CE and ICP sample introduction that incorporates a dedicated Flow Focusing® based nebulizer as aerosol generation unit was presented by Kovachev et al. [147], and on-line coupling of CE with ICP-MS was developed by Liu et al. [148] using a sprayer with a novel direct-injection high-efficiency nebulizer (DIHEN) chamber as the interface. HG technique is also often integrated into CE hyphenated systems to provide a kind interface method. For example, a microfluidic chip-based capillary electrophoresis (µchip-CE) HG system was interfaced with a microwave induced plasma optical emission spectrometry (MIP-OES) by Matusiewicz and Ślachciński [149] to provide As(III) and As(V) species separation capabilities. Although CE provides an effective measure to fulfill species separation, there still exist major challenges that limit its practical acceptance. For example, no sufficient care on possible changes in speciation during electrophoresis, no appropriate treatment on method validation and system suitability aspects, etc [150].

It is noted that although there has been significant progress in speciation analysis based on the hyphenated chromatographic separation with atomic spectrometry or mass spectrometry detectors, and these hyphenated methods can provide the most complete information on the species distributions and even structures, they also have themselves disadvantages. A limitation related to the hyphenated techniques is the low sample volume introduced into the system which leads to the necessity of a very sensitive detector. It sometimes seems that non-chromatographic techniques are more suitable if sample volume is not a limitation, and thus less sensitive and less expensive detectors can be used due to the possibility of separation and pre-concentration the desired species. In addition, investment and operational costs associated with hyphenated techniques sometimes also play important roles to restrict the spread of speciation analysis as a usual task.

3. Detection Techniques for Speciation Analysis

The selection of detection techniques depends on the concentration level of the species presented in the sample and also the type of matrix and its composition. In terms of the detection approaches for speciation analysis, they must be selective and extremely sensitive since the species of interest usually accounts for only a small fraction of the total amount. The frequently used detection methods with high selectivity and sensitivity for As, Hg, Se and Sb species can be classified into atomic spectrometry and mass spectrometry methods.

3.1. Atomic Spectrometry Methods

Atomic spectrometry are subdivided into AFS, AAS, and AES (or OES), among which AFS is the most often used method, and represents a suitable alternative to the other atomic spectrometric and mass spectrometric techniques [151]. The direct coupling between HPLC and detectors will probably suffer from the interferences from the sample matrices. Therefore, when AFS is used for speciation analysis of As, Se, Sb and Hg, HG technique for As, Se, Sb, and cold vapor (CV) generation for Hg are commonly used as online post-column derivatization method to separate the analytes from sample matrices [152]. The integration of HG/CV based on the reaction of BH_4^- with the acidized sample prior to detector is proved to be an effective measure to reduce interferences and background signal from the sample matrices. The detection limits lower than µg/L will be obtained using HPLC-HG-AFS for As speciation analysis [153]. However, it is noted that transition metals presented in samples will cause serious interferences in HG process. Some improving measures such as mask may be taken into consideration [77,78].

Although there are some reports about the applications of AFS for the speciation analysis of As, Hg, Se, and Sb in recent years [70,108,154–158], the development of atomic spectrometry methods has not been as fast as one would like because they usually need to be used together with HG or CV technique, during which the post-column treatment generally is required by the nature of this technique. In other word, HG is most suitable for low valence hydride-forming species, i.e., As(III), Sb(III), Hg(II) and Se(IV). However, the other inorganic or organic species can not or only present low reaction efficiency. In order to fulfill on-line and simultaneously speciation analysis, some pretreatment measures need to be adopted. For example, in order to simultaneously separate and determine organic species, on-line thermal microwave or UV irradiation prior to HG in the presence of strong oxidizing agents is developed to decompose the organic species. The latter is the most often used and inexpensive method for no cooling system is required after decomposition. For example, de Quadros et al. [159] developed a procedure for simultaneous determination of Hg(II), MeHg, EtHg by photodecomposition of organomercury compounds and reduction of Hg(II) to mercury vapor under microwave/ultraviolet (MW/UV) irradiation. Of course, some other new methods such as post-column oxidation using Fe_3O_4 magnetic nanoparticles [160] were also developed to on-line convert hydride generation/cold vapor generation inactive species into their active species. For example, Sun et al. [161] developed an on-line digestion device based on the nano-TiO_2-catalyzed photo-oxidation of As species. Illuminating for 3 min can quantitatively converted As(III), As(V), MMA and DMA into As(V) at 1% $K_2S_2O_8$ (w/v).

It is noted that the higher chemical valence of analytes would be dominant after the eluted organic compounds are oxidized either via a UV or microwave digestion process. Therefore, a pretreatment to transfer into lower valence compounds is required, that is As(V)→As(III), Sb(V)→Sb(III) and Se(VI)→Se(IV). For example, As(V) has low HG efficiency, and thus in order to improve the analytical sensitive, an acidic thiourea solution was used on-line by Yu et al. [162] and thioglycolic acid was used by Musil and Matoušek [163] to pre-reduce As(V) prior to HG reaction. However, resulting from the differences in chemical properties of each element and their associated compounds, the reactivity of these different compounds varies greatly. For example, KI can reduce As(V) and Sb(V) to As(III) and Sb(III) at room temperature, whereas it is impossible to reduce Se(VI) to Se(IV) under the same conditions.

Although there are some reports on the analysis of As, Hg, Se and Sb species by AAS [164–167] or AES [168–170] in recent years, AFS is described to be superior to AAS and similar to ICP-MS regarding sensitivity and linear calibration range for As and Se species in routine analysis. Analytical features such as low detection limits and wide linear calibration ranges, simplicity, lower acquisition and running costs make AFS a suitable atomic detector in speciation studies.

3.2. Mass Spectrometry Methods

The unquestionable advantages of ICP-MS over other species detectors are its high sensitivity and multi-element on-line detection capacity. In addition, the application of MS allows not only to obtain the information on the qualitative and quantitative contents of the sample, but also to determine the structure and molar masses of the analytes. The coupling of different separation techniques with ICP-MS has become common practice for the speciation analysis of trace As, Hg, Se and Sb [171,172]. Unlike HG/CV-AFS, no oxidation and pre-reduction steps are required for ICP-MS, unless HG is introduced in the system.

Even though the interface of ICP-MS detector with HPLC is relatively simple, the main problem is that the mobile phase used must be compatible with detection system. Sodium or potassium phosphate buffer mobile phases often utilized in IEC are not appropriate for a MS detector. As discussed above, non-volatile buffer salts can be collected on the lenses and skimmer cones resulting in signal drift and a high maintenance level for cleaning the inner surfaces of the MS detector, and thus the use of volatile buffer systems or ones that have low residue is required [97]. Organic modifiers are often used in the mobile phase of RPC, and large volumes of organic solvent reaching the ICP probably results in an unstable plasma. In this sense, methanol is more widely used than acetonitrile for RPC mobile phases [109,111]. Meanwhile, desolvation the liquid aerosol before it reaches the ICP, simple flow splitting after the HPLC column, or the use of a small bore or microbore column is also adopted to reduce the amount of organic solvent introduced into the detector [98,173,174].

Although ICP-MS exhibits very good analytical performances for ultra-trace determination, one of its disadvantages is vulnerable to interferences with the molecular ion signals by atomic argon (Ar) and chlorine which can hinder the measurement of Se and As species. For example, when ICP-MS is used as a detector for As determination, it frequently suffers from chloride interference as $^{38}Ar^{37}Cl^+$, $^{40}Ar^{35}Cl^+$ (the m/z 75 is the same as ^{75}As) are generated if samples contain high amount of chloride [175,176]. However, the introduction of ICP-MS equipped with collision/reaction cell (CRC) or dynamic reaction cell (DRC) is an effective approach to overcome these problems linked with polyatomic interferences, among which the DRC technique is introduced by using the reacting gas, such as ammonia, hydrogen, oxygen, etc. The reacting gas overcomes these interferences by atom transfer or charge transfer reactions to break the polyatomic ions into atoms or ions with different m/z [121,177,178]. For example, a DRC for spectral interferences elimination by using oxygen and ammonia as reaction gases was developed by Marcinkowska et al. [178] for multielemental speciation analysis of Cr(VI), As(III) and As(V) in water by advanced hyphenated technique HPLC/ICP-DRC-MS. Moreover, with the introduction of an additional quadrupole, ICP-tandem MS (ICP-MS/MS) provides more reaction/collision modes for interference elimination [179,180]. ICP-MS/MS can be seen as a conventional ICP-CRC-MS unit with an additional quadrupole located before the CRC. Only ions of a given m/z are allowed to enter the CRC, by which it contributes to a better control over the reactions taking place in the cell. For example, arsenic species in seafood were determined by Schmidt et al. [103] by LC-ICP-MS/MS using O_2 as reaction gas for the conversion of ^{75}As to $^{75}As^{16}O$. ICP-MS/MS was used by Gao et al. [158] for the detection of selenium species in rice after separated by IP-RPC. Two reaction gas modes (H_2, O_2) and a collision mode (He) were investigated and found that H_2 mode was the best choice for eliminating interferences and obtaining a higher signal-to-noise ratio.

MS detection allows the use of isotope dilution analysis (IDA) for speciation analysis due to its specific detection based on the ratio m/z [181]. ID-MS is considered to be an effective method offering accurate determination of elemental species with only small uncertainties. For example, post column isotope dilution with Se-78 spike was performed by Jeong et al. [182] for quantitative speciation of Se in human blood serum and urine. Internal standardization based on the species-unspecific isotope dilution analysis technique was proposed by Castillo et al. [183] to overcome the matrix effects and signal drift originated in the speciation of As in urine, by which it allows the calculation of the corrected overall species concentrations without requiring any methodological calibration. Moreover, in order to avoid the deterioration of sensitivity, accuracy, and long-term stability of system due to the direct introduction of salt- or organic-rich effluent into the instrument, a suitable interfacing technique is highly desirable to couple HPLC with ICP-MS for the detection of elemental species in complex matrices. Accordingly, the generation of volatile analytes by derivatization has been extensively and increasingly reported so as to improve the analytical sensitivity and eliminate the spectral/non-spectral interferences from the sample matrices and effluents [184,185]. As stated ahead, online hydride/vapor generation technique can effectively solve this problem. However, the species which can react with BH_4^- to generation hydride/vapor are limited. For example, it is thought that Se(VI) is not reducible into hydride according to the studies on the reduction kinetics of inorganic Se species with $NaBH_4$. Consequently, inorganic Se(VI) and Se(IV) analysis by HG technique must be carried out by first determining Se(IV) and then transforming Se(VI) to Se(IV) prior to the determination. Meanwhile, the stability of plasma may worsen when determined by HG-ICP-MS because online HG system delivers not only hydride vapor but also large amounts of hydrogen into the ICP. Therefore, the other alternative vapor generation techniques are developed. For example, an on-line sequential photocatalyst-assisted digestion and vaporization device was coupled between LC and ICP-MS by Tsai et al. [186] for Se speciation analysis.

It is noted that although modern techniques using MS detection can help to obtain a better understanding of the experimental data and species identification, many analytical laboratories cannot support such instruments due to their high price and expensive maintenance. Therefore, the hyphenation of chromatography with atomic spectrometry seems to be a well substitute of mass spectrometry.

4. Conclusion and Perspective

As far as the separation and detection of element speciation in environmental and biological samples are concerned, different approaches can be used based on on-line or off-line procedures. The hyphenated techniques, in which effective separation methods are coupled on-line with diverse selective and sensitive detectors, are attractive tools in the speciation analysis of As, Hg, Se and Se. Their main advantages include extremely low limits of detection and quantification, insignificant influence of interferences on the determination process, as well as very high precision and repeatability. Although powerful techniques based on MS are nowadays extensively used for the speciation analysis of trace elements, it is considered as an expensive instrument to purchase and maintain, and only few laboratories can support the high cost of such techniques. The hyphenation of chromatography to atomic spectrometry detectors especially the AFS is still liable and low-cost alternative for routine laboratories. Meanwhile, HG in conjunction with AFS detection deserves more research because it can be hyphenated easily to LC, and provides detection limits of the same order of those obtained with MS techniques. Therefore, it is predictable that HPLC coupled with HG-AFS will be promising for speciation analysis of As, Hg, Se and Sb in environmental and biological samples, and has vast potential for further development.

Author Contributions: X.Y. and C.L. contributed to literature search and writing of the manuscript; Y.G. and T.D. revised the manuscript with critical reviews and comments.

Funding: This work was supported by the National Natural Science Foundation of China (grant numbers U1607129, U1607123 and 21773170) and the Yangtze Scholars and Innovative Research Team of the Chinese University (grant number IRT_17R81).

Conflicts of Interest: The authors declare no conflict of interest.

References

1. Dumout, E.; Vanhaecke, F.; Cornelis, R. Selenium speciation from food source to metabolites: A critical review. *Anal. Bioanal. Chem.* **2006**, *385*, 1304–1323. [CrossRef] [PubMed]
2. Vadala, R.; Mottese, A.F.; Bua, G.D.; Salvo, A.; Mallamace, D.; Corsaro, C.; Vasi, S.; Giofre, S.V.; Alfa, M.; Cicero, N.; et al. Statistical analysis of mineral concentration for the geographic identification of garlic samples from Sicily (Italy), Tunisia and Spain. *Foods* **2016**, *5*, 20. [CrossRef] [PubMed]
3. Albergamo, A.; Rotondo, A.; Salvo, A.; Pellizzeri, V.; Bua, D.G.; Maggio, A.; Cicero, N.; Dugo, G. Metabolite and mineral profiling of "Violetto di Niscemi" and "Spinoso di Menfi" globe artichokes by H-1-NMR and ICP-MS. *Nat. Prod. Res.* **2017**, *31*, 990–999. [CrossRef] [PubMed]
4. Nordberg, M.; Duffus, J.; Templeton, D.M. Glossary of terms used in toxicokinetics (IUPAC Recommendations 2003). *Pure Appl. Chem.* **2004**, *76*, 1033–1082. [CrossRef]
5. Templeton, D.M.; Ariese, F.; Cornelis, R.; Danielsson, L.G.; Muntau, H.; van Leeuwen, H.P.; Lobinski, R. Guidelines for terms related to chemical speciation and fractionation of elements. Definitions, structural aspects, and methodological approaches (IUPAC Recommendations 2000). *Pure Appl. Chem.* **2000**, *72*, 1453–1470. [CrossRef]
6. Tessier, A.; Campbell, P.G.C.; Bisson, M. Sequential extraction procedure for the speciation of particulate trace metals. *Anal. Chem.* **1979**, *51*, 844–851. [CrossRef]

7. Zhang, S.H.; Wang, Y.; Pervaiz, A.; Kong, L.H.; He, M.C. Comparison of diffusive gradients in thin-films (DGT) and chemical extraction methods for predicting bioavailability of antimony and arsenic to maize. *Geoderma* 2018, *332*, 1–9. [CrossRef]
8. Aguilar-Carrillo, J.; Herrera, L.; Gutierrez, E.J.; Reyes-Dominguez, I.A. Solid-phase distribution and mobility of thallium in mining-metallurgical residues: Environmental hazard implications. *Environ. Pollut.* 2018, *243*, 1833–1845. [CrossRef] [PubMed]
9. Izquierdo, M.; Tye, A.M.; Chenery, S.R. Using isotope dilution assays to understand speciation changes in Cd, Zn, Pb and Fe in a soil model system under simulated flooding conditions. *Geoderma* 2017, *295*, 41–52. [CrossRef]
10. Salvo, A.; La Torre, G.L.; Mangano, V.; Casale, K.E.; Bartolomeo, G.; Santini, A.; Granata, T.; Dugo, G. Toxic inorganic pollutants in foods from agricultural producing areas of Southern Italy: Level and riskassessment. *Ecotoxicol. Environ. Saf.* 2018, *148*, 114–124. [CrossRef] [PubMed]
11. Kumarathilaka, P.; Seneweera, S.; Meharg, A.; Bundschuh, J. Arsenic speciation dynamics in paddy rice soil-water environment: Sources, physico-chemical, and biological factors—A review. *Water Res.* 2018, *140*, 403–414. [CrossRef] [PubMed]
12. Zhu, S.L.; Zhang, Z.L.; Zagar, D. Mercury transport and fate models in aquatic systems: A review and synthesis. *Sci. Total Environ.* 2018, *639*, 538–549. [CrossRef] [PubMed]
13. Natasha; Shahid, M.; Niazi, N.K.; Khalid, S.; Murtaza, B.; Bibi, I.; Rashid, M.I. A critical review of selenium biogeochemical behavior in soil-plant system with an inference to human health. *Environ. Pollut.* 2018, *234*, 915–934. [CrossRef] [PubMed]
14. Huang, K.; Xu, Y.; Packianathan, C.; Gao, F.; Chen, C.; Zhang, J.; Shen, Q.R.; Rosen, B.P.; Zhao, F.J. Arsenic methylation by a novel ArsM As(III) S-adenosylmethionine methyltransferase that requires only two conserved cysteine residues. *Mol. Microbiol.* 2018, *107*, 265–276. [CrossRef] [PubMed]
15. Lazaro, W.L.; Diez, S.; da Silva, C.J.; Ignacio, A.R.A.; Guimaraes, J.R.D. Seasonal changes in periphytic microbial metabolism determining mercury methylation in a tropical wetland. *Sci. Total Environ.* 2018, *627*, 1345–1352. [CrossRef]
16. Ruszczynska, A.; Konopka, A.; Kurek, E.; Elguera, J.C.T.; Bulska, E. Investigation of biotransformation of selenium in plants using spectrometric methods. *Spectrochim. Acta B* 2017, *130*, 7–16. [CrossRef]
17. Takahashi, K.; Suzuki, N.; Ogra, Y. Effect of administration route and dose on metabolism of nine bioselenocompounds. *J. Trace Elem. Med. Biol.* 2018, *49*, 113–118. [CrossRef] [PubMed]
18. Terol, A.; Ardini, F.; Basso, A.; Grotti, M. Determination of selenium urinary metabolites by high temperature liquid chromatography-inductively coupled plasma mass spectrometry. *J. Chromatogr. A* 2015, *1380*, 112–119. [CrossRef] [PubMed]
19. Amayo, K.O.; Raab, A.; Krupp, E.M.; Feldmann, J. Identification of arsenolipids and their degradation products in cod-liver oil. *Talanta* 2014, *118*, 217–223. [CrossRef] [PubMed]
20. Sele, V.; Sloth, J.J.; Holmelid, B.; Valdersnes, S.; Skov, K.; Amlund, H. Arsenic-containing fatty acids and hydrocarbons in marine oils—Determination using reversed-phase HPLC-ICP-MS and HPLC-qTOE-MS. *Talanta* 2014, *121*, 89–96. [CrossRef] [PubMed]
21. Rumpler, A.; Edmonds, J.S.; Katsu, M.; Jensen, K.B.; Goessler, W.; Raber, G.; Gunnlaugsdottir, H.; Francesconi, K.A. Arsenic-containing long-chain fatty acids in cod-liver oil: A result of biosynthetic infidelity? *Angew. Chem. Int. Ed.* 2008, *47*, 2665–2667. [CrossRef] [PubMed]
22. Contreras-Acuña, M.; García-Barrera, T.; García-Sevillano, M.A.; Gómez-Ariza, J.L. Speciation of arsenic in marine food (*Anemonia sulcata*) by liquid chromatography coupled to inductively coupled plasma mass spectrometry and organic mass spectrometry. *J. Chromatogr. A* 2013, *1282*, 133–141. [CrossRef] [PubMed]
23. Peng, H.Y.; Hu, B.; Liu, Q.Q.; Yang, Z.L.; Lu, X.F.; Huang, R.F.; Li, X.F.; Zuidhof, M.J.; Le, X.C. Liquid chromatography combined with atomic and molecular mass spectrometry for speciation of arsenic in chicken liver. *J. Chromatogr. A* 2014, *1370*, 40–49. [CrossRef] [PubMed]
24. Kot, A.; Namiesnik, J. The role of speciation in analytical chemistry. *TrAC-Trend Anal. Chem.* 2000, *19*, 69–79. [CrossRef]
25. Sadee, B.; Foulkes, M.E.; Hill, S.J. Coupled techniques for arsenic speciation in food and drinking water: A review. *J. Anal. Atom. Spectrom.* 2015, *30*, 102–118. [CrossRef]
26. Nearing, M.M.; Koch, I.; Reimer, K.J. Complementary arsenic speciation methods: A review. *Spectrochim. Acta B* 2014, *99*, 150–162. [CrossRef]

27. Huber, J.; Leopold, K. Nanomaterial-based strategies for enhanced mercury trace analysis in environmental and drinking waters. *TrAC-Trend Anal. Chem.* **2016**, *80*, 280–292. [CrossRef]
28. Amde, M.; Yin, Y.G.; Zhang, D.; Liu, J.F. Methods and recent advances in speciation analysis of mercury chemical species in environmental samples: A review. *Chem. Speciat. Bioavailab.* **2016**, *28*, 51–65. [CrossRef]
29. Pyrzynska, K.; Sentkowska, A. Liquid chromatographic analysis of selenium species in plant materials. *TrAC-Trend Anal. Chem.* **2019**, *111*, 128–138. [CrossRef]
30. Pettine, M.; McDonald, T.J.; Sohn, M.; Anquandah, G.A.K.; Zboril, R.; Sharma, V.K. A critical review of selenium analysis in natural water samples. *Trends Environ. Anal.* **2015**, *5*, 1–7. [CrossRef]
31. Ferreira, S.L.C.; dos Anjos, J.P.; Felix, C.S.A.; da Silva, M.M.; Palacio, E.; Cerda, V. Speciation analysis of antimony in environmental samples employing atomic fluorescence spectrometry—Review. *TrAC-Trend Anal. Chem.* **2019**, *110*, 335–343. [CrossRef]
32. Miravet, R.; Hernandez-Nataren, E.; Sahuquillo, A.; Rubio, R.; Lopez-Sanchez, J.F. Speciation of antimony in environmental matrices by coupled techniques. *TrAC-Trend Anal. Chem.* **2010**, *29*, 28–39. [CrossRef]
33. Carvalho, D.C.; Coelho, N.M.M.; Melo Coelho, L.; Borges, S.S.S.; Neri, T.S.; Alves, V.N. Strategies to increase selectivity of analytical methods for As, Cr and Se speciation in biological samples: A review. *Sample Prep.* **2014**, *2*, 1–12. [CrossRef]
34. Vieira, M.A.; Grinberg, P.; Bobeda, C.R.R.; Reyes, M.N.M.; Campos, R.C. Non-chromatographic atomic spectrometric methods in speciation analysis: A review. *Spectrochim. Acta B* **2009**, *64*, 459–476. [CrossRef]
35. Gonzalvez, A.; Cervera, M.L.; Armenta, S.; de la Guardia, M. A review of non-chromatographic methods for speciation analysis. *Anal. Chim. Acta* **2009**, *636*, 129–157. [CrossRef] [PubMed]
36. Ibrahim, A.S.A.; Al-Farawati, R.; Hawas, U.; Shaban, Y. Recent microextraction techniques for determination and chemical speciation of selenium. *Open Chem.* **2017**, *15*, 103–122. [CrossRef]
37. Werner, J.; Grzeskowiak, T.; Zgola-Grzeskowiak, A.; Stanisz, E. Recent trends in microextraction techniques used in determination of arsenic species. *TrAC-Trend Anal. Chem.* **2018**, *105*, 121–136. [CrossRef]
38. Pena-Pereira, F.; Lavilla, I.; Bendicho, C. Miniaturized preconcentration methods based on liquid-liquid extraction and their application in inorganic ultratrace analysis and speciation: A review. *Spectrochim. Acta B* **2009**, *64*, 1–15. [CrossRef]
39. Panhwar, A.H.; Tuzen, M.; Kazi, T.G. Ultrasonic assisted dispersive liquid-liquid microextraction method based on deep eutectic solvent for speciation, preconcentration and determination of selenium species (IV) and (VI) in water and food samples. *Talanta* **2017**, *175*, 352–358. [CrossRef] [PubMed]
40. Akramipour, R.; Golpayegani, M.R.; Gheini, S.; Fattahi, N. Speciation of organic/inorganic mercury and total mercury in blood samples using vortex assisted dispersive liquid-liquid microextraction based on the freezing of deep eutectic solvent followed by GFAAS. *Talanta* **2018**, *186*, 17–23. [CrossRef] [PubMed]
41. Haghnazari, L.; Mirzaei, N.; Arfaeinia, H.; Karimyan, K.; Sharafi, H.; Fattahi, N. Speciation of As(III)/As(V) and total inorganic arsenic in biological fluids using new mode of liquid-phase microextraction and electrothermal atomic absorption spectrometry. *Biol. Trace Elem. Res.* **2018**, *183*, 173–181. [CrossRef] [PubMed]
42. Zeng, C.J.; Yan, Y.Y.; Tang, J.; Wu, Y.H.; Zhong, S.S. Speciation of Arsenic(III) and Arsenic(V) based on Triton X-100 hollow fiber liquid phase microextraction coupled with flame atomic absorption spectrometry. *Spectrosc. Lett.* **2017**, *50*, 220–226. [CrossRef]
43. Turker, A.R. Speciation of trace metals and metalloids by solid phase extraction with spectrometric detection: A critical review. *Turk. J. Chem.* **2016**, *40*, 847–867. [CrossRef]
44. Su, C.K.; Chen, W.C. 3D-printed, TiO_2 NP-incorporated minicolumn coupled with ICP-MS for speciation of inorganic arsenic and selenium in high-salt-content samples. *Microchim. Acta* **2018**, *185*, 1–8. [CrossRef] [PubMed]
45. Panhwar, A.H.; Tuzen, M.; Hazer, B.; Kazi, T.G. Solid phase microextraction method using a novel polystyrene oleic acid imidazole polymer in micropipette tip of syringe system for speciation and determination of antimony in environmental and food samples. *Talanta* **2018**, *184*, 115–121. [CrossRef] [PubMed]
46. Wang, H.; Hen, B.B.; Zhu, S.Q.; Yu, X.X.; He, M.; Hu, B. Chip-based magnetic solid-phase microextraction online coupled with micro HPLC-ICP-MS for the determination of mercury species in cells. *Anal. Chem.* **2016**, *88*, 796–802. [CrossRef] [PubMed]

47. Ali, J.; Tuzen, M.; Kazi, T.G.; Hazer, B. Inorganic arsenic speciation in water samples by miniaturized solid phase microextraction using a new polystyrene polydimethyl siloxane polymer in micropipette tip of syringe system. *Talanta* **2016**, *161*, 450–458. [CrossRef] [PubMed]
48. Nyaba, L.; Matong, J.M.; Dimpe, K.M.; Nomngongo, P.N. Speciation of inorganic selenium in environmental samples after suspended dispersive solid phase microextraction combined with inductively coupled plasma spectrometric determination. *Talanta* **2016**, *159*, 174–180. [CrossRef] [PubMed]
49. Fan, Z.F. Determination of antimony(III) and total antimony by single-drop microextraction combined with electrothermal atomic absorption spectrometry. *Anal. Chim. Acta* **2007**, *585*, 300–304. [CrossRef] [PubMed]
50. Tolessa, T.; Tan, Z.Q.; Yin, Y.G.; Liu, J.F. Single-drop gold nanoparticles for headspace microextraction and colorimetric assay of mercury (II) in environmental waters. *Talanta* **2018**, *176*, 77–84. [CrossRef] [PubMed]
51. Jia, X.Y.; Zhao, J.Y.; Ren, H.Y.; Wang, J.N.; Hong, Z.X.; Zhang, X. Zwitterion-functionalized polymer microspheres-based solid phase extraction method on-line combined with HPLC-ICP-MS for mercury speciation. *Talanta* **2019**, *196*, 592–599. [CrossRef] [PubMed]
52. Londonio, A.; Hasuoka, P.E.; Pacheco, P.; Gil, R.A.; Smichowski, P. Online solid phase extraction-HPLC-ICP-MS system for mercury and methylmercury preconcentration using functionalised carbon nanotubes for their determination in dietary supplements. *J. Anal. Atom. Spectrom.* **2018**, *33*, 1737–1744. [CrossRef]
53. Li, P.; Chen, Y.J.; Hu, X.; Lian, H.Z. Magnetic solid phase extraction for the determination of trace antimony species in water by inductively coupled plasma mass spectrometry. *Talanta* **2015**, *134*, 292–297. [CrossRef] [PubMed]
54. Zhang, L.; Morita, Y.; Sakuragawa, A.; Isozaki, A. Inorganic speciation of As(III, V), Se(IV, VI) and Sb(III, V) in natural water with GF-AAS using solid phase extraction technology. *Talanta* **2007**, *72*, 723–729. [CrossRef] [PubMed]
55. Peng, H.Y.; Zhang, N.; He, M.; Chen, B.B.; Hu, B. Simultaneous speciation analysis of inorganic arsenic, chromium and selenium in environmental waters by 3-(2-aminoethylamino) propyltrimethoxysilane modified multi-wall carbon nanotubes packed microcolumn solid phase extraction and ICP-MS. *Talanta* **2015**, *131*, 266–272. [CrossRef] [PubMed]
56. Zhao, L.Y.; Zhu, Q.Y.; Mao, L.; Chen, Y.J.; Lian, H.Z.; Hu, X. Preparation of thiol- and amine-bifunctionalized hybrid monolithic column via "one-pot" and applications in speciation of inorganic arsenic. *Talanta* **2019**, *192*, 339–346. [CrossRef] [PubMed]
57. Zheng, C.B.; Hu, L.G.; Hou, X.D.; He, B.; Jiang, G.B. Headspace solid-phase microextraction coupled to miniaturized microplasma optical emission spectrometry for detection of mercury and lead. *Anal. Chem.* **2018**, *90*, 3683–3691. [CrossRef] [PubMed]
58. Yang, Y.; Tan, Q.; Lin, Y.; Tian, Y.F.; Wu, L.; Hou, X.D.; Zheng, C.B. Point discharge optical emission spectrometer as a gas chromatography (GC) detector for speciation analysis of mercury in human hair. *Anal. Chem.* **2018**, *90*, 11996–12003. [CrossRef] [PubMed]
59. Lin, Y.; Yang, Y.; Li, Y.X.; Yang, L.; Hou, X.D.; Feng, X.B.; Zheng, C.B. Ultrasensitive speciation analysis of mercury in rice by headspace solid phase microextraction using porous carbons and gas chromatography-dielectric barrier discharge optical emission spectrometry. *Environ. Sci. Technol.* **2016**, *50*, 2468–2476. [CrossRef] [PubMed]
60. Mester, Z. Gas phase sampling of volatile (organo)metallic compounds above solid samples. *J. Anal. Atom. Spectrom.* **2002**, *17*, 868–871. [CrossRef]
61. Zhang, W.F.; Hu, Y.A.; Cheng, H.F. Optimization of microwave-assisted extraction for six inorganic and organic arsenic species in chicken tissues using response surface methodology. *J. Sep. Sci.* **2015**, *38*, 3063–3070. [CrossRef] [PubMed]
62. Zounr, R.A.; Tuzen, M.; Khuhawar, M.Y. Ultrasound assisted deep eutectic solvent based on dispersive liquid liquid microextraction of arsenic speciation in water and environmental samples by electrothermal atomic absorption spectrometry. *J. Mol. Liq.* **2017**, *242*, 441–446. [CrossRef]
63. Shirkhanloo, H.; Khaligh, A.; Mousavi, H.Z.; Rashidi, A. Ultrasound assisted-dispersive-ionic liquid-micro-solid phase extraction based on carboxyl-functionalized nanoporous graphene for speciation and determination of trace inorganic and organic mercury species in water and caprine blood samples. *Microchim. J.* **2017**, *130*, 245–254. [CrossRef]

64. Altunay, N.; Gurkan, R. Separation/preconcentration of ultra-trace levels of inorganic Sb and Se from different sample matrices by charge transfer sensitized ion-pairing using ultrasonic-assisted cloud point extraction prior to their speciation and determination by hydride generation AAS. *Talanta* **2016**, *159*, 344–355. [PubMed]
65. Lou, C.G.; Liu, W.Q.; Liu, X.D. Quantitative analysis of arsenic speciation in guano and ornithogenic sediments using microwave-assisted extraction followed by high-performance liquid chromatography coupled to hydride generation atomic fiuorescence spectrometry. *J. Chromatogr. B* **2014**, *969*, 29–34. [CrossRef] [PubMed]
66. Saucedo-Velez, A.A.; Hinojosa-Reyes, L.; Villanueva-Rodriguez, M.; Caballero-Quintero, A.; Hernandez-Ramirez, A.; Guzman-Mar, J.L. Speciation analysis of organoarsenic compounds in livestock feed by microwave-assisted extraction and high performance liquid chromatography coupled to atomic fluorescence spectrometry. *Food Chem.* **2017**, *232*, 493–500. [CrossRef] [PubMed]
67. Cao, Y.P.; Yan, L.Z.; Huang, H.L.; Deng, B.Y. Selenium speciation in radix puerariae using ultrasonic assisted extraction combined with reversed phase high performance liquid chromatography-inductively coupled plasma-mass spectrometry after magnetic solid-phase extraction with 5-sulfosalicylic acid functionalized magnetic nanoparticles. *Spectrochim. Acta B* **2016**, *122*, 172–177.
68. Musil, S.; Petursdottir, A.H.; Raab, A.; Gunnlaugsdottir, H.; Krupp, E.; Feldmann, J. Speciation without chromatography using selective hydride generation: Inorganic arsenic in rice and samples of marine origin. *Anal. Chem.* **2014**, *86*, 993–999. [CrossRef] [PubMed]
69. Welna, M.; Pohl, P. Potential of the hydride generation technique coupled to inductively coupled plasma optical emission spectrometry for non-chromatographic As speciation. *J. Anal. Atom. Spectrom.* **2017**, *32*, 1766–1779. [CrossRef]
70. Hu, P.Y.; Wang, X.; Yang, L.; Yang, H.Y.; Tang, Y.Y.; Luo, H.; Xiong, X.L.; Jiang, X.; Huang, K. Speciation of mercury by hydride generation ultraviolet atomization-atomic fluorescence spectrometry without chromatographic separation. *Microchem. J.* **2018**, *143*, 228–233. [CrossRef]
71. Vieira, M.A.; Ribeiro, A.S.; Curtius, A.J.; Sturgeon, R.E. Determination of total mercury and methylmercury in biological samples by photochemical vapor generation. *Anal. Bioanal. Chem.* **2007**, *388*, 837–847. [CrossRef] [PubMed]
72. Mendez, H.; Lavilla, I.; Bendicho, C. Mild sample pretreatment procedures based on photolysis and sonolysis-promoted redox reactions as a new approach for determination of Se(IV), Se(VI) and Se(-II) in model solutions by the hydride generation technique with atomic absorption and fluorescence detection. *J. Anal. Atom. Spectrom.* **2004**, *19*, 1379–1385.
73. Chen, Y.W.; Zhou, M.D.; Tong, J.; Belzile, N. Application of photochemical reactions of Se in natural waters by hydride generation atomic fluorescence spectrometry. *Anal. Chim. Acta* **2005**, *545*, 142–148. [CrossRef]
74. Chen, Y.W.; Zhou, X.L.; Tong, J.; Truong, Y.; Belzile, N. Photochemical behavior of inorganic and organic selenium compounds in various aqueous solutions. *Anal. Chim. Acta* **2005**, *545*, 149–157. [CrossRef]
75. Shuvaeva, O.V.; Gustaytis, M.A.; Anoshin, G.N. Mercury speciation in environmental solid samples using thermal release technique with atomic absorption detection. *Anal. Chim. Acta* **2008**, *621*, 148–154. [CrossRef] [PubMed]
76. Kaercher, L.E.; Goldschmidt, F.; Paniz, J.N.G.; Flores, É.M.M.; Dressler, V.L. Determination of inorganic and total mercury by vapor generation atomic absorption spectrometry using different temperatures of the measurement cell. *Spectrochim. Acta Part B* **2005**, *60*, 705–710. [CrossRef]
77. Liao, M.X.; Deng, T.L. Arsenic species analysis in porewaters and sediments using hydride generation atomic fluorescence spectrometry. *J. Environ. Sci.* **2006**, *18*, 995–999. [CrossRef]
78. Xi, J.C.; He, M.C.; Wang, K.P.; Zhang, G.Z. Comparison of masking agents for antimony speciation analysis using hydride generation atomic fluorescence spectrometry. *Front. Environ. Sci. Eng.* **2015**, *9*, 970–978. [CrossRef]
79. Teran-Baamonde, J.; Bouchet, S.; Tessier, E.; Amouroux, D. Development of a large volume injection method using a programmed temperature vaporization injector-gas chromatography hyphenated to ICP-MS for the simultaneous determination of mercury, tin and lead species at ultra-trace levels in natural waters. *J. Chromatogr. A* **2018**, *1547*, 77–85. [CrossRef] [PubMed]

80. Giraaldez, I.; Ruiz-Azcona, P.; Vidal, A.; Morales, E. Speciation of selenite and selenoamino acids in biota samples bdual stir bar sorptive extraction-single desorption-capillary gas chromatography/mass spectrometry. *Microchim. J.* **2015**, *122*, 197–204. [CrossRef]
81. Rahman, G.M.M.; Wolle, M.M.; Fahrenholz, T.; Kingston, H.M.; Pamuku, M. Measurement of mercury species in whole blood using speciated isotope dilution methodology integrated with microwave-enhanced solubilization and spike equilibration, headspace-solid-phase microextraction, and GC-ICP-MS analysis. *Anal. Chem.* **2014**, *86*, 6130–6137. [CrossRef] [PubMed]
82. Gajdosechova, Z.; Pagliano, E.; Zborowski, A.; Mester, Z. Headspace in-tube microextraction and GC-ICP-MS determination of mercury species in petroleum hydrocarbons. *Energy Fuels* **2018**, *32*, 10493–10501. [CrossRef]
83. Cai, Y.; Monsalud, S.; Jaffé, R.; Jones, R.D. Gas chromatographic determination of organomercury following aqueous derivatization with sodium tetraethylborate and sodium tetraphenylborate: Comparative study of gas chromatography coupled with atomic fluorescence spectrometry, atomic emission spectrometry and mass spectrometry. *J. Chromatogr. A* **2000**, *876*, 147–155. [PubMed]
84. Nevado, J.J.B.; Martín-Doimeadios, R.C.R.; Krupp, E.M.; Bernardo, F.J.G.; Fariñas, N.R.; Moreno, M.J.; Wallace, D.; Ropero, M.J.P. Comparison of gas chromatographic hyphenated techniques for mercury speciation analysis. *J. Chromatogr. A* **2011**, *1218*, 4545–4551. [CrossRef] [PubMed]
85. Jung, M.Y.; Kang, J.H.; Jung, H.J.; Ma, S.Y. Inorganic arsenic contents in ready-to-eat rice products and various Korean rice determined by a highly sensitive gas chromatography-tandem mass spectrometry. *Food Chem.* **2018**, *240*, 1179–1183. [CrossRef] [PubMed]
86. Kang, J.H.; Jung, H.J.; Jung, M.Y. One step derivatization with British Anti-Lewsite in combination with gas chromatography coupled to triple-quadrupole tandem mass spectrometry for the fast and selective analysis of inorganic arsenic in rice. *Anal. Chim. Acta* **2016**, *934*, 231–238. [CrossRef] [PubMed]
87. Gionfriddo, E.; Naccarato, A.; Sindona, G.; Tagarelli, A. A reliable solid phase microextraction-gas chromatography-triple quadrupole mass spectrometry method for the assay of selenomethionine and selenomethylselenocysteine in aqueous extracts: Difference between selenized and not-enriched selenium potatoes. *Anal. Chim. Acta* **2012**, *747*, 58–66. [CrossRef] [PubMed]
88. Ghasemi, E.; Sillanpaa, M.; Najafi, N.M. Headspace hollow fiber protected liquid-phase microextraction combined with gas chromatography-mass spectroscopy for speciation and determination of volatile organic compounds of selenium in environmental and biological samples. *J. Chromatogr. A* **2011**, *118*, 380–386. [CrossRef] [PubMed]
89. Smith, L.M.; Maher, W.A.; Craig, P.J.; Jenkins, R.O. Speciation of volatile antimony compounds in culture headspace gases of Cryptococcus humicolus using solid phase microextraction and gas chromatography-mass spectrometry. *Appl. Organomet. Chem.* **2002**, *16*, 287–293. [CrossRef]
90. Rekhi, H.; Rani, S.; Sharma, N.; Malik, A.K. A review on recent applications of high-performance liquid chromatography in metal determination and speciation analysis. *Crit. Rev. Anal. Chem.* **2017**, *47*, 524–537. [CrossRef] [PubMed]
91. Son, S.H.; Lee, W.B.; Kim, D.; Lee, Y.; Nam, S.H. An alternative analytical method for determining arsenic species in rice by using ion chromatography and inductively coupled plasma-mass spectrometry. *Food Chem.* **2019**, *270*, 353–358. [CrossRef] [PubMed]
92. Shi, Q.L.; Ju, M.Y.; Zhu, X.X.; Gan, H.; Gu, R.L.; Wu, Z.N.; Meng, Z.Y.; Dou, G.F. Pharmacokinetic properties of arsenic species after intravenous and intragastrical administration of arsenic trioxide solution in cynomolgus macaques using HPLC-ICP-MS. *Molecules* **2019**, *24*, 241. [CrossRef] [PubMed]
93. Guo, L.X.; Zhang, G.W.; Wang, J.T.; Zhong, Y.P.; Huang, Z.G. Determination of arsenic species in ophiocordyceps sinensis from major habitats in China by HPLC-ICP-MS and the edible hazard assessment. *Molecules* **2018**, *23*, 1012. [CrossRef] [PubMed]
94. Cui, S.; Kim, C.K.; Lee, K.S.; Min, H.S.; Lee, J.H. Study on the analytical method of arsenic species in marine samples by ion chromatography coupled with mass spectrometry. *Microchem. J.* **2018**, *143*, 16–20. [CrossRef]
95. Doker, S.; Yilmaz, M. Speciation of arsenic in spring, well, and tap water by high-performance liquid chromatography-inductively coupled plasma-mass spectrometry. *Anal. Lett.* **2018**, *51*, 254–264. [CrossRef]
96. Yu, H.M.; Du, H.; Wu, L.; Li, R.L.; Sun, Q.; Hou, X.D. Trace arsenic speciation analysis of bones by high performance liquid chromatography-inductively coupled plasma mass spectrometry. *Microchim. J.* **2018**, *141*, 176–180. [CrossRef]

97. Zhao, F.; Liu, Y.M.; Zhang, X.Q.; Dong, R.; Yu, W.J.; Liu, Y.F.; Guo, Z.M.; Liang, X.M.; Zhu, J.H. Enzyme-assisted extraction and liquid chromatography-inductively coupled plasma mass spectrometry for the determination of arsenic species in fish. *J. Chromatogr. A* **2018**, *1573*, 48–58. [CrossRef] [PubMed]
98. Cheng, H.Y.; Shen, L.H.; Liu, J.H.; Xu, Z.G.; Wang, Y.C. Coupling nanoliter high-performance liquid chromatography to inductively coupled plasma mass spectrometry for arsenic speciation. *J. Sep. Sci.* **2018**, *41*, 1524–1531. [CrossRef] [PubMed]
99. Schmidt, L.; Landero, J.A.; Novo, D.L.; Duarte, F.A.; Mesko, M.F.; Caruso, J.A.; Flores, E.M.M. A feasible method for As speciation in several types of seafood by LC-ICP-MS/MS. *Food Chem.* **2018**, *255*, 340–347. [CrossRef] [PubMed]
100. Esperanza, M.G.; Barrientos, E.Y.; Wrobel, K.; Aguilar, F.J.A.; Escobosa, A.R.; Wrobel, K. Determination of total arsenic and speciation analysis in Mexican maize tortillas by hydride generation-microwave plasma atomic emission spectrometry and high performance liquid chromatography-inductively coupled plasma-mass spectrometry. *Anal. Methods* **2017**, *9*, 2059–2068. [CrossRef]
101. Chen, S.Z.; Guo, Q.Z.; Liu, L.P. Determination of arsenic species in edible mushrooms by high-performance liquid chromatography coupled to inductively coupled plasma mass spectrometry. *Food Anal. Method* **2017**, *10*, 740–748. [CrossRef]
102. Han, T.T.; Ji, H.W.; Li, H.X.; Cui, H.; Song, T.; Duan, X.J.; Zhu, Q.L.; Cai, F.; Zhang, L. Speciation analysis of arsenic compounds in seafood by ion chromatography-atomic fluorescence spectrometry. *J. Ocean Univ. China* **2017**, *16*, 455–460. [CrossRef]
103. Schmidt, L.; Landero, J.A.; Santos, R.F.; Mesko, M.F.; Mello, P.A.; Flores, E.M.M.; Caruso, J.A. Arsenic speciation in seafood by LC-ICP-MS/MS: Method development and influence of culinary treatment. *J. Anal. Atom. Spectrom.* **2017**, *32*, 1490–1499. [CrossRef]
104. Firat, M.; Bakirdere, S.; Sel, S.; Chormey, D.S.; Elkiran, O.; Erulas, F.; Turak, F. Arsenic speciation in water and biota samples at trace levels by ion chromatography inductively coupled plasma-mass spectrometry. *Int. J. Environ. Anal. Chem.* **2017**, *97*, 684–693. [CrossRef]
105. Lin, C.H.; Chen, Y.; Su, Y.A.; Luo, Y.T.; Shih, T.T.; Sun, Y.C. Nanocomposite-coated microfluidic-based photocatalyst-assisted reduction device to couple high-performance liquid chromatography and inductively coupled plasma-mass spectrometry for online determination of inorganic arsenic species in natural water. *Anal. Chem.* **2017**, *89*, 5892–5900. [CrossRef] [PubMed]
106. Ozcan, S.; Bakirdere, S.; Ataman, O.Y. Speciation of arsenic in fish by high-performance liquid chromatography-inductively coupled plasma-mass spectrometry. *Anal. Lett.* **2016**, *49*, 2501–2512. [CrossRef]
107. Jia, X.Y.; Gong, D.R.; Wang, J.N.; Huang, F.Y.; Duan, T.C.; Zhang, X. Arsenic speciation in environmental waters by a new specific phosphine modified polymer microsphere preconcentration and HPLC-ICP-MS determination. *Talanta* **2016**, *160*, 437–443. [CrossRef] [PubMed]
108. Gao, X.S.; Dai, J.Y.; Zhao, H.Y.; Zhu, J.; Luo, L.; Zhang, R.; Zhang, Z.; Li, L. Synthesis of MoS_2 nanosheets for mercury speciation analysis by HPLC-UV-HG-AFS. *RSC Adv.* **2018**, *8*, 18364–18371. [CrossRef]
109. Liu, H.; Luo, J.Y.; Ding, T.; Gu, S.Y.; Yang, S.H.; Yang, M.H. Speciation analysis of trace mercury in sea cucumber species of apostichopus japonicus using high-performance liquid chromatography Conjunction with inductively coupled plasma mass spectrometry. *Biol. Trace Elem. Res.* **2018**, *186*, 554–561. [CrossRef] [PubMed]
110. Liu, Y.M.; Zhang, F.P.; Jiao, B.Y.; Rao, J.Y.; Leng, G. Automated dispersive liquid-liquid microextraction coupled to high performance liquid chromatography-cold vapour atomic fluorescence spectroscopy for the determination of mercury species in natural water samples. *J. Chromatogr. A* **2017**, *1493*, 1–9. [CrossRef] [PubMed]
111. Yao, C.H.; Jiang, S.J.; Sahayam, A.C.; Huang, Y.L. Speciation of mercury in fish oils using liquid chromatography inductively coupled plasma mass spectrometry. *Microchem. J.* **2017**, *133*, 556–560. [CrossRef]
112. Zhu, S.Q.; Chen, B.B.; He, M.; Huang, T.; Hu, B. Speciation of mercury in water and fish samples by HPLC-ICP-MS after magnetic solid phase extraction. *Talanta* **2017**, *171*, 213–219. [CrossRef] [PubMed]
113. Li, L.; Wang, Z.H.; Zhang, S.X.; Wang, M.L. Directly-thiolated graphene based organic solvent-free cloud point extraction-like method for enrichment and speciation of mercury by HPLC-ICP-MS. *Microchem. J.* **2017**, *132*, 299–307. [CrossRef]
114. Zhang, S.X.; Luo, H.; Zhang, Y.Y.; Li, X.Y.; Liu, J.S.; Xu, Q.; Wang, Z.H. In situ rapid magnetic solid-phase extraction coupled with HPLC-ICP-MS for mercury speciation in environmental water. *Microchem. J.* **2016**, *126*, 25–31. [CrossRef]

115. Fang, Y.; Pan, Y.S.; Li, P.; Xue, M.; Pei, F.; Yang, W.J.; Ma, N.; Hu, Q.H. Simultaneous determination of arsenic and mercury species in rice by ion-pairing reversed phase chromatography with inductively coupled plasma mass spectrometry. *Food Chem.* **2016**, *213*, 609–615. [CrossRef] [PubMed]
116. Le Roux, S.; Baker, P.; Crouch, A. Determination of mercury in selected polluted sediments using HPLC-ICP-MS in Westbank Area, Western Cape, South Africa. *S. Afr. J. Chem.* **2016**, *69*, 124–131. [CrossRef]
117. Bakirdere, S.; Volkan, M.; Ataman, O.Y. Selenium speciation in chicken breast samples from inorganic and organic selenium fed chickens using high performance liquid chromatography-inductively coupled plasma-mass spectrometry. *J. Food Compos. Anal.* **2018**, *71*, 28–35. [CrossRef]
118. Hu, T.; Liu, L.P.; Chen, S.Z.; Wu, W.L.; Xiang, C.G.; Guo, Y.B. Determination of selenium species in cordyceps militaris by high-performance liquid chromatography coupled to hydride generation atomic fluorescence spectrometry. *Anal. Lett.* **2018**, *51*, 2316–2330. [CrossRef]
119. Gao, H.H.; Chen, M.X.; Hu, X.Q.; Chai, S.S.; Qin, M.L.; Cao, Z.Y. Separation of selenium species and their sensitive determination in rice samples by ion-pairing reversed-phase liquid chromatography with inductively coupled plasma tandem mass spectrometry. *J. Sep. Sci.* **2018**, *41*, 432–439. [CrossRef] [PubMed]
120. Yazdi, M.; Yamini, Y. Inorganic selenium speciation in water and biological samples by three phase hollow fiber-based liquid phase microextraction coupled with HPLC-UV. *New J. Chem.* **2017**, *41*, 2378–2385. [CrossRef]
121. Wiktor, L.; Barbara, M.; Dariusz, K.; Piotr, K.; Danuta, B. Study on Speciation of As, Cr, and Sb in bottled flavored drinking water samples using advanced analytical techniques IEC/SEC-HPLC/ICP-DRC-MS and ESI-MS/MS. *Molecules* **2019**, *24*, 668. [CrossRef]
122. Marcinkowska, M.; Lorenc, W.; Baralkiewicz, D. Study of the impact of bottles material and color on the presence of As-III, As-V, Sb-III, Sb-V and Cr-VI in matrix-rich mineral water—Multielemental speciation analysis by HPLC/ICP-DRC-MS. *Microchem. J.* **2017**, *132*, 1–7. [CrossRef]
123. Lin, Y.A.; Jiang, S.J.; Sahayam, A.C. Determination of antimony compounds in waters and juices using ion chromatography-inductively coupled plasma mass spectrometry. *Food Chem.* **2017**, *230*, 76–81. [CrossRef] [PubMed]
124. Marcinkowska, M.; Komorowicz, I.; Barałkiewicz, D. New procedure for multielemental speciation analysis of five toxic species: As(III), As(V), Cr(VI), Sb(III) and Sb(V) in drinking water samples by advanced hyphenated technique HPLC/ICP-DRC-MS. *Anal. Chim. Acta* **2016**, *920*, 102–111. [CrossRef] [PubMed]
125. Quiroz, W.; Astudillo, F.; Bravo, M.; Cereceda-Balic, F.; Vidal, V.; Palomo-Marin, M.R.; Rueda-Holgado, F.; Pinilla-Gil, E. Antimony speciation in soils, sediments and volcanic ashes by microwave extraction and HPLC-HG-AFS detection. *Microchem. J.* **2016**, *129*, 111–116. [CrossRef]
126. Jablonska-Czapla, M.; Szopa, S. Arsenic, antimony and chromium speciation using HPLC-ICP-MS in selected river ecosystems of Upper Silesia, Poland—A preliminary study and validation of methodology. *Water Sci. Technol.-Water Supply* **2016**, *16*, 354–361. [CrossRef]
127. Wei, C.J.; Liu, J.X. A new hydride generation system applied in determination of arsenic species with ion chromatography–hydride generation-atomic fluorescence spectrometry (IC–HG-AFS). *Talanta* **2007**, *73*, 540–545. [CrossRef] [PubMed]
128. Chen, X.P.; Han, C.; Cheng, H.Y.; Wang, Y.C.; Liu, J.H.; Xua, Z.G.; Hu, L. Rapid speciation analysis of mercury in seawater and marine fish by cation exchange chromatography hyphenated with inductively coupled plasma mass spectrometry. *J. Chromatogr. A* **2013**, *1314*, 86–93. [CrossRef] [PubMed]
129. Zhang, Q.H.; Yanga, G.P. Selenium speciation in bay scallops by high performance liquid chromatography separation and inductively coupled plasma mass spectrometry detection after complete enzymatic extraction. *J. Chromatogr. A* **2014**, *1325*, 83–91. [CrossRef] [PubMed]
130. Schaeffer, R.; Soeroes, C.; Ipolyi, I.; Fodor, P.; Thomaidis, N.S. Determination of arsenic species in seafood samples from the Aegean Sea by liquid chromatography-(photo-oxidation)-hydride generation-atomic fluorescence spectrometry. *Anal. Chim. Acta* **2005**, *547*, 109–118. [CrossRef]
131. Sánchez-Rodas, D.; Mellano, F.; Martínez, F.; Palencia, P.; Giráldez, I.; Morales, E. Speciation analysis of Se-enriched strawberries (*Fragaria ananassa Duch*) cultivated on hydroponics by HPLC-TR-HG-AFS. *Microchem. J.* **2016**, *127*, 120–124. [CrossRef]
132. Chu, Y.L.; Jiang, S.J. Speciation analysis of arsenic compounds in edible oil by ion chromatography–inductively coupled plasma mass spectrometry. *J. Chromatogr. A* **2011**, *1218*, 5175–5179. [CrossRef] [PubMed]

133. Wolle, M.M.; Rahman, G.M.M.; Kingston, H.M.; Pamuku, M. Speciation analysis of arsenic in prenatal and children's dietary supplements using microwave-enhanced extraction and ion chromatography–inductively coupled plasma mass spectrometry. *Anal. Chim. Acta* **2014**, *818*, 23–31. [CrossRef] [PubMed]
134. Wojcieszek, J.; Kwiatkowski, P.; Ruzik, L. Speciation analysis and bioaccessibility evaluation of trace elements in goji berries (*Lycium Barbarum* L.). *J. Chromatogr. A* **2017**, *1492*, 70–78. [CrossRef] [PubMed]
135. Jia, Y.Y.; Wang, L.; Ma, L.; Yang, Z.G. Speciation analysis of six arsenic species in marketed shellfish: Extraction optimization and health risk assessment. *Food Chem.* **2018**, *244*, 311–316. [CrossRef] [PubMed]
136. Reyes, L.H.; Mar, J.L.G.; Rahman, G.M.M.; Seybert, B. Simultaneous determination of arsenic and selenium species in fish tissues using microwave–assisted enzymatic extraction and ion chromatography–inductively coupled plasma mass spectrometry. *Talanta* **2009**, *78*, 983–990. [CrossRef] [PubMed]
137. Nan, K.; He, M.; Chen, B.B.; Chen, Y.J.; Hu, B. Arsenic speciation in tree moss by mass spectrometry based hyphenated techniques. *Talanta* **2018**, *183*, 48–54. [CrossRef] [PubMed]
138. Sentkowska, A.; Pyrzynska, K. Hydrophilic interaction liquid chromatography in the speciation analysis of selenium. *J. Chromatogr. B* **2018**, *1074*, 8–15. [CrossRef] [PubMed]
139. Le, X.C.; Li, X.F.; Lai, V.; Ma, M.; Yalcin, S.; Feldmann, J. Simultaneous speciation of selenium and arsenic using elevated temperature liquid chromatography separation with inductively coupled plasma mass spectrometry detection. *Spectrochim. Acta B* **1998**, *53*, 899–909. [CrossRef]
140. Ammann, A.A. Arsenic speciation by gradient anion exchange narrow bore ion chromatography and high resolution inductively coupled plasma mass spectrometry detection. *J. Chromatogr. A* **2010**, *1217*, 2111–2116. [CrossRef] [PubMed]
141. Milstein, L.S.; Essader, A.; Pellizzari, E.D.; Fernando, R.A.; Raymer, J.H.; Levine, K.E.; Akinbo, O. Development and application of a robust speciation method for determination of six arsenic compounds present in human urine. *Environ. Health Perspect.* **2003**, *111*, 293–296. [CrossRef] [PubMed]
142. Timerbaev, A.R. Element speciation analysis using capillary electrophoresis: Twenty years of development and applications. *Chem. Rev.* **2013**, *113*, 778–812. [CrossRef] [PubMed]
143. Liu, L.H.; He, B.; Yun, Z.J.; Sun, J.; Jiang, G.B. Speciation analysis of arsenic compounds by capillary electrophoresis on-line coupled with inductively coupled plasma mass spectrometry using a novel interface. *J. Chromatogr. A* **2013**, *1304*, 227–233. [CrossRef] [PubMed]
144. Li, J.H.; Liu, J.Y.; Lu, W.H.; Gao, F.F.; Wang, L.Y.; Ma, J.P.; Liu, H.T.; Liao, C.Y.; Chen, L.X. Speciation analysis of mercury by dispersive solid-phase extraction coupled with capillary electrophoresis. *Electrophoresis* **2018**, *39*, 1763–1770. [CrossRef] [PubMed]
145. Yang, F.F.; Li, J.H.; Lu, W.H.; Wen, Y.Y.; Cai, X.Q.; You, J.M.; Ma, J.P.; Ding, Y.J.; Chen, L.X. Speciation analysis of mercury in water samples by dispersive liquid-liquid microextraction coupled to capillary electrophoresis. *Electrophoresis* **2014**, *35*, 474–481. [CrossRef] [PubMed]
146. Li, P.J.; He, M.; Chen, B.B.; Hu, B. Automated dynamic hollow fiber liquid-liquid-liquid microextraction combined with capillary electrophoresis for speciation of mercury in biological and environmental samples. *J. Chromatogr. A* **2015**, *1415*, 48–56. [CrossRef] [PubMed]
147. Kovachev, N.; Aguirre, M.Á.; Hidalgo, M.; Simitchiev, K.; Stefanova, V.; Kmetov, V.; Canals, A. Elemental speciation by capillary electrophoresis with inductively coupled plasma spectrometry: A new approach by Flow Focusing® nebulization. *Microchem. J.* **2014**, *117*, 27–33. [CrossRef]
148. Liu, L.H.; Yun, Z.J.; He, B.; Jiang, G.B. Efficient interface for online coupling of capillary electrophoresis with inductively coupled plasma-mass spectrometry and its application in simultaneous speciation analysis of arsenic and selenium. *Anal. Chem.* **2014**, *86*, 8167–8175. [CrossRef] [PubMed]
149. Matusiewicz, H.; Ślachciński, M. Development of a new hybrid technique for inorganic arsenic speciation analysis by microchip capillary electrophoresis coupled with hydride generation microwave induced plasma spectrometry. *Microchem. J.* **2012**, *102*, 61–67. [CrossRef]
150. Timerbaev, A.R. Element speciation analysis by capillary electrophoresis: What are the hints on becoming a standard analytical methodology. *Anal. Chim. Acta* **2001**, *433*, 165–180. [CrossRef]
151. Clough, R.; Harrington, C.F.; Hill, S.J.; Madrid, Y.; Tyson, J.F. Atomic spectrometry update: Review of advances in elemental speciation. *J. Anal. Atom. Spectrom.* **2018**, *33*, 1103–1149. [CrossRef]
152. D'Ulivo, A.; Baiocchi, C.; Pitzalis, E.; Onor, M.; Zamboni, R. Chemical vapor generation for atomic spectrometry. A contribution to the comprehension of reaction mechanisms in the generation of volatile hydrides using borane complexes. *Spectrochim. Acta B* **2004**, *59*, 471–486. [CrossRef]

153. Grijalba, A.C.; Fiorentini, E.F.; Martinez, L.D.; Wuilloud, R.G. A comparative evaluation of different ionic liquids for arsenic species separation and determination in wine varietals by liquid chromatography-hydride generation atomic fluorescence spectrometry. *J. Chromatogr. A* **2016**, *1462*, 44–54. [CrossRef] [PubMed]
154. Liu, C.X.; Xiao, Z.M.; Jia, Z.; Tian, J.; Liu, X.L.; Fan, X. Quantitative determination of arsenic species in feed using liquid chromatography-hydride generation atomic fluorescence spectrometry. *Chin. J. Anal. Chem.* **2018**, *46*, 537–542.
155. Wang, Y.; Li, Y.Q.; Lv, K.; Chen, X.L.; Yu, X.Y. A simple and sensitive non-chromatographic method for quantification of four arsenic species in rice by hydride generation-atomic fluorescence spectrometry. *Spectrochim. Acta B* **2018**, *149*, 197–202. [CrossRef]
156. Zhang, Y.L.; Miro, M.; Kolev, S.D. A novel on-line organic mercury digestion method combined with atomic fluorescence spectrometry for automatic mercury speciation. *Talanta* **2018**, *189*, 220–224. [CrossRef] [PubMed]
157. Grijalba, A.C.; Fiorentini, E.F.; Wuilloud, R.G. Ionic liquid-assisted separation and determination of selenium species in food and beverage samples by liquid chromatography coupled to hydride generation atomic fluorescence spectrometry. *J. Chromatogr. A* **2017**, *1491*, 117–125. [CrossRef] [PubMed]
158. dos Santos, G.S.; Silva, L.O.B.; Santos, A.F.; da Silva, E.G.P.; dos Santos, W.N.L. Analytical strategies for determination and environmental impact assessment of inorganic antimony species in natural waters using hydride generation atomic fluorescence spectrometry (HG-AFS). *J. Braz. Chem. Soc.* **2018**, *29*, 185–190. [CrossRef]
159. de Quadros, D.P.C.; Campanella, B.; Onor, M.; Bramanti, E.; Borges, D.L.G.; D'Ulivo, A. Mercury speciation by high-performance liquid chromatography atomic fluorescence spectrometry using an integrated microwave/UV interface. Optimization of a single step procedure for the simultaneous photo-oxidation of mercury species and photo-generation of Hg^0. *Spectrochim. Acta B* **2014**, *101*, 312–319.
160. Ai, X.; Wang, Y.; Hou, X.D.; Yang, L.; Zheng, C.B.; Wu, L. Advanced oxidation using Fe_3O_4 magnetic nanoparticles and its application in mercury speciation analysis by high performance liquid chromatography-cold vapor generation atomic fluorescence spectrometry. *Analyst* **2013**, *138*, 3494–3501. [CrossRef] [PubMed]
161. Sun, Y.C.; Chen, Y.J.; Tsai, Y.N. Determination of urinary arsenic species using an on-line nano-TiO_2 photooxidation device coupled with microbore LC and hydride generation-ICP-MS system. *Microchem. J.* **2007**, *86*, 140–145. [CrossRef]
162. Yu, X.P.; Deng, T.L.; Guo, Y.F.; Wang, Q. Arsenic species analysis in freshwater using liquid chromatography combined to hydride generation atomic fluorescence spectrometry. *J. Anal. Chem.* **2014**, *69*, 83–88. [CrossRef]
163. Musil, S.; Matoušek, T. On-line pre-reduction of pentavalent arsenicals by thioglycolic acid for speciation analysis by selective hydride generation–cryotrapping–atomic absorption spectrometry. *Spectrochim. Acta B* **2008**, *63*, 685–691. [CrossRef] [PubMed]
164. Caylak, O.; Elci, S.G.; Hol, A.; Akdogan, A.; Divrikli, U.; Elci, L. Use of an aminated Amberlite XAD-4 column coupled to flow injection cold vapour generation atomic absorption spectrometry for mercury speciation in water and fish tissue samples. *Food Chem.* **2019**, *274*, 487–493. [CrossRef] [PubMed]
165. Wang, X.J.; Chen, P.; Cao, L.; Xu, G.L.; Yang, S.Y.; Fang, Y.; Wang, G.Z.; Hong, X.C. Selenium speciation in rice samples by magnetic ionic liquid-based up-and-down-shaker-assisted dispersive liquid-liquid microextraction coupled to graphite furnace atomic absorption spectrometry. *Food Anal. Method* **2017**, *10*, 1653–1660. [CrossRef]
166. dos Santos, Q.O.; Silva, M.M.; Lemos, V.A.; Ferreira, S.L.C.; de Andrade, J.B. An online preconcentration system for speciation analysis of arsenic in seawater by hydride generation flame atomic absorption spectrometry. *Microchem. J.* **2018**, *143*, 175–180. [CrossRef]
167. Maratta, A.; Carrizo, B.; Bazan, V.L.; Villafane, G.; Martinez, L.D.; Pacheco, P. Antimony speciation analysis by hydride trapping on hybrid nanoparticles packed in a needle trap device with electro-thermal atomic absorption spectrometry determination. *J. Anal. Atom. Spectrom.* **2018**, *33*, 2195–2202. [CrossRef]
168. Welna, M.; Pohl, P.; Szymczycha-Madeja, A. Non-chromatographic speciation of inorganic arsenic in rice by hydride generation inductively coupled plasma optical emission spectrometry. *Food Anal. Method* **2019**, *12*, 581–594. [CrossRef]
169. Mo, J.M.; Li, Q.; Guo, X.H.; Zhang, G.X.; Wang, Z. Flow injection photochemical vapor generation coupled with miniaturized solution-cathode glow discharge atomic emission spectrometry for determination and speciation analysis of mercury. *Anal. Chem.* **2017**, *89*, 10353–10360. [CrossRef] [PubMed]

170. Dundar, M.S.; Kaptan, F.; Caner, C.; Altundag, H. Speciation of antimony using dithizone ligand via cloud point extraction and determination by USN-ICP-OES. *Atom. Spectrosc.* **2018**, *39*, 100–105.
171. Marcinkowska, M.; Baralkiewicz, D. Multielemental speciation analysis by advanced hyphenated technique—HPLC/ICP-MS: A review. *Talanta* **2016**, *161*, 177–204. [CrossRef] [PubMed]
172. Popp, M.; Hann, S.; Koellensperger, G. Environmental application of elemental speciation analysis based on liquid or gas chromatography hyphenated to inductively coupled plasma mass spectrometry—A review. *Anal. Chim. Acta* **2010**, *668*, 114–129. [CrossRef] [PubMed]
173. Terol, A.; Marcinkowska, M.; Ardini, F.; Grotti, M. Fast determination of toxic arsenic species in food samples using narrow-bore high-performance liquid-chromatography inductively coupled plasma mass spectrometry. *Anal. Sci.* **2016**, *32*, 911–915. [CrossRef] [PubMed]
174. Cheng, H.Y.; Zhang, W.W.; Wang, Y.C.; Liu, J.H. Interfacing nanoliter liquid chromatography and inductively coupled plasma mass spectrometry with an in-column high-pressure nebulizer for mercury speciation. *J. Chromaatogr. A* **2018**, *1575*, 59–65. [CrossRef] [PubMed]
175. Bolea-Fernandez, E.; Balcaen, L.; Resano, M.; Vanhaecke, F. Interference-free determination of ultra-trace concentrations of arsenic and selenium using methyl fluoride as a reaction gas in ICP-MS/MS. *Anal. Bioanal. Chem.* **2015**, *407*, 919–929. [CrossRef] [PubMed]
176. Stiboller, M.; Raber, G.; Gjengedal, E.L.F.; Eggesbo, M.; Francesconi, K.A. Quantifying inorganic arsenic and other water-soluble arsenic species in human milk by HPLC/ICPMS. *Anal. Chem.* **2017**, *89*, 6266–6272. [CrossRef] [PubMed]
177. Izabela, K.; Adam, S.; Danuta, B. Total arsenic and arsenic species determination in freshwater fish by ICP-DRC-MS and HPLC/ICP-DRC-MS techniques. *Molecules* **2019**, *24*, 607. [CrossRef]
178. Marcinkowska, M.; Komorowicz, I.; Baralkiewicz, D. Study on multielemental speciation analysis of Cr(VI), As(III) and As(V) in water by advanced hyphenated technique HPLC/ICP-DRC-MS. Fast and reliable procedures. *Talanta* **2015**, *144*, 233–240. [CrossRef] [PubMed]
179. Bolea-Fernandez, E.; Balcaen, L.; Resano, M.; Vanhaecke, F. Overcoming spectral overlap via inductively coupled plasma-tandem mass spectrometry (ICPMS/MS). A tutorial review. *J. Anal. Atom. Spectrom.* **2017**, *32*, 1660–1679. [CrossRef]
180. Balcaen, L.; Bolea-Fernandez, E.; Resano, M.; Vanhaecke, F. Inductively coupled plasma-tandem mass spectrometry (ICP-MS/MS): A powerful and universal tool for the interference-free determination of (ultra) trace elements—A tutorial review. *Anal. Chim. Acta* **2015**, *894*, 7–19. [CrossRef] [PubMed]
181. Rodriguez-Gonzalez, P.; Alonso, J.I.G. Recent advances in isotope dilution analysis for elemental speciation. *J. Anal. Atom. Spectrom.* **2010**, *25*, 239–259. [CrossRef]
182. Jeong, J.S.; Lee, J.; Park, Y.N. Quantitative speciation of selenium in human blood serum and urine with AE-RP- and AF-HPLC-ICP/MS. *Bull. Korean Chem. Soc.* **2013**, *34*, 3817–3824. [CrossRef]
183. Castillo, A.; Boix, C.; Fabregat, N.; Roig-Navarro, A.F.; Rodriguez-Castrillon, J.A. Rapid screening of arsenic species in urine from exposed human by inductively coupled plasma mass spectrometry with germanium as internal standard. *J. Anal. Atom. Spectrom.* **2012**, *27*, 354–358. [CrossRef]
184. Petursdottir, A.H.; Gunnlaugsdottir, H. Selective and fast screening method for inorganic arsenic in seaweed using hydride generation inductively coupled plasma mass spectrometry (HG-ICP-MS). *Microchem. J.* **2019**, *144*, 45–50. [CrossRef]
185. Matousek, T.; Wang, Z.F.; Douillet, C.; Musil, S.; Styblo, M. Direct speciation analysis of arsenic in whole blood and blood plasma at low exposure levels by hydride generation-cryotrapping-inductively coupled plasma mass spectrometry. *Anal. Chem.* **2017**, *89*, 9633–9637. [CrossRef] [PubMed]
186. Tsai, Y.N.; Lin, C.H.; Hsu, I.H.; Sun, Y.C. Sequential photocatalyst-assisted digestion and vapor generation device coupled with anion exchange chromatography and inductively coupled plasma mass spectrometry for speciation analysis of selenium species in biological samples. *Anal. Chim. Acta* **2014**, *806*, 165–171. [CrossRef] [PubMed]

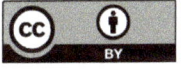 © 2019 by the authors. Licensee MDPI, Basel, Switzerland. This article is an open access article distributed under the terms and conditions of the Creative Commons Attribution (CC BY) license (http://creativecommons.org/licenses/by/4.0/).

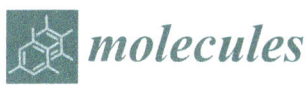

Article

Understanding the Solution Behavior of Epinephrine in the Presence of Toxic Cations: A Thermodynamic Investigation in Different Experimental Conditions

Francesco Crea [1,*], Concetta De Stefano [1], Anna Irto [1], Gabriele Lando [1], Stefano Materazzi [2], Demetrio Milea [1], Alberto Pettignano [3] and Silvio Sammartano [1]

1 Dipartimento di Scienze Chimiche, Biologiche, Farmaceutiche ed Ambientali, Università degli Studi di Messina, V.le F. Stagno d'Alcontres, 31, I-98166 Messina, Italy; cdestefano@unime.it (C.D.S.); airto@unime.it (A.I.); glando@unime.it (G.L.); dmilea@unime.it (D.M.); ssammartano@unime.it (S.S.)
2 Dipartimento di Chimica, Università "La Sapienza" di Roma, Piazzale A. Moro 5, I-00185 Rome, Italy; stefano.materazzi@uniroma1.it
3 Dipartimento di Fisica e Chimica, Università degli Studi di Palermo, V.le delle Scienze, ed. 17, I-90128 Palermo, Italy; alberto.pettignano@unipa.it
* Correspondence: fcrea@unime.it

Received: 31 December 2019; Accepted: 21 January 2020; Published: 24 January 2020

Abstract: The interactions of epinephrine ((R)-(−)-3,4-dihydroxy-α-(methylaminomethyl)benzyl alcohol; Eph^-) with different toxic cations (methylmercury(II): CH_3Hg^+; dimethyltin(IV): $(CH_3)_2Sn^{2+}$; dioxouranium(VI): UO_2^{2+}) were studied in $NaCl_{aq}$ at different ionic strengths and at $T = 298.15$ K ($T = 310.15$ K for $(CH_3)_2Sn^{2+}$). The enthalpy changes for the protonation of epinephrine and its complex formation with UO_2^{2+} were also determined using isoperibolic titration calorimetry: $\Delta H_{HL} = -39 \pm 1$ kJ mol^{-1}, $\Delta H_{H2L} = -67 \pm 1$ kJ mol^{-1} (overall reaction), $\Delta H_{ML} = -26 \pm 4$ kJ mol^{-1}, and $\Delta H_{M2L2(OH)2} = 39 \pm 2$ kJ mol^{-1}. The results were that UO_2^{2+} complexation by Eph^- was an entropy-driven process. The dependence on the ionic strength of protonation and the complex formation constants was modeled using the extended Debye–Hückel, specific ion interaction theory (SIT), and Pitzer approaches. The sequestering ability of adrenaline toward the investigated cations was evaluated using the calculation of $pL_{0.5}$ parameters. The sequestering ability trend resulted in the following: $UO_2^{2+} \gg (CH_3)_2Sn^{2+} > CH_3Hg^+$. For example, at $I = 0.15$ mol dm^{-3} and pH = 7.4 (pH = 9.5 for CH_3Hg^+), $pL_{0.5} = 7.68$, 5.64, and 2.40 for UO_2^{2+}, $(CH_3)_2Sn^{2+}$, and CH_3Hg^+, respectively. Here, the pH is with respect to ionic strength in terms of sequestration.

Keywords: epinephrine; toxic cations; enthalpy and entropy changes; dependence on ionic strength; sequestering ability

---

1. Introduction

Catecholamines, such as dopamine, epinephrine (or adrenaline), and norepinephrine, are hormones produced by the medullary portion of the adrenal glands, which are small triangular organs located above the kidneys. They are released in blood in response to physical or emotional stress and help to transmit nerve impulses to the brain, increase the availability of glucose and fatty acids to promote energy production, and dilate the bronchioles and pupils. After performing their activities, catecholamines are metabolized into inactive forms: dopamine is transformed in homovanilic acid (HVA), norepinephrine turns into normetanephrine and vanilmandelic acid (VMA), and epinephrine becomes metanephrine and VMA. Both hormones and their metabolites are excreted by urine, in which they are usually present in small variable concentrations, which appreciably increase during and immediately after exposure to stress [1,2].

Pheochromocytomas and other types of neuroendocrine tumors, however, can produce large amounts of catecholamines, leading to their increased concentration levels in both blood and urine (together with their metabolites). This may result in persistent and severe episodic hypertension, severe headache, tachycardia, excessive sweating, nausea, anxiety, and tingling in the extremities.

Epinephrine ((R)-(−)-3,4-dihydroxy-α-(methylaminomethyl)benzyl alcohol, also known as adrenaline, Scheme 1), is synthesized by an enzymatic process that converts tyrosine into a series of intermediates and ultimately epinephrine. In particular, epinephrine acts on nearly all body tissues and increases heart rate and the force of heart contractions, facilitating blood flow to the muscles and the brain. Epinephrine relaxes smooth muscle and helps the conversion of glycogen into glucose in the liver, increasing the blood sugar level: it also causes acceleration in breathing and in medicine is used in treatments for cardiac arrest, asthma, and glaucoma [3–5].

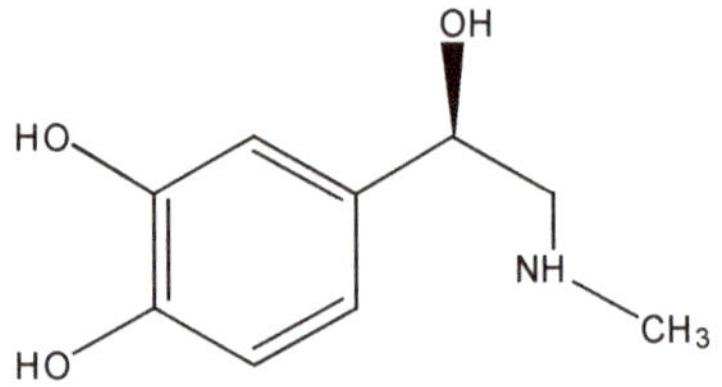

Scheme 1. (R)-(−)-3,4-Dihydroxy-α-(methylaminomethyl)benzyl alcohol.

The behavior of epinephrine in physiological conditions is dependent on the different forms in which it can be present, i.e., on its chemical speciation. As an example, epinephrine can have an influence on platelet aggregation, for which epinephrine is an agonist [6], but this phenomenon is influenced by the interaction between divalent and trivalent metal ions such as calcium, copper, manganese, magnesium, cadmium, and aluminum.

As it has been reported in many papers, the behavior of catecholamines in aqueous solution depends on many parameters, such as pH, temperature, ionic medium, ionic strength, and exposure to light and oxygen (they tend to be quickly oxidized) [1,7–12].

The acid–base properties and solubility of epinephrine in different experimental conditions have already been documented in the literature [13–17]. Taking into account that the pharmacological action of epinephrine can be influenced by the presence of metal cations present in the same environment, we decided to investigate the complexation of this hormone toward some selected toxic cations by using (Ion Selective Electrode) ISE-[H$^+$] potentiometry, UV spectrophotometry, calorimetry, and thermogravimetry at ionic strength values ranging from 0 to 1.0 I/mol dm^{-3} at T = 298.15 K and T = 310.15 K. Due to their importance from both a biological and environmental point of view, the selected cations were $(CH_3)_2Sn^{2+}$, UO_2^{2+}, and CH_3Hg^+, whose properties and activities are already well known [18–34].

In this investigation, the speciation models of the cation–epinephrine systems and the corresponding formation constants of the species in different experimental conditions were determined following well-established criteria for the selection of the best speciation models, which have already been reported in previous papers [35–39].

The dependence of the formation constants on ionic strength was studied by means of a Debye–Hückel type equation, as well as through Pitzer and specific ion interaction theory (SIT) approaches [40–48].

The enthalpy and entropy change values of protonation for epinephrine and complex formation for the metal–ligand species of UO_2^{2+} were also determined using isoperibol calorimetry.

Using a simple Boltzmann-type equation, the sequestering ability of epinephrine toward the investigated toxic cations was quantified in different experimental conditions by means of the $pL_{0.5}$ parameter.

The information obtained from the speciation studies can be useful in modeling the behavior of such molecules in quite different experimental conditions, such as those of many natural waters and biological fluids.

2. Results and Discussion

2.1. Acid–Base Properties of Epinephrine and Investigated Cations

The acid–base properties of the cations investigated in this work (i.e., their hydrolytic behavior), as well as those of epinephrine (i.e., its protonation), must be known in the exact experimental conditions of the considered systems. The hydrolysis constants of $(CH_3)_2Sn^{2+}$, UO_2^{2+}, and CH_3Hg^+ in $NaCl_{(aq)}$ at $0 < I/\text{mol dm}^{-3} \leq 1.0$ and $T = 298.15$ K ($T = 310.15$ K for $(CH_3)_2Sn^{2+}$) were taken from References [49–51] and are reported in Tables S1–S3. In the case of methylmercury(II), its chloride interactions were explicitly taken into account, considering the formation of CH_3HgCl species through their corresponding stability constants in calculations (Table S3).

Concerning the protonation constants of epinephrine, it is worth mentioning here that, as with other catecholamines, its acid–base properties are not easy to determine, since they tend to be oxidized in aqueous solution, especially at pH > 10.0–10.5 [1,9,10,52]. Moreover, epinephrine has four potentially functional groups, that can undergo acid-base reactions, but only two are in the pH range of biological interest. For this reason, it has often been considered to be a bidentate ligand, though some studies have reported some values related to the third protonation step (log K_a ~ 13) [13,53,54] associated with the protonation/dissociation of the second phenolic group. Log K_a values of ~ 13.5–14 have been attributed to the hydroxyl group of the alkyl chain [13,53,54]. The values used in this work have been previously determined by this group together with their dependence on ionic strength and temperature in different models. Protonation constants at infinite dilution and the corresponding parameters for their dependence on ionic strength in the EDH and SIT models (Equations (4)–(7)) for values in molar and molal concentration scales, respectively, in $NaCl_{(aq)}$ at $T = 298.15$ and 310.15 K are reported in Table S4 [17].

2.2. Epinephrine–Cation Interactions

Chemical speciation studies of cation/ligand systems, such as those investigated in this work, are particularly difficult, not only for the accurate determination of the stability constants of formed complexes, but also for their identification, i.e., for the definition of reliable speciation models. In this vein, some general rules and guidelines may be very helpful [35–39], such as the following:

(i) The simplicity of the proposed model. The simpler the better, both in terms of number and nature of species considered;
(ii) The formation percentages of the species considered in the investigated conditions. Sometimes minor species are included in models to improve the quality of fits, but their significance has to be verified, possibly in a broad range of experimental conditions and/or using different techniques;
(iii) The likelihood of the proposed species. *Similar* ligands generally form *similar* species and show *similar* binding modes. Theoretical and/or experimental evidence about coordination may be supportive; and
(iv) "Statistical significance" of species and models. Experimental data are, nowadays, almost exclusively elaborated by software based on nonlinear least squares minimization. A derived fit's parameters (e.g., variances/standard deviations of fits, uncertainties associated with refined variables), which are obtained for various models, should be compared (by relative tests) to check for statistically significant differences.

Evidently, all this cannot prescind from a consistent number of experiments opportunely designed to cover a wide range of conditions (in terms of total concentrations, concentration ratios, and pH, as well as ionic media, temperatures, and ionic strengths, if pertinent).

2.2.1. CH_3Hg^+/Eph^- Complexes

Investigations of a CH_3Hg^+/Eph^- system were carried out up to pH = 11 without observing the formation of sparingly soluble species. The stability constants of the CH_3Hg^+/Eph^- species, determined in $NaCl_{(aq)}$ at different ionic strengths and at T = 298.15 K, are reported in Table 1.

Table 1. Experimental stability constants of CH_3Hg^+/Eph^- complexes in $NaCl_{aq}$ at different ionic strengths and at T = 298.15 K.

I/mol dm^{-3}	log β_{110} [1,3]	log β_{111} [1,3]	log β_{11-1} [1,3]	log β_{MLCl} [2,3]
0.151	8.56 ± 0.03	17.33 ± 0.04	−0.79 ± 0.04	9.17 ± 0.07
0.502	8.38 ± 0.06	17.24 ± 0.03	−1.08 ± 0.03	8.70 ± 0.04
0.753	8.20 ± 0.04	17.14 ± 0.03	−1.27 ± 0.02	8.49 ± 0.05
0.998	8.15 ± 0.06	16.99 ± 0.04	−1.44 ± 0.04	8.44 ± 0.07

[1] log β_{pqr} refers to equilibrium: p M^{m+} + q L^{z-} + r H^+ = $M_pL_qH_r^{(mp-zq+r)}$; [2] log β_{MLCl} refers to equilibrium: M^+ + L^- + Cl^- = $MLCl^-$; [3] ±95% confidence interval.

The speciation of methylmercury(II) in sodium chloride aqueous solutions was characterized by the formation of MOH and MCl species (Table S3). The latter species was quite stable, so that, in the presence of epinephrine, the formation of ternary MLCl$^-$ was observed in the pH range 8.0–10.5, as is shown in the speciation diagrams in Figure 1a,b.

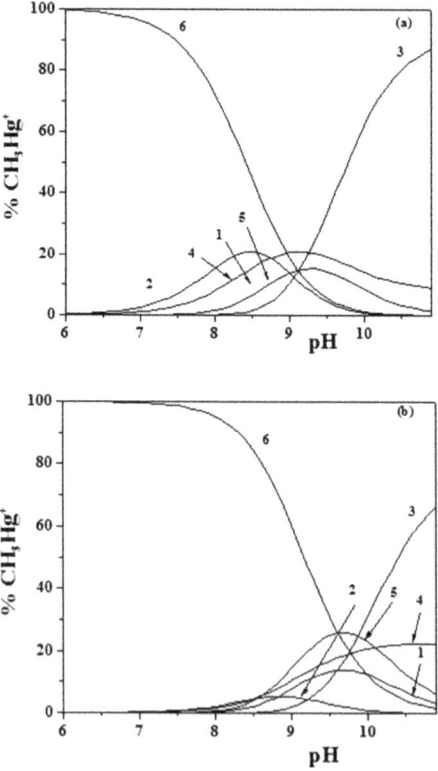

Figure 1. (a,b) Distribution diagram of the species for the CH_3Hg^+/Eph^- system: C_{CH3Hg+} = 1 mmol dm^{-3}; C_{Eph} = 3 mmol dm^{-3} ((a) I = 0.15 mol dm^{-3}; (b) I = 1 mol dm^{-3} (Stoichiometry of the species: 1: ML; 2: MLH; 3: MLOH; 4: MOH; 5: MLCl; 6: MCl); M = CH_3Hg^+; L = Eph^-).

Concerning the other species determined (i.e., MLH$^+$, ML^0, and MLOH$^-$), ML^0 was formed almost in the same pH range as the MLCl$^-$ species, while MLH$^+$ occurred at lower pH values (about 7), and MLOH$^-$ occurred above pH ~8.5. Comparing the diagrams in Figure 1a,b, obtained at $I = 0.15$ and $I = 1.0$ mol dm^{-3}, respectively, the effect of the ionic strength on the distribution of the species can be observed, which resulted in a shift of the maximum formation percentages toward higher pH values at higher ionic strengths.

From the analysis of the distribution diagrams in Figure 1a,b, it is also evident how the formation of CH$_3$Hg$^+$/Eph^- species became significant at pH ~9.0–9.5. This is an indication that, in physiological conditions (e.g., in blood plasma at pH ~7.4), the behavior of adrenaline is scarcely influenced by the presence of CH$_3$Hg$^+$.

2.2.2. (CH$_3$)$_2$Sn^{2+}/Eph^- Complexes

The interactions between dimethyltin(IV) and epinephrine were studied at $T = 310.15$ K and in NaCl$_{(aq)}$ at different ionic strengths by means of potentiometry, though some checks were also made at $I = 0.15$ mol dm^{-3} using UV-VIS spectrophotometric titrations (Table S5).

In the experimental conditions adopted, the formation of the MLH^{2+}, ML$^+$, and MLOH^0 species was observed. The corresponding stability constants are reported in Table 2.

Table 2. Experimental stability constants of (CH$_3$)$_2$Sn^{2+}/Eph^- complexes in NaCl$_{aq}$ at different ionic strengths and $T = 310.15$ K.

I/mol dm^{-3}	log β_{110} [1]	log β_{111} [1]	log $\beta_{11\text{-}1}$ [1]
0.099	15.79 ± 0.02	20.46 ± 0.02	7.95 ± 0.01
0.149	15.60 ± 0.02	20.28 ± 0.02	7.81 ± 0.01
0.247	15.30 ± 0.01	19.98 ± 0.02	7.57 ± 0.01
0.492	14.73 ± 0.01	19.43 ± 0.02	7.13 ± 0.01
0.734	14.26 ± 0.02	18.98 ± 0.02	6.77 ± 0.01
0.974	13.83 ± 0.03	18.56 ± 0.03	6.43 ± 0.02

[1] log β_{pqr} refers to equilibrium: p M^{m+} + q L^{z-} + r H$^+$ = M$_p$L$_q$H$_r$$^{(mp-zq+r)}$; ±95% confidence interval.

As it was already said, UV-VIS spectrophotometric titrations at $I = 0.15$ mol dm^{-3} and $T = 310.15$ K were also carried out, confirming the speciation model obtained using potentiometric data and obtaining stability constants that were highly comparable to the potentiometric results: log β_{110} = 15.74 ± 0.04, log β_{111} = 20.11 ± 0.03, and log $\beta_{11\text{-}1}$ = 8.19 ± 0.02.

An example of spectrophotometric titration is reported in Figure 2 (experimental conditions: c_M = 0.03 mmol dm^{-3}; c_{Eph} = 0.09 mmol dm^{-3}), in which spectra were collected from pH = 2.38 to pH = 11.21 without the formation of sparingly soluble species being observed.

Increasing pH and a bathochromic shift of the band at λ_{max} = 279 nm were observed up to λ ~295 nm, together with a hypsochromic shift for the band at λ = 248 nm. The molar extinction coefficients (ε/mol^{-1} cm^{-1} dm^{-3}) of the free and protonated adrenaline species were already determined in a prior paper [17] (Figure S1), while those relative to the (CH$_3$)$_2$Sn^{2+} complexes are studied here and are reported in Figure 3. Comparing the determined data using the different analytical techniques and taking into account the different concentration range used, we can consider them to be in very good agreement.

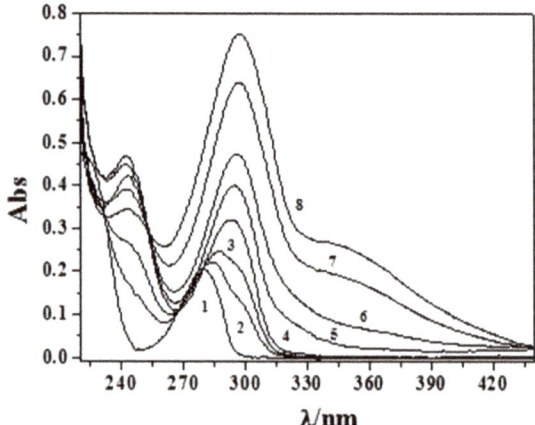

Figure 2. Titration curves at some different pH values at $I = 0.15$ mol dm^{-3} and $T = 310.15$ K for the $(CH_3)_2Sn^{2+}/Eph^-$ system. Experimental conditions: $c_M = 0.03$ mmol dm^{-3} and $c_L = 0.09$ mmol dm^{-3} (1: pH = 2.38; 2: pH = 7.37; 3: pH = 8.14; 4: pH = 9.14; 5: pH = 10.06; 6: pH = 10.36; 7: pH = 10.92; 8: pH = 11.21).

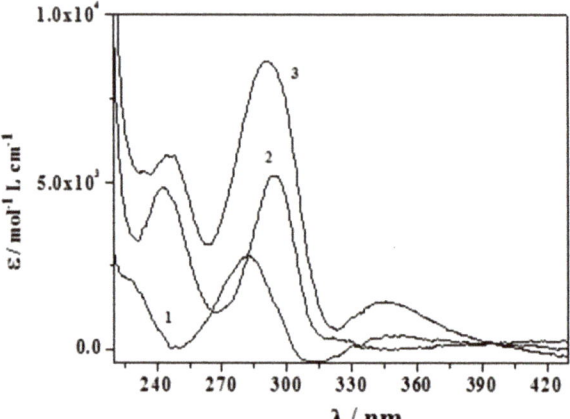

Figure 3. Here, ε/mol^{-1} L cm^{-1} versus λ/nm for the $(CH_3)_2Sn^{2+}/Eph^-$ species in NaCl$_{aq}$ at $I = 0.15$ mol dm^{-3} and $T = 310.15$ K (Stoichiometry of the species. 1: MLH; 2: ML; 3: MLOH; M = $(CH_3)_2Sn^{2+}$; L = Eph^-).

Figures 4 and 5 report the distribution diagrams of the $(CH_3)_2Sn^{2+}/Eph^-$ species in NaCl$_{(aq)}$ at $I = 0.15$ mol dm^{-3} and $T = 310.15$ K in a 1:1 molar ratio at two different concentrations.

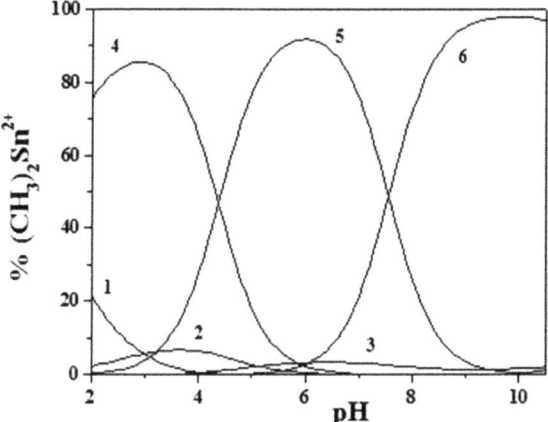

Figure 4. Distribution diagram of the species for the $(CH_3)_2Sn^{2+}/Eph^-$ system at $I = 0.15$ mol dm^{-3}, $T = 310.15$ K, and $c_M = c_L = 3.00$ mmol dm^{-3} (from potentiometric data). (Stoichiometry of the species. 1: M; 2: M(OH); 3: M(OH)$_2$; 4: MLH; 5: ML; and 6: MLOH. M = $(CH_3)_2Sn^{2+}$; L = Eph^-).

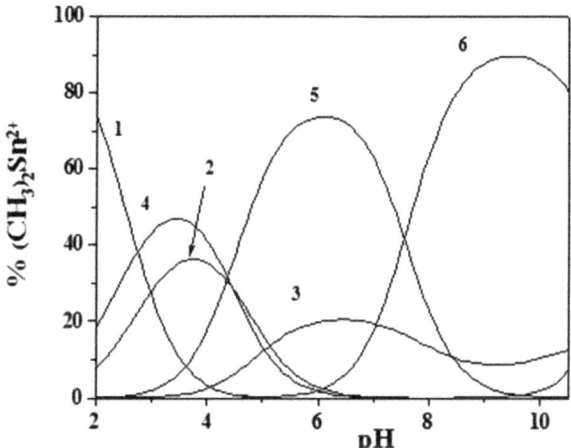

Figure 5. Distribution diagram of the species for the $(CH_3)_2Sn^{2+}/Eph^-$ system at $I = 0.15$ mol dm^{-3}, $T = 310.15$ K, and $c_M = c_L = 0.06$ mmol dm^{-3} (from UV spectrophotometric data). (Stoichiometry of the species. 1: M; 2: M(OH); 3: M(OH)$_2$; 4: MLH; 5: ML; 6: MLOH. M = $(CH_3)_2Sn^{2+}$; L = Eph^-).

As can be observed, a higher presence of both the free metal ion (at low pH) and the hydrolytic species of $(CH_3)_2Sn^{2+}$ occurred at low component concentrations (UV-VIS spectrophotometric measurements). Nevertheless dimethyltin(IV)/epinephrine species were significant in all of the investigated pH range, an indication that this cation may influence epinephrine behavior in physiological conditions.

2.2.3. UO_2^{2+}/Eph^- Complexes

As reported in the experimental section, dioxouranium(VI) was used in the form of $UO_2(Ac)_2$ salt, meaning that acetate was always present during the experiments at a concentration always double that of UO_2^{2+}. Since this cation tends to form quite stable complexes with many carboxylic ligands, including acetate, the stability constants of UO_2^{2+}/Ac^- complexes must be taken into account during data analysis. Corresponding values were taken from a previous work [55] and are reported in Table S6. An analysis of experimental data for the UO_2^{2+}/Eph^- system at T = 298.15 K in $NaCl_{(aq)}$ at different ionic strengths was performed up to pH ~8.5, since the formation of sparingly soluble species was observed in all conditions at higher pH values. The resulting elaboration was particularly difficult due to the tendency of UO_2^{2+} to form further species with stoichiometries different from mononuclear/monomeric ones. By applying the above-cited criteria for the selection of the most suitable speciation model, the formation of many different species was considered and tested. Finally, the accepted speciation scheme accounted for the formation of four species, namely the mononuclear ML^+ and MLOH and the dinuclear $M_2L_2^{2+}$ and $M_2L_2(OH)_2$. The corresponding stability constants at different ionic strengths are reported in Table 3.

Table 3. Experimental stability constants of UO_2^{2+}/Eph^- complexes in $NaCl_{aq}$ at different ionic strengths and T = 298.15 K.

I/mol dm^{-3}	log β_{110} [1]	log β_{11-1} [1]	log β_{220} [1]	log β_{22-2} [1]
0.146	12.35 ± 0.02	6.75 ± 0.01	27.46 ± 0.05	16.46 ± 0.02
0.491	12.16 ± 0.01	6.57 ± 0.01	26.97 ± 0.02	16.13 ± 0.01
0.736	12.03 ± 0.01	6.44 ± 0.02	26.99 ± 0.02	16.12 ± 0.01
0.982	11.96 ± 0.01	6.46 ± 0.03	26.96 ± 0.03	16.10 ± 0.01

[1] log β_{pqr} refers to equilibrium: p M^{m+} + q L^{z-} + r H^+ = $M_pL_qH_r^{(mp-zq+r)}$; ±95% confidence interval.

Figures 6 and 7 better evidence the effect of ionic strength and of the ligand-to-metal ratio on the distribution of the species for the UO_2^{2+}/Eph^- system. As was observed, dioxouranium(VI) complexation by epinephrine became significant at pH > 4.0, with all corresponding species reaching high formation percentages. At pH ~7.4, UO_2^{2+} speciation was dominated by the formation of the $M_2L_2(OH)_2$ species, which reached percentages higher than 40%.

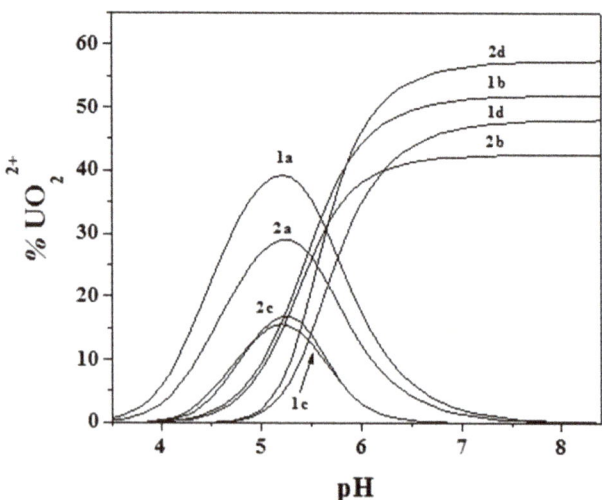

Figure 6. Distribution diagram of the species for the UO_2^{2+}/Eph^- system: c_{UO22+} = 1 mmol dm^{-3} e; c_{Eph} = 3 mmol dm^{-3} (1: I = 0.15 mol dm^{-3}; 2: I = 1 mol dm^{-3}; (Stoichiometry of the species. a: ML; b: MLOH; c: M_2L_2; d: $M_2L_2(OH)_2$. M = UO_2^{2+}; L = Eph^-).

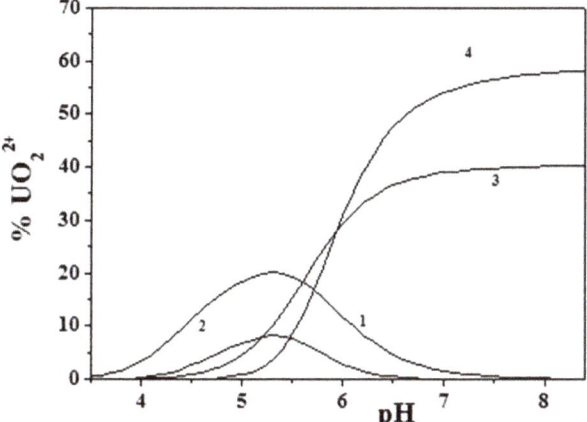

Figure 7. Distribution diagram of the species for the UO_2^{2+}/Eph^- system at $I = 0.15$ mol dm^{-3}. $c_{UO22+} = 2$ mmol dm^{-3} and $c_{Eph} = 2$ mmol dm^{-3} (Stoichiometry of the species. 1: ML; 2: M_2L_2; 3: MLOH; 4: $M_2L_2(OH)_2$. M = UO_2^{2+}; L = Eph^-).

Changes in ionic strength (Figure 6) only affected the formation percentages of the species and had little/no effect on the pH range in which they were present, which also happened when varying the ligand-to-metal ratio (Figure 7).

2.3. Calorimetric Analysis

By means of an isoperibol titration calorimeter, the enthalpy changes for the protonation epinephrine and its complex formation with UO_2^{2+} were determined in NaCl$_{(aq)}$ at $I = 0.5$ mol dm^{-3} and $T = 298.15$ K by the heat of reactions collected during the titrations.

Concerning the determination of the protonation enthalpy changes of epinephrine, solutions containing Eph^- (4–5 mmol dm^{-3}) and the ionic medium were previously neutralized with standard NaOH solution and then titrated with standard HCl solutions, as is described in the experimental section. The ligand concentrations reported above were used in order to obtain suitable amounts of the LH^0 and LH^{2+} species during the calorimetric titrations, allowing for the measurement of the ΔH/kJ mol^{-1} (expressed as overall formation enthalpies according to L^- + i H^+ = $LH_i^{(i-1)}$, where L = generic ligand; H = proton). The protonation enthalpy changes of epinephrine are reported in Table 4 and were in good agreement with analogous values reported in the literature for similar molecules, such as dopamine ($\Delta H = -46$ and -83 kJ mol^{-1} for LH^0 and LH_2^+, respectively) [53,56].

Table 4. ΔH, ΔG, and $T\Delta S$ values for Eph^- protonation and its complexes with UO_2^{2+} in NaCl$_{aq}$ at $I = 0.5$ mol dm^{-3} and $T = 298.15$ K.

Species [1]	ΔH [2]	ΔG [2]	$T\Delta S$ [2]
LH	−39 ± 1	−57.69 ± 0.05	19 ± 3
LH$_2$	−67 ± 1	−107.39 ± 0.05	40 ± 3
ML	−26 ± 4	−69.16 ± 0.02	43 ± 10
M$_2$L$_2$(OH)$_2$	39 ± 2	−92.21 ± 0.02	131 ± 6

[1] log β_{pqr} refers to equilibrium: p M^{m+} + q L^{z-} + r H$^+$ = $M_pL_qH_r^{(mp-zq+r)}$; [2] in kJ mol^{-1}; ±95% confidence interval.

The protonation enthalpy changes determined, as described above, were then used as input in calculations for the determination of formation enthalpy changes of UO_2^{2+}/Eph^- species, together with those related to UO_2^{2+} hydrolysis and its acetate complexes (taken from the literature) [55,57]. The formation thermodynamic parameters are reported in Table 4 only for the ML and $M_2L_2(OH)_2$ species, since no reliable data could be obtained for other complex species in the experimental conditions adopted. The reliability of the results obtained is also supported by the low values of both the standard deviation for the global fit of experimental data (σ = 0.054) and the mean deviation of the variation of the heats of reaction (∂Q = 0.146). As can be observed, the formation of the ML species was exothermic, while the overall formation reaction of $M_2L_2(OH)_2$ was endothermic. Even considering the reaction relative to the hydrolysis and dimerization of the ML complex as it formed $M_2L_2(OH)_2$ species (according to the reaction 2 ML = $M_2L_2(OH)_2$ + 2 H$^+$), it was ΔH = 91 kJ mol^{-1}. These values, when analyzed with all of the thermodynamic parameters reported in Table 4, clearly indicate how the main contribution to complex formation is entropic in nature.

2.4. Ionic Strength Dependence

The dependence of formation constants on ionic strength was investigated by means of an extended Debye–Hückel (EDH)-type equation, SIT (specific ion interaction theory), and the Pitzer approach. Further details are given in their dedicated section.

The stability constants of cation/epinephrine complexes in Tables 1–3 were fitted to Equation (4) to obtain their corresponding values at infinite dilution and their C parameters (EDH) to model their dependent ionic strength on a molar scale, as reported in Table 5.

Table 5. Stability constants of M^{n+}/Eph^- at infinite dilution and corresponding parameters for their dependence on ionic strength in $NaCl_{aq}$ using the extended Debye–Hückel (EDH) and specific ion interaction theory (SIT) models at T = 298.15 K.

	CH_3Hg^+			
	$\log \beta_{110}$ [1,3]	$\log \beta_{111}$ [1,3]	$\log \beta_{11-1}$ [1,3]	$\log \beta_{MLCl}$ [2,3]
$\log \beta^0_{pqr}$	8.98 ± 0.07	17.73 ± 0.05	−0.62 ± 0.05	9.47 ± 0.08
C [4]	−0.49 ± 0.11	−0.32 ± 0.07	−0.86 ± 0.08	−0.71 ± 0.12
$\Delta \varepsilon$ [5]	−0.48 ± 0.08	−0.34 ± 0.04	−0.85 ± 0.06	−0.71 ± 0.10
	UO_2^{2+}			
	$\log \beta_{110}$ [1,3]	$\log \beta_{11-1}$ [1,3]	$\log \beta_{220}$ [1,3]	$\log \beta_{22-2}$ [1,3]
$\log \beta^0_{pqr}$	12.86 ± 0.03	7.24 ± 0.01	28.16 ± 0.06	17.40 ± 0.03
C [4]	−0.09 ± 0.03	0.02 ± 0.03	−0.02 ± 0.08	0.33 ± 0.03
$\Delta \varepsilon$ [5]	−0.09 ± 0.02	0.03 ± 0.04	−0.04 ± 0.04	0.32 ± 0.02
	$(CH_3)_2Sn^{2+}$ [6]			
	$\log \beta_{110}$ [1,3]	$\log \beta_{111}$ [1,3]	$\log \beta_{11-1}$ [1,3]	
$\log \beta^0_{pqr}$	16.37 ± 0.04	20.81 ± 0.06	8.50 ± 0.04	
C [4]	−1.79 ± 0.08	−1.95 ± 0.08	−1.30 ± 0.06	
$\Delta \varepsilon$ [5]	−1.75 ± 0.08	−1.91 ± 0.10	−1.26 ± 0.06	

[1] log β_{pqr} refers to equilibrium: p M^{m+} + q L^{z-} + r H^+ = $M_pL_qH_r^{(mp-zq+r)}$; [2] log β_{MLCl} refers to equilibrium: M^+ + L^- + Cl^- = $MLCl^-$; [3] ±95% confidence interval; [4] EDH equation (Equation (4)) in mol dm^{-3}; [5] SIT equations (Equations (4) and (7)) in mol kg^{-1}; [6] at T = 310.15 K.

The same table also reports the analogous $\Delta \varepsilon$ values (SIT) obtained from the fitting of constants after their conversion to the molal concentration scale [58–60]. These parameters could be used for the calculation of the complex formation constants of M^{n+}/Eph^- species at ionic strengths different from those experimentally investigated (from infinite dilution up to $I \sim 1.0$) on the molar and/or molal concentration scales. Some calculated values are reported in Tables S7–S9.

As reported in the experimental section, $\Delta \varepsilon$ values account for all the classical SIT coefficients (ε) of species involved in the considered equilibrium. The calculation of $\Delta \varepsilon$ instead of classical SIT coefficients is particularly indicated when one or more ε values are not available (so that the system of equations related to various equilibria results is undetermined, hampering the calculation of other single ε values), as it is preferable to resorting to assumptions/approximations that could lead to erroneous results (as could happen, for example, when the activity coefficients of neutral species are fixed as γ = 1). Nevertheless, when it is possible, the calculation of classical SIT coefficients is desired, as they are of more general utility. In this vein, the SIT coefficients of single UO_2^{2+}/Eph^- species were calculated in this work (Table 6), while this is not possible for CH_3Hg^+/Eph^- and $(CH_3)_2Sn^{2+}/Eph^-$ systems.

Table 6. Classical SIT interaction coefficients for UO_2^{2+}/Eph^- species at $T = 298.15$ K.

M^{m+}	X^{z-}	Neutral Species	ε_{MX}	k_m [5]
H^+	Cl^-	–	0.12 [1]	–
Na^+	Eph^-	–	−0.219 [2]	–
UO_2^{2+}	Cl^-	–	0.25 [3]	–
UO_2Eph^+	Cl^-	–	0.12 ± 0.01 [4]	–
–	–	UO_2EphOH	–	0.11 ± 0.02 [4]
$(UO_2)_2(Eph)_2^{2+}$	Cl^-	–	0.11 ± 0.02 [4]	–
–	–	$(UO_2)_2(Eph)_2(OH)_2$	–	−0.05 ± 0.01 [4]

[1] Reference [61]; [2] Reference [17]; [3] Reference [55]; [4] ±95% confidence interval; [5] Setschenow coefficient of neutral species [62,63].

Analogous considerations can be done when adopting the Pitzer approach. Instead of making unsuitable approximations and/or assumptions, the simplified Pitzer equation (Equation (20)) can be used instead of classical Pitzer formalism (Equations (10)–(18)). The simplified Pitzer coefficients for the dependence of the stability constants of all the epinephrine/cation species (including protonation constants) determined in this work are reported in Table 7.

Table 7. Simplified Pitzer coefficients for the dependence on ionic strength of M^{n+}/Eph^- species in $NaCl_{aq}$ at $T = 298.15$ K.

	H^+			
	$\log K_{011}$ [1,2]	$\log K_{012}$ [1,2]		
$\log K^0_{01r}$	10.41 ± 0.04	8.65 ± 0.02		
p_1	0.21 ± 0.03	0.93 ± 0.10		
p_3	0.11 ± 0.02	0.35 ± 0.11		
	CH_3Hg^+			
	$\log \beta_{110}$ [2,3]	$\log \beta_{111}$ [2,3]	$\log \beta_{11-1}$ [2,3]	$\log \beta_{MLCl}$ [2,4]
$\log \beta^0_{pqr}$	8.98 ± 0.06	17.74 ± 0.06	−0.62 ± 0.04	9.47 ± 0.09
p_1	0.17 ± 0.10	−0.22 ± 0.13	−0.60 ± 0.08	−0.25 ± 0.12
p_3	−1.31 ± 0.24	0.37 ± 0.18	−1.15 ± 0.26	−0.86 ± 0.32
	UO_2^{2+}			
	$\log \beta_{110}$ [2,3]	$\log \beta_{11-1}$ [2,3]	$\log \beta_{220}$ [2,3]	$\log \beta_{22-2}$ [2,3]
$\log \beta^0_{pqr}$	12.86 ± 0.04	7.24 ± 0.02	28.16 ± 0.04	17.40 ± 0.04
p_1	−0.02 ± 0.12	0.15 ± 0.10	0.58 ± 0.18	0.72 ± 0.12
p_3	1.52 ± 0.21	1.38 ± 0.30	0.70 ± 0.25	2.41 ± 0.31
	$(CH_3)_2Sn^{2+}$ [5]			
	$\log \beta_{110}$ [2,3]	$\log \beta_{111}$ [2,3]	$\log \beta_{11-1}$ [2,3]	
$\log \beta^0_{pqr}$	16.36 ± 0.05	20.80 ± 0.07	8.50 ± 0.06	
p_1	−1.64 ± 0.13	−1.78 ± 0.16	−1.20 ± 0.09	
p_3	0.64 ± 0.23	−0.36 ± 0.18	1.01 ± 0.15	

[1] $\log K_{01r}$ refers to equilibrium: $H^+ + H_{r-1}L^{(z-r-1)-} = H_rL^{(z-r)-}$; [2] ±95% confidence interval; [3] $\log \beta_{pqr}$ refers to equilibrium: $p M^{m+} + q L^{z-} + r H^+ = M_pL_qH_r^{(mp-zq+r)}$; [4] $\log \beta_{MLCl}$ refers to equilibrium: $M^+ + L^- + Cl^- = MLCl^-$; [5] at $T = 310.15$ K.

As noted, fits were performed, refining only p_1 and p_3 parameters and neglecting p_2. The rationale behind this choice was that p_2, dependent on I^2, accounts for the C^Φ and Ψ coefficients in classical Pitzer equations, which can usually be neglected at relatively low ionic strengths (usually at $I < 1$ mol kg^{-1}). Moreover, it is known that classical Pitzer coefficients are very highly correlated, so that their simultaneous refinement dramatically increases the risk of overparametrization [64]. That is why, when possible, and when no statistically significant improvements of fit quality can be obtained, it is preferable to reduce the number of Pitzer coefficients that are calculated, as was done in this work.

However, in addition to the simplified Pitzer approach, classical Pitzer coefficients were determined for the protonation constants of epinephrine (with a standard deviation on the whole fit of $\sigma = 0.083$) and for the UO$_2^{2+}$/Eph$^-$ species ($\sigma = 0.054$), analogously to what was done for the SIT model. These values are reported in Table 8.

Table 8. Classical Pitzer interaction coefficients for H$^+$/Eph$^-$ and UO$_2^{2+}$/Eph$^-$ species at $T = 298.15$ K.

M^{m+}	X^{z-}	Neutral Species	$\beta^{(0)}$	$\beta^{(1)}$	$C^{(\varphi)}$	k_m [4]
H^{+} [1]	Cl$^-$	–	0.1775 [2]	0.2945 [2]	0.00080 [2]	–
Na$^+$	Cl$^-$	–	0.0765 [2]	0.2664 [2]	0.00127 [2]	–
Na$^+$	Eph$^-$	–	−0.1252	0.6187	–	–
–	–	HEph	–	–	–	−0.108
H$_2$Eph$^+$	Cl$^-$	–	−0.0264	−0.0263	–	–
UO$_2^{2+}$	Cl$^-$	–	0.4274 [3]	1.644 [3]	−0.03686 [3]	–
UO$_2$Eph$^+$	Cl$^-$	–	0.3241	0.7930	–	–
–	–	UO$_2$EphOH	–	–	–	0.11
(UO$_2$)$_2$(Eph)$_2^{2+}$	Cl$^-$	–	0.0139	3.933	–	–
–	–	(UO$_2$)$_2$(Eph)$_2$(OH)$_2$	–	–	–	−0.05

[1] $\theta_{HNa} = 0.036$ and $\psi_{HNaCl} = -0.004$ in the calculations, from Reference [45]; [2] Reference [45]; [3] Reference [51]; [4] Setschenow coefficient of neutral species [62].

2.5. Sequestering Ability

For accurate comparisons between different metal/ligand systems in terms of sequestration, comparing the stability of some common species to the same stoichiometry is not always sufficient, because secondary interactions of both the metal and the ligand under consideration with other components in the systems can influence the effective strength of the interaction between them.

Other difficulties are observed when the sequestering ability has to be estimated at different pH values, ionic strengths, and temperatures. To facilitate this kind of evaluation, the use of the parameter pL$_{0.5}$ has been proposed. This represents the total concentration of ligands necessary to sequester 50% of a metal cation present in trace concentration (~10^{-10} mol dm^{-3}) in a given solution. This parameter is described through a sigmoidal-type Boltzmann equation:

$$x_M = \frac{1}{1 + 10^{(pL - pL_{0.5})}}, \quad (1)$$

where x_M is the mole fraction of metal complexed by the ligand, pL = -log c_L, and pL$_{0.5}$ = -log c_L when $x_M = 0.5$. The sequestering ability can be graphically represented by a dose–response curve characterized by asymptotes equal to 1 for pL$\to -\infty$ and 0 for pL $\to +\infty$, which are obtained by plotting the mole fraction of the metal complexed versus the pL values. The higher the value of pL$_{0.5}$, the greater the sequestering ability is. With this method of calculation (further details can be found in Reference [33]), pL$_{0.5}$ allows for an evaluation of the sequestering ability of a ligand in any condition, such as at different pHs, ionic strengths, ionic media and temperatures and/or in the presence of any interfering ligands and/or metal cations, as often occurs in real multicomponent systems. Moreover, it is independent of the analytical concentration of the metal ion (since it is considered to be a trace concentration).

The pL$_{0.5}$ values for the sequestration of epinephrine by the metal ions were investigated and calculated in various conditions, and they are reported in Table 9.

Table 9. Here, pL$_{0.5}$ values for the M^{n+}/Eph$^-$ systems calculated in different experimental conditions.

I/mol dm^{-3}	pH	pL$_{0.5}$
	UO$_2^{2+}$ [1]	
0.15	5.5	4.35
0.15	7.4	7.68
0.15	8.2	8.89
0.5	7.4	7.79
0.75	7.4	7.85
1	7.4	7.89
	CH$_3$Hg$^+$ [1]	
0.15	9.5	2.40
0.5	9.5	2.95
0.75	9.5	2.77
1	9.5	2.64
	(CH$_3$)$_2$Sn^{2+} [2]	
0.15	4.0	4.76
0.15	7.4	5.64
0.15	8.2	5.97
0.15	10.0	5.99
0.50	7.4	5.15
1.00	7.4	4.59

[1] at T = 298.15 K; [2] at T = 310.15 K.

The sequestering ability of epinephrine toward CH$_3$Hg$^+$ became significant above pH ~9.0–9.5, since at lower pH values this cation is almost entirely complexed by chloride ions (see Figure 1a,b), especially at high ionic strength. At the same pH value, the sequestering ability of Eph$^-$ toward UO$_2^{2+}$ was fairly constant, with a mean value of pL$_{0.5}$ = 7.80 ± 0.09 at pH = 7.4. For (CH$_3$)$_2$Sn^{2+} at T = 310.15 K, a variation of about one order of magnitude with ionic strength was observed at pH = 7.4 (see Figure 8).

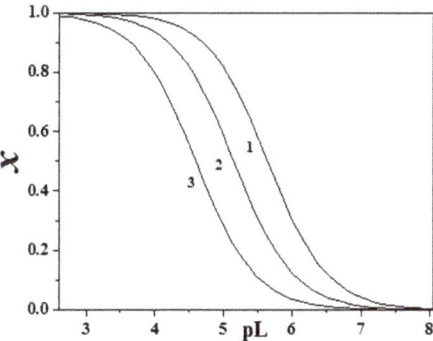

Figure 8. Sequestering ability of Eph$^-$ toward (CH$_3$)$_2$Sn^{2+} at T = 310.15 K, pH = 7.4 (1: I = 0.15 mol dm^{-3}, pL$_{0.5}$ = 5.64; 2: I = 0.50 mol dm^{-3}, pL$_{0.5}$ = 5.15; 3: I = 1.00 mol dm^{-3}, pL$_{0.5}$ = 4.59).

In the case of CH$_3$Hg$^+$, an initial increase of the pL$_{0.5}$ with the ionic strength was observed up to about I = 0.5 mol dm^{-3}, while it started to decrease above this value (see Figure 9). This was justified by the formation of a CH_3HgCl^0 species, which lowered the free cation concentration and consequently the extent of its interaction with epinephrine.

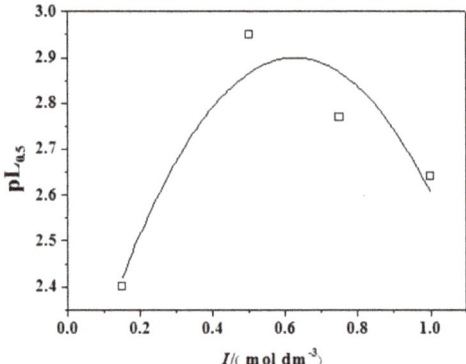

Figure 9. Trend of the $pL_{0.5}$ values for the CH_3Hg^+/Eph^- system at different ionic strengths and $T = 298.15$ K.

However, the effect of pH on $pL_{0.5}$ was more significant than that of ionic strength (see Figures S2 and S3 for $(CH_3)_2Sn^{2+}$ and UO_2^{2+}, respectively), with the sequestering ability generally increasing with pH due to the ligand deprotonation, though the greater cation hydrolysis competed with sequestration (epinephrine increased pH). In any case, in the analysis of $pL_{0.5}$ values calculated in various conditions, the following trend could be generally observed concerning the sequestering ability of Eph^- toward the investigated cations: $UO_2^{2+} >> (CH_3)_2Sn^{2+} >> CH_3Hg^+$.

2.6. Thermogravimetric Characterization

A series of UO_2^{2+}/Eph^--precipitated compounds was investigated by thermogravimetric analysis (TGA) to determine stoichiometry and thermal stability. This information can be useful in comparing the solution and solid state properties of characterized complexes.

The TGA profiles in an oxidant purging atmosphere (air flow) always showed a similar stability of the precipitated solids up to 275 °C, followed by two well-defined weight loss steps (see, as an example, Figure 10). The first one occurred in the temperature range 275–400 °C, and the second, final process occurred in the temperature range 400–580 °C. The percent weight loss from the TGA curves was calculated and related to the molecular weight of the ligand to propose the stoichiometry of the analyzed precipitates. These results allowed for a determination of the number of ligand molecules lost in the initial TGA step and the final decomposition (to give uranyl oxide).

The UO_2^{2+}/Eph^- ratios in the precipitated solids were very different and were systematically dependent on the solution conditions (i.e., ionic strength). However, the calculated stoichiometry of the analyzed precipitates highlighted an unusual coordination that is realistically not possible, since the experimental evidence showed that the dependence of the stoichiometric uranyl/ligand ratios on the ionic strength of the starting solution led to an UO_2^{2+}/Eph^- ratio up to 1:13. The calculations performed on the precipitate obtained at $I = 0.15$ mol dm^{-3} (pH of formation ~8.5) allowed us to calculate a metal-to-ligand molar ratio of 3:10, assuming the formation of U_3O_8 at the end of the thermal decomposition. An elaboration performed on the precipitate, obtained at $I = 0.75$ mol dm^{-3}, led to a metal-to-ligand molar ratio of 1:7.

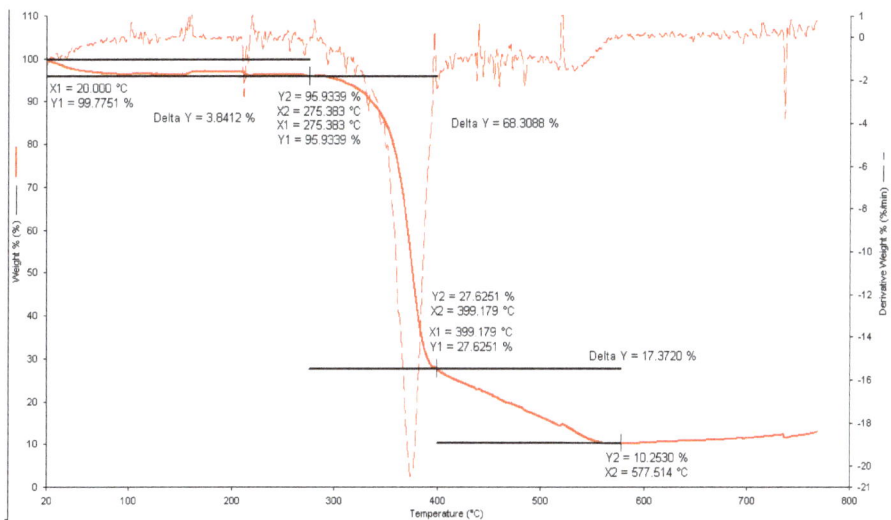

Figure 10. Thermogravimetric curve for the UO_2^{2+}/Eph^- precipitate obtained at $I = 0.15$ mol dm^{-3}. Component concentration in the solution: $C_{UO2^{2+}} = 2$ mmol dm^{-3} and $C_{Eph} = 4$ mmol dm^{-3}. Solid line: % weight loss versus $T/°C$; dashed line: derivative weight loss versus $T/°C$.

The experimental evidence led to the conclusion that all of these precipitates were the result of a coprecipitation process that was the consequence of the stability of aggregates in solution due to increasing solution interactions, which were favored by the increasing ionic strength. The experimental evidence also elicited that the formation and precipitation of solid state structures was relatively fast, and the precipitated solids were consequently influenced.

2.7. Literature Comparisons

To our knowledge, no thermodynamic studies on the interaction of epinephrine with the cations under investigation have ever been reported in literature. The only information for the UO_2^{2+}/Eph^- system has been with regard to spectral studies. Some papers have reported results on epinephrine interactions with different ions, but only at a single ionic strength and temperature. Some of them are shown in Table 10.

The main difficulty in a direct comparison to the results obtained here was due to the different approaches used for the determination of the acid–base properties of epinephrine. In some cases, it has been considered to be a triprotic ligand (L^{2-}) using the calculation of the third protonation constant (with a log K^H value of about 13–14), which is out of the pH range of physiological interest [13,53,54,56]. In other cases [17], only the protonation constants of one phenolic group and of the amine group of the alkyl chain have been considered. Other aspects that must be taken into account during comparisons are the different ionic media and ionic strengths used and the pH range of investigation, which can influence the obtained results. The literature has essentially been with regard to the interaction of epinephrine with divalent metal cations (Mn^{2+}, Co^{2+}, Ni^{2+}, Zn^{2+}, Cu^{2+}, Cd^{2+}, Pb^{2+}, Hg^{2+}), even if some data are also available for lanthanide complexes.

Table 10. Literature data for some M^{n+}/Eph^- systems.

M^{m+}	I^1	Medium	T/K	Species [2]					Ref.
				$\log \beta_{110}$	$\log \beta_{111}$	$\log \beta_{121}$	$\log \beta_{122}$	$\log \beta_{120}$	
Ni^{2+}	0.5	$NaNO_3$	293.15	–	17.43	22.9	32.0	12.5	[14]
	0.1	KCl	298.15	10.40	–	–	–	–	[65]
	0.2	KCl	298.15	9.43	18.87	24.7	34.5	14.2	[15] [3]
Cu^{2+}	0.5	$NaNO_3$	293.15	–	22.64	–	43.1	23.9	[14]
	0.1	KCl	298.15	14.95	–	–	–	27.45	[66]
	0.2	KCl	298.15	15.6	23.57	34.2	44.0	24.0	[15]
Zn^{2+}	0.5	$NaNO_3$	293.15	–	18.26	–	–	–	[14]
	0.1	KCl	298.15	10.92	–	–	–	20.12	[65]
	0.2	KCl	298.15	–	19.75	28.35	37.99	18.19	[15]
Cd^{2+}	0.5	$NaNO_3$	293.15	–	16.45	–	–	–	[14]
Pb^{2+}	0.5	$NaNO_3$	293.15	–	21.06	–	–	–	[14]
Mn^{2+}	0.1	KCl	298.15	8.80	–	–	–	15.1	[65]
	0.2	KCl	298.15	7.69	17.56	22.5	–	12.46	[15]
Co^{2+}	0.1	KCl	298.15	9.61	–	–	–	16.71	[65]
	0.2	KCl	298.15	9.23	18.60	25.25	35.07	15.15	[15]
La^{3+}	0.2	KCl	298.15	–	5.96	–	10.5	–	[67]
Y^{3+}	0.2	KCl	298.15	–	7.40	–	13.78	–	[54]
Pr^{3+}	0.15	NaCl	310.15	9.76	–	–	–	18.21	[68]
Hg^{2+}	0.1	$NaNO_3$	298.15	8.20	–	–	–	15.36	[65]

[1] in mol dm^{-3}; [2] $\log \beta_{pqr}$ refers to equilibrium: p M^{m+} + q L^{z-} + r H^+ = $M_pL_qH_r^{(mp-zq+r)}$; [3] for Ni^{2+}/Eph^- systems, the ML$_2$OH species was also proposed: $\log \beta = 6.74$.

In a comparison between the speciation models and the stability constants reported in Table 10, a fairly good agreement in terms of simplicity of the speciation schemes (characterized by simple mononuclear species) can be observed. The behavior of the UO_2^{2+}/Eph^- system has been different in terms of formation of binuclear species with stoichiometry: M_2L_2 and $M_2L_2(OH)_2$, as is usual for the chemistry of UO_2^{2+}. Similar considerations can be done comparing the stability constants of the most common MLH species.

Again, no data have been published for both the dependence of the stability constants on ionic strength and for the determination of the complex formation enthalpy changes. The only available data that are useful for comparison are with regard to the protonation enthalpy changes of dopamine [53,56]. Considering the similarity of its structure to epinephrine, it is possible to state that the results here obtained can be considered to be in good agreement.

Taking into account the order of magnitude of the stability of complexes formed by epinephrine with the cations here investigated and comparing it to information from the literature, it is possible to hypothesize that for our systems as well, the interaction should occur via the phenolic oxygen(s) of the two phenolic groups, excluding the amine group of the lateral chain [13,65–67,69–71]. There has been various evidence that has supported this assumption, as has been reported by Moustafa [71], who carried out FT-IR spectra on an Hg^{2+}/Eph^- complex. He observed that, in this complex, characteristic bands of epinephrine at 3331 cm^{-1} and 1340 cm^{-1}, which were ascribable to the stretching and bending of the catechol groups, disappeared in the spectrum of the binary metal complex due to the displacement of the hydrogens by the metal ion and consequent coordination through the oxygen of the phenolic groups. Moustafa also showed that in the FT-IR spectra of the binary Hg^{2+}/Eph^- complex, the presence of a characteristic band of adrenaline at 3448 cm^{-1} was due to an –OH of the side chain ethanolamine. This is a further indication that only two phenolic groups are involved in coordinating with metal ions. Besides, Jameson and Neille [65] have stated that Ni^{2+}/Eph^- complexes have anomalous behavior, explaining that there is chelation through the interaction of the phenolic and secondary amine groups, even if it occurs only at given metal-to-ligand molar ratios.

3. Materials and Methods

3.1. Chemicals

Epinephrine solutions were prepared by weighing the ligand without further purification. The purity was checked potentiometrically by alkalimetric titrations and was >99%. Sodium chloride aqueous solutions were prepared by weighing pure salt previously dried in an oven at $T = 383.15$ K for 2 h. Sodium hydroxide and hydrochloric acid solutions were prepared from concentrated ampoules and standardized against potassium hydrogen phthalate and sodium carbonate, respectively. Solutions of $(CH_3)_2Sn^{2+}$ and CH_3Hg^+ were prepared from the corresponding chlorides or nitrate salts and were used without further purification. For UO_2^{2+}, diacetate salt was used, and the purity was determined through the gravimetric determination of uranium after ignition to the oxide U_3O_8 [55]. All products were purchased from Sigma-Aldrich (Milan, Italy) (only dimethyltin(IV) was from Alfa-Aesar (Gandle, Germany)) and its various brands at their highest available purity. All solutions were prepared with analytical-grade water ($\rho = 18$ MΩ cm^{-1}) using grade A glassware and were preserved from atmospheric CO_2 by means of soda lime traps.

3.2. Apparatus and Procedure

3.2.1. Potentiometric Titrations

The interactions of epinephrine with the selected cations were studied potentiometrically by means of an apparatus consisting of an 809 model Metrohm Titrando system connected to a half-cell Ross Type glass electrode (model 8101 from Thermo-Orion (Waltham, MA, USA)) coupled with a standard Ag/AgCl reference electrode. The system, which was connected to a personal computer and controlled by a Metrohm TiAMO 2.2 computer program, allowed us to carry out automatic titrations through the addition of the desired amounts of titrant when the equilibrium state was reached and to record the e.m.f. (electromotive force) of the solution under investigation. The estimated accuracy was ±0.15 mV and ±0.003 mL for the e.m.f and titrant volume readings, respectively. The measurements were carried out under magnetic stirring in thermostat cells at $T = 298.15$ and 310.15 ± 0.1 K by means of water circulation in the outer chamber of the titration cell (from a thermocryostat (model D1-G Haake)). Purified $N_{2(g)}$ was bubbled into the solutions in order to exclude the presence of $CO_{2(g)}$ and $O_{2(g)}$. The titrant solutions consisted of different amounts of the desired cation, epinephrine, an excess of hydrochloric acid, and NaCl to obtain the desired ionic strength values. In order to investigate the possible formation of both mono- and polynuclear species, solutions were prepared in a wide range of cation-to-ligand molar ratios and were titrated with standard, carbonate-free NaOH up to alkaline pH values or until the formation of sparingly soluble species. As an example, Table 1 reports the experimental conditions employed in the investigations of the $(CH_3)_2Sn^{2+}/Eph^-$ system (component concentrations, ligand/cation molar ratios, titrant concentrations, pH ranges of investigation, mean number of experimental points collected for each titration, and number of measurements for each experimental condition). They are for $I = 0.15$ mol dm^{-3}, but similar conditions were also used at the other investigated ionic strengths, as well as for the $CH_3Hg^+/$ and UO_2^{2+}/Eph^- systems. For each experiment, independent titrations of strong acid (HCl) solutions with NaOH solutions were carried out under the same experimental conditions of the metal/ligand system, with the aim of determining the electrode potential (E^0) and the acidic junction potential ($E_j = j_a [H^+]$). In this way, the pH scale used was a free concentration scale, pH $\equiv -\log [H^+]$, where $[H^+]$ is the free proton concentration (not activity). The reliability of the calibration in the alkaline range was checked by calculating the ionic product of water (pK_w).

3.2.2. Spectrophotometric Titrations

The spectrophotometric measurements, carried out at $T = 310.15 \pm 0.1$ K, were performed by a Varian Cary 50 (Agilent Scientific Instruments (Santa Clara, CA, USA)) UV-VIS spectrophotometer equipped with an optic fiber probe with a fixed 1-cm path length. A wavelength range from λ = 200 to 450 nm was investigated. The spectrophotometer was connected to a Personal Computer, and Varian Cary WinUV (3.00 version) software was used for the data acquisition (absorbance (A) versus wavelength (λ/nm)). During these measurements, a 602 Biotrode combined metro-sensor glass electrode (from Metrohm (Herisau, Switzerland)) was inserted into the thermostat measurement cell (total volume of 25 or 50 mL). The electrode was connected to a 713-model Metrohm potentiometer, and the addition of titrant was carried out by a 665-model Metrohm automatic burette. This allowed us to record simultaneously for each addition of titrant: absorbance (A) versus wavelength (λ/nm) (from the spectrophotometric apparatus) and e.m.f. (mV) versus the volume of titrant (mL) (from the potentiometric apparatus). The solutions under investigation consisted of different amounts of dimethyltin(IV), epinephrine, and background salt to reach pre-established ionic strength values (see Table S5 for experimental conditions). The homogeneity of the solution during the titration was performed with a magnetic stirring bar, and before each experiment, $N_{2(g)}$ was bubbled in the solution for at least 5 min in order to exclude the presence of $CO_{2(g)}$ and $O_{2(g)}$.

3.2.3. Calorimetric Titrations

Calorimetric titrations were performed at T = 298.150 ± 0.001 K by a Calorimetry Sciences Corporation (CSC, Lindon, UT, USA) Model 4285 calorimeter equipped with a Mod. 7211 constant temperature bath, both for the determination of the protonation enthalpy changes of epinephrine and the corresponding values for complexation with UO_2^{2+}. In the first case, 25 or 50 mL of solution containing epinephrine in variable concentrations (from 4 to 5 mmol dm^{-3}), previously neutralized with NaOH and NaCl$_{(aq)}$ in order to obtain a pre-established ionic strength value (I = 0.5 mol dm^{-3}), were titrated with HCl (c_H = 0.5133 mol dm^{-3}), which was delivered by a 2.5-cm^3-capacity Hamilton syringe, model 1002TLL (Sigma Aldrich, Milan, Italy). The pH range investigated was from pH ~10.5 up to pH ~4.8 (see Table S10 for experimental conditions). For each experimental condition, measurements were repeated at least three times. For the enthalpy change values of the complexation of epinephrine with UO_2^{2+}, a different procedure was used. The titrand solutions consisted of epinephrine in variable concentrations (from 4 to 6 mmol dm^{-3}) previously neutralized with NaOH (for protonation measurements and NaCl$_{(aq)}$) in order to have a pre-established ionic strength value (I = 0.5 mol dm^{-3}). The titrant was the salt of the metal ion, in this case $UO_2(Ac)_2$ (dioxouranium diacetate salt). The enthalpy of dilution was measured before each experiment. The accuracy of the calorimetric apparatus was Q ± 0.008 J, and the accuracy of the titrant volume was ±0.001 cm^3. This was checked by titrating a THAM (tris-(hydroxymethyl)amino-methane) buffer with HCl. The enthalpy changes used in the calculations for the ionization of water at different ionic strengths were taken from De Stefano et al. [72].

3.2.4. Thermogravimetric Measurements

A thermoanalytic characterization was performed using Perkin-Elmer TGA7 (Waltham, MA, USA) equipment. The investigated samples (approximately 2–10 mg) were heated in platinum crucibles in the temperature range 20–850 °C under an atmosphere of air (gaseous mixture of nitrogen and oxygen with 80% and 20% v/v, respectively) at a flow rate of 100 mL min^{-1} and a scanning rate of 10 °C min^{-1}. These conditions allowed for the best resolution of the thermogravimetric curves.

3.3. Calculations

3.3.1. Computer Programs

BSTAC and STACO computer programs were used for the refinement of all the parameters (formation constants, analytical concentration of reagents, formal electrode potential) of the alkalimetric titrations. The least squares computer program LIANA, which refines the parameters of a generic $y = f(x)$ linear or nonlinear equation, was used to fit the Debye–Hückel, Pitzer, and SIT parameters and to calculate the formation constants at infinite dilution through an extrapolation of the experimental ones at different ionic strengths. Details for the BSTAC, STACO, and LIANA computer programs are reported in Reference [73]. UV spectra were analyzed by the Hypspec2014 computer program [74], which allows for the calculation of stability constants and the molar absorbance spectrum of each absorbing species using the experimental absorbance intensity, the analytical concentration of reagents, and the proposed chemical model as input. The advantage of this program is that for aqueous solutions containing few components, it allows for the simultaneous treatment of potentiometric and spectrophotometric data. The ES4ECI program [75] was used for the calculation of the formation percentages of the species present in solution at equilibrium and to draw both the speciation and the sequestration diagrams in different conditions. The ES5CM computer program [76] was used for the elaboration of calorimetric data from the isoperibol titration calorimetry. The input data for the elaboration of the calorimetric data contained the hydrolysis constants of uranyl and their corresponding enthalpy change values, the protonated species of epinephrine, the UO_2 acetate species, and the formation constants of the UO_2^{2+}/Eph^- complexes (determined by potentiometry). This software allows for the determination of enthalpy changes in solution from calorimetric data. The main characteristics of the program for the calculation of the ΔH for the equilibria involved in solution were (i) the calculation of the concentrations of all the species at each point of the calorimetric titration and (ii) the resolution of the linear equations system:

$$-Q_{corr,h} = \sum_i \Delta H_i^0 \delta n_{ih}, \tag{2}$$

where Q_{corr} is the heat of the reaction collected and corrected for the dilution and for the contribution to the heat of the reaction due to the species for which the ΔH^0 is known; δ_n is the concentration variation for the ith species; and h is the index for the point of titration.

Within the manuscript, if not differently specified, hydrolysis ($q = 0, r < 0$) constants of cations, protonation ($p = 0$) constants of the ligands (L^{z-}), and complex formation constants are given according to the overall equilibrium:

$$p\ M^{m+} + q\ L^{z-} + r\ H^+ = M_pL_qH_r^{(mp-zq+r)} \qquad \log \beta_{pqr}. \tag{3}$$

Ligand protonation constants may also be given according to the stepwise equilibrium:

$$H^+ + LH_{r-1}^{(z-r-1)-} = LH_r^{(z-r)-} \qquad \log K_{01r}. \tag{4}$$

Protonation, hydrolysis and complex formation constants, concentrations, and ionic strengths are expressed in the molar (c, mol dm^{-3}) or molal (m, mol kg^{-1}(H$_2$O)) concentration scales. Molar to molal conversions were performed using appropriate procedures that have already been reported in previous papers [58–60]. In the manuscript, if not differently reported, the errors associated with formation constants, enthalpy and entropy change values, and the parameters for dependence on ionic strength are expressed as a 95% confidence interval (C.I.).

3.3.2. Dependence on Ionic Strength

The dependence of the formation constants on ionic strength was studied by means of different approaches, namely the extended Debye–Hückel (EDH), specific ion interaction theory (SIT), and Pitzer approaches (general information can be found, e.g., in References [40–46], while for some examples of their applications one can refer to [64,77–80]).

Extended Debye–Hückel (EDH) and Specific Ion Interaction Theory (SIT) Approaches

The extended Debye–Hückel-type equation used was

$$\log \beta_{pqr} = \log \beta_{pqr}^0 - A\ z^* \frac{\sqrt{I}}{1 + 1.5\ \sqrt{I}} + C\ I, \tag{5}$$

where β_{pqr} and β^0_{pqr} refer to the formation constant of the $M_pL_qH_r$ species at a given ionic strength and at infinite dilution, respectively;

$$A = 0.51 + \frac{0.856 \cdot (T - 298.15) + 0.00385 \cdot (T - 298.15)^2}{1000}; \tag{6}$$

$$z^* = \sum z^2_{react} - \sum z^2_{prod}; \tag{7}$$

and C is an empirical parameter that accounts for the dependence of the formation constants on ionic strength in the molar concentration scale [81]. When stability constants and ionic strengths are expressed in the molal concentration scale, Equation (4) becomes the classical and widely used SIT (specific ion interaction theory) equation, in which C is replaced by $\Delta\varepsilon$, where

$$\Delta\varepsilon = \sum \varepsilon_{react} - \sum \varepsilon_{prod} \tag{8}$$

and ε is the SIT coefficient for the interaction of all ionic species involved in the considered equilibrium with all the ions (of opposite sign) of the ionic medium. In all equilibria involving uncharged species, their activity coefficients must also be taken into account by the Setschenow equation [62,82],

$$\log \gamma = k_{c,m} I, \tag{9}$$

in which k_c and k_m are the Setschenow coefficients of the neutral species in a given medium in the molar and molal concentration scales, respectively.

Analogously, for all equilibria involving water (e.g., in hydrolysis reactions), its activity must be considered in calculations. In this manuscript, the simple relationship

$$a_w = -0.015 \, I \tag{10}$$

was used for these purposes (valid in NaCl$_{(aq)}$ at T = 298.15 K) [83].

Pitzer Approach

Together with SIT, the Pitzer approach is among the most widely used approaches to model the dependence of activity coefficients (and stability constants) on medium and ionic strength. For a cation "M^{z+}" or an anion "X^{z-}" in ionic media containing other cations "c" and anions "a", this is

$$\ln \gamma_M = z^2_+ f^\gamma + 2 \sum_a m_a(B_{Ma} + E\, C_{Ma}) + \sum_a \sum_c m_c m_a(z^2_+ B'_{ca} + z_+ C_{ca}) + \\ \sum_c m_c(2\Theta_{Mc} + \sum_a m_a \Psi_{Mca}) + \sum_a \sum_{a'} m_a m_{a'} \Psi_{Maa'}, \tag{11}$$

$$\ln \gamma_X = z^2_- f^\gamma + 2 \sum_c m_c(B_{Xc} + E\, C_{Xc}) + \sum_a \sum_c m_c m_a(z^2_- B'_{ca} + z_- C_{ca}) + \\ \sum_a m_a(2\Theta_{Xa} + \sum_c m_c \Psi_{Xac}) + \sum_c \sum_{c'} m_c m_{ac'} \Psi_{Xcc'} \tag{12}$$

with

$$E = 1/2 \sum_i m_i |z_i|, \tag{13}$$

$$f^\gamma = -A_\Phi \left[\frac{\sqrt{I}}{1 + 1.2\sqrt{I}} + \frac{2}{1.2} \ln(1 + 1.2\sqrt{I})\right], \tag{14}$$

$$B_{MX} = \beta^{(0)}_{MX} + \beta^{(1)}_{MX} f(\alpha_1 \sqrt{I}) + \beta^{(2)}_{MX} f(\alpha_2 \sqrt{I}), \tag{15}$$

$$B'_{MX} = \frac{\beta^{(1)}_{MX} f'(\alpha_1 \sqrt{I}) + \beta^{(2)}_{MX} f'(\alpha_2 \sqrt{I})}{I}, \quad (16)$$

$$C_{MX} = \frac{C^\Phi_{MX}}{2\sqrt{|z_M z_X|}}, \quad (17)$$

$$f(x) = \frac{2[1-(1+x)\exp(-x)]}{x^2}, \quad (18)$$

$$f'(x) = \frac{-2\left[1-\left(1+x+\frac{x^2}{2}\right)\exp(-x)\right]}{x^2}, \quad (19)$$

where A_Φ = 0.392 and 0.399 at T = 298.15 and 310.15 K, respectively; α_1 and α_2 can vary, though very often they are α_1 = 2.0 and α_2 = 0.0 ((kg mol^{-1})$^{1/2}$) for all electrolytes except 2:2 (in which α_1 = 1.4 and α_2 = 12); and $\beta^{(0)}$, $\beta^{(1)}$, $\beta^{(2)}$, C^Φ, Θ, and Ψ are the so-called Pitzer interaction coefficients. Finally, in the Pitzer model, the activity coefficient of a neutral species in a given medium is accounted for by

$$\log \gamma = 2 \lambda I. \quad (20)$$

In order to bypass difficulties related to a quite complex mathematical formulation (or when some interaction coefficients are not available), some simplified forms of Pitzer equations can be used to model the dependence of stability constants on ionic strength:

$$\log \beta_{pqr} = \log \beta^0_{pqr} + \frac{z^* f^\gamma + 2p_1 I + p_2 I^2 + p_3\left[2I\,f(2\sqrt{I})\right] + \frac{1}{2}z^*\left[2I\,f'(2\sqrt{I})\right]\beta^{(1)}_{MX}}{\ln 10}, \quad (21)$$

where p_1 and p_2 represent, for all species involved in the formation equilibrium, the summation sign of all the classical Pitzer coefficients dependent on I (i.e., $\beta^{(0)}$, Θ, λ) and I^2 (i.e., C^Φ, Ψ), respectively, while p_3 is given by all $\beta^{(1)}$ values.

4. Conclusions

The interaction of epinephrine with CH_3Hg^+, $(CH_3)_2Sn^{2+}$, and UO_2^{2+} was investigated in different experimental conditions in $NaCl_{aq}$ solutions, and the main results can be summarized as follows:

i. The speciation models were characterized by simple mononuclear species, except for UO_2^{2+}, where we observed the formation of the binuclear species M_2L_2 and $M_2L_2(OH)_2$, which have already been obtained in several other UO_2^{2+}/oxygen donor ligand systems;

ii. The investigations, carried out in $NaCl_{aq}$, allowed us to obtain the ternary $(CH_3Hg)EphCl^0$ species for the CH_3Hg^+/Eph^- system;

iii. The CH_3Hg^+/Eph^- species had the lowest stability compared to the $(CH_3)_2Sn^{2+}/Eph^-$ and UO_2^{2+}/Eph^- systems;

iv. For the $(CH_3)_2Sn^{2+}/Eph^-$ system, complexation started at acidic pH values (about 4);

v. The stability and the formation percentage of these species were higher than those of the CH_3Hg^+/Eph^- system;

vi. The speciation model was formed by simple mononuclear species (MLH, ML, and MLOH), as was confirmed by UV spectrophotometry;

vii. Despite a fairly high stability of the complexes, the hydrolytic species of dimethyltin(IV) played a fundamental role in the speciation of the system;

viii. For the UO_2^{2+}/Eph^- system, the formation of binuclear complexes was observed together with the mononuclear ones;

ix. Complexation by epinephrine strongly reduced UO_2^{2+} hydrolysis along the entire investigated pH range;

x. By means of isoperibol calorimetry, enthalpy and entropy changes for both the protonation of epinephrine and its complexes with UO_2^{2+} were determined;

xi. The obtained results highlighted that the process of formation of the UO_2^{2+}/Eph^- species was exothermic in nature and that the entropic contribution was the driving force of the reactions;

xii. The dependence of the stability constants on ionic strength was investigated using EDH, SIT, and Pitzer models;

xiii. The effective sequestering ability of adrenaline toward the investigated cations was quantified by means of the $pL_{0.5}$ parameter;

xiv. Ionic strength had a lower effect on the sequestering ability than did pH;

xv. For the CH_3Hg^+/Eph^- system, $pL_{0.5}$ increased up to $I = 0.5$ mol dm^{-3}, and then it started to decrease from this value up to $I = 1.0$ mol dm^{-3} (as a result of chloride interactions with methylmercury).

Supplementary Materials: The following are available online at http://www.mdpi.com/1420-3049/25/3/511/s1, Table S1: Hydrolysis constants of $(CH_3)_2Sn^{2+}$ in $NaCl_{aq}$ at different ionic strengths and $T = 310.15$ K; Table S2. Hydrolysis constants of UO_2^{2+} in $NaCl_{aq}$ at different ionic strengths and $T = 298.15$ K; Table S3: Hydrolysis constants and chloride complex ^{1} of CH_3Hg^+ in $NaCl_{aq}$ at different ionic strengths and $T = 298.15$ K; Table S4: Protonation constants of epinephrine at infinite dilution and parameters for their dependence on ionic strength in $NaCl_{aq}$ using EDH and SIT models at $T = 298.15$ and 310.15 K; Table S5: Example of experimental conditions adopted for the $(CH_3)_2Sn^{2+}/Eph^-$ system in $NaCl_{aq}$ at $I = 0.15$ mol dm^{-3} and at $T = 310.15$ K; Table S6: Stability constants of UO_2^{2+}/Ac^- species in $NaCl_{aq}$ at different ionic strengths and $T = 298.15$ K; Table S7: Stability constants of CH_3Hg^+/Eph^- complexes in $NaCl_{aq}$ at different ionic strengths and $T = 298.15$ K, calculated using the EDH and SIT models; Table S8: Stability constants of $(CH_3)_2Sn^{2+}/Eph^-$ complexes in $NaCl_{aq}$ at different ionic strengths and $T = 310.15$ K, calculated using the EDH and SIT models; Table S9: Stability constants of UO_2^{2+}/Eph^- complexes in $NaCl_{aq}$ at different ionic strengths and $T = 298.15$ K, calculated using the EDH and SIT models; Table S10: Example of experimental conditions adopted for calorimetric titrations in $NaCl_{aq}$ at $I = 0.50$ mol dm^{-3} and at $T = 298.15$ K; Figure S1: Molar absorptivity coefficients of adrenaline versus λ/nm ($C_L = 0.09$ mmol L^{-1}) in $NaCl_{aq}$ at $I = 0.15$ mol dm^{-3} and $T = 310.15$ K; Figure S2: Sequestering ability of Eph^- toward $(CH_3)_2Sn^{2+}$ at $T = 310.15$ K and $I = 0.15$ mol dm^{-3}; Figure S3: Sequestering ability of Eph^- toward UO_2^{2+} at $I = 0.15$ mol dm^{-3} and at different pH values.

Author Contributions: Conceptualization, F.C., A.I., and D.M.; methodology, F.C., C.D.S., and G.L.; software, S.S. and A.P.; validation, F.C., D.M., A.I., and A.P.; formal analysis, F.C., A.I., and S.M.; investigation, F.C. and A.I.; data curation, F.C., A.I., D.M., and A.P.; writing—original draft preparation, F.C. and D.M.; writing—review and editing, F.C., G.L., and D.M.; supervision, C.D.S. and S.S.; project administration, F.C., C.D.S., and S.S.; funding acquisition, C.D.S. and S.S. All authors have read and agreed to the published version of the manuscript.

Funding: We thank MIUR (Ministero dell'Istruzione, dell'Università e della Ricerca) for financial support (cofounded PRIN project with Prot. 2015MP34H3).

Conflicts of Interest: The authors declare no conflicts of interest.

References

1. Szulczewski, D.H.; Hong, W.H. Epinephrine. In *Analytical Profiles of Drug Substances*; Academic Press: Cambridge, MA, USA, 1978; pp. 193–229.
2. Schweigert, N.; Zehnder, A.J.; Eggen, R.I. Chemical properties of catechols and their molecular modes of toxic action in cells, from microorganisms to mammals. *Environ. Microbiol.* **2001**, *3*, 81–91. [CrossRef]
3. Cahill, L.; Alkire, M.T. Epinephrine enhancement of human memory consolidation: Interaction with arousal at encoding. *Neurobiol. Learn. Mem.* **2003**, *79*, 194–198. [CrossRef]
4. Flint, R.W., Jr.; Bunsey, M.D.; Riccio, D.C. Epinephrine-induced enhancement of memory retrieval for inhibitory avoidance conditioning in preweanling Sprague-Dawley rats. *Dev. Psychobiol.* **2007**, *49*, 303–311. [CrossRef]
5. Jurado-Berbel, P.; Costa-Miserachs, D.; Torras-Garcia, M.; Coll-Andreu, M.; Portell-Cortes, I. Standard object recognition memory and "what" and "where" components: Improvement by post-training epinephrine in highly habituated rats. *Behav. Brain Res.* **2010**, *207*, 44–50. [CrossRef] [PubMed]

6. Piperea-Sianu, A.; Sirbu, I.; Mati, E.; Piperea-Sianu, D.; Mircioiu, C. Study of Synergic Effect between Some Metal Ions and Adrenaline on Human Blood Platelets Aggregation. *Farmacia* **2015**, *63*, 828–834.
7. Campuzano, H.C.; Wilkerson, J.E.; Horvath, S.M. Fluorometric analysis of epinephrine and norepinephrine. *Anal. Biochem.* **1975**, *64*, 578–587. [CrossRef]
8. Grunert, R.; Wollmann, H. The effect of ultraviolet and visible light on drugs of the phenylalkylamine series with a view toward their stability in plastic containers. *Pharmazie* **1982**, *37*, 798–799. [PubMed]
9. Bonhomme, L.; Benhamou, D.; Comoy, E.; Preaux, N. Stability of epinephrine in alkalinized solutions. *Ann. Emerg. Med.* **1990**, *19*, 1242–1244. [CrossRef]
10. Grant, T.A.; Carroll, R.G.; Church, W.H.; Henry, A.; Prasad, N.H.; Abdel-Rahman, A.A.; Allison, E.J., Jr. Environmental temperature variations cause degradations in epinephrine concentration and biological activity. *Am. J. Emerg. Med.* **1994**, *12*, 319–322. [CrossRef]
11. Nagy, P.I.; Takacs-Novak, K. Tautomeric and conformational equilibria of biologically important (hydroxyphenyl)alkylamines in the gas phase and in aqueous solution. *Phys. Chem. Chem. Phys.* **2004**, *6*, 2838–2848. [CrossRef]
12. Adeniyi, W.K.; Wright, A.R. Novel fluorimetric assay of trace analysis of epinephrine in human serum. *Spectrochim. Acta A Mol. Biomol. Spectrosc.* **2009**, *74*, 1001–1004. [CrossRef] [PubMed]
13. Antikainen, P.J.; Witikainen, U. A comparative study on the ionization of catechol amines in aqueous solutions. *Acta Chem. Scand.* **1973**, *27*, 2075–2082. [CrossRef] [PubMed]
14. Grgas-Kužnar, B.; Simeon, V.; Weber, O.A. Complexes of adrenaline and related compounds with Ni^{2+}, Cu^{2+}, Zn^{2+}, Cd^{2+} and Pb^{2+}. *J. Inorg. Nucl. Chem.* **1974**, *36*, 2151–2154. [CrossRef]
15. Gergely, A.; Kiss, T.; Deák, G.; Sóvágó, I. Complexes of 3,4-dihydroxyphenyl derivatives IV. Equilibrium studies on some transition metal complexes formed with adrenaline and noradrenaline. *Inorg. Chim. Acta* **1981**, *56*, 35–40. [CrossRef]
16. Ibrahim, O.B.; Mohamed, M.A.; Refat, M.S. Study the chemical composition and biological outcomes resulting from the interaction of the hormone adrenaline with heavy elements: Infrared, Raman, electronic, 1H NMR, XRD and SEM studies. *J. Mol. Struct.* **2014**, *1056*, 13–24. [CrossRef]
17. Bretti, C.; Cigala, R.M.; Crea, F.; De Stefano, C.; Vianelli, G. Solubility and modeling acid-base properties of adrenaline in NaCl aqueous solutions at different ionic strengths and temperatures. *Eur. J. Pharm. Sci.* **2015**, *78*, 37–46. [CrossRef]
18. Choppin, G.R.; Allard, B. Complexes of actinides with naturally occurring organic compounds. In *Handbook on the Physics and Chemistry of Actinides*; Freeman, A.J., Keller, C., Eds.; Elsevier Science: Amsterdam, The Netherlands, 1985; p. 407.
19. Rashan, L.J.; AlAllaf, T.A.K. New dimethyltin (IV) compounds and their complexes with nitrogen containing ligands of antitumour activity. *Eur. J. Cancer* **1997**, *33*, 817. [CrossRef]
20. Carrier, G.; Bouchard, M.; Brunet, R.C.; Caza, M. A toxicokinetic model for predicting the tissue distribution and elimination of organic and inorganic mercury following exposure to methyl mercury in animals and humans. II. Application and validation of the model in humans. *Toxicol. Appl. Pharm.* **2001**, *171*, 50–60. [CrossRef]
21. Ullrich, S.M.; Tanton, T.W.; Abdrashitova, S.A. Mercury in the Aquatic Environment: A Review of Factors Affecting Methylation. *Crit. Rev. Environ. Sci. Technol.* **2001**, *31*, 241–293. [CrossRef]
22. Moulin, V.; Moulin, C. Radionuclide speciation in the environment: A review. *Radiochim. Acta* **2001**, *89*, 773–778. [CrossRef]
23. Guillaumont, R.; Fanghänel, T.; Fuger, J.; Grenthe, I.; Neck, V.; Palmer, D.A.; Rand, M.H. *Update on the Chemical Thermodynamics of Uranium, Neptunium, Plutonium, Americium and Technetium*; Elsevier: Amsterdam, The Netherlands, 2003.
24. Salbu, B.; Lind, O.C.; Skipperud, L. Radionuclide speciation and its relevance in environmental impact assessments. *J. Environ. Radioact.* **2004**, *74*, 233–242. [CrossRef] [PubMed]
25. Crea, F.; Foti, C.; Sammartano, S. Sequestering ability of polycarboxylic ligands towards dioxouranium(VI). *Talanta* **2008**, *75*, 775–785. [CrossRef]
26. Cigala, R.M.; De Stefano, C.; Giacalone, A.; Gianguzza, A.; Sammartano, S. Hydrolysis of Monomethyl-, Dimethyl-, and Trimethyltin(IV) Cations in Fairly Concentrated Aqueous Solutions at $I = 1 \text{ mol·L}^{-1}(NaNO_3)$ and $T = 298.15$ K. Evidence for the Predominance of Polynuclear Species. *J. Chem. Eng. Data* **2011**, *56*, 1108–1115. [CrossRef]

27. Berto, S.; Crea, F.; Daniele, P.G.; Gianguzza, A.; Pettignano, A.; Sammartano, S. Advances in investigation of dioxouranium(VI) complexes of interest for natural fluids. *Coord. Chem. Rev.* **2012**, *256*, 63–81. [CrossRef]
28. Cataldo, S.; De Stefano, C.; Gianguzza, A.; Pettignano, A. Sequestration of $(CH_3)Hg^+$ by amino-polycarboxylic chelating agents. *J. Mol. Liq.* **2012**, *172*, 46–52. [CrossRef]
29. Cataldo, S.; Gianguzza, A.; Pettignano, A.; Piazzese, D.; Sammartano, S. Complex Formation of Copper(II) and Cadmium(II) with Pectin and Polygalacturonic Acid in Aqueous Solution. An ISE-H^+ and ISE-Me^{2+} Electrochemical Study. *Int. J. Electrochem. Sci.* **2012**, *7*, 6722–6737.
30. Cataldo, S.; De Stefano, C.; Gianguzza, A.; Pettignano, A.; Sammartano, S. Sequestration of alkyltin(IV) cations by complexation with amino-polycarboxylic chelating agents. *J. Mol. Liq.* **2013**, *187*, 74–82. [CrossRef]
31. Cataldo, S.; Gianguzza, A.; Pettignano, A.; Villaescusa, I. Mercury(II) removal from aqueous solution by sorption onto alginate, pectate and polygalacturonate calcium gel beads. A kinetic and speciation based equilibrium study. *React. Funct. Polym.* **2013**, *73*, 207–217. [CrossRef]
32. Lavoie, R.A.; Jardine, T.D.; Chumchal, M.M.; Kidd, K.A.; Campbell, L.M. Biomagnification of mercury in aquatic food webs: A worldwide meta-analysis. *Environ. Sci. Technol.* **2013**, *47*, 13385–13394. [CrossRef]
33. Crea, F.; De Stefano, C.; Foti, C.; Milea, D.; Sammartano, S. Chelating agents for the sequestration of mercury(II) and monomethyl mercury(II). *Curr. Med. Chem.* **2014**, *21*, 3819–3836. [CrossRef]
34. Piazzese, D.; Cataldo, S.; Muratore, N. Voltammetric Investigation on Uranyl Sorption by Alginate Based Material. Influence of Hydrolysis and pH Dependence. *Int. J. Electrochem. Sci.* **2015**, *10*, 7423–7439.
35. Crea, F.; Milea, D.; Sammartano, S. Enhancement of hydrolysis through the formation of mixed hetero-metal species: Dioxouranium(VI)-cadmium(II) mixtures. *Ann. Chim. (Rome)* **2005**, *95*, 767–778. [CrossRef] [PubMed]
36. Crea, F.; Milea, D.; Sammartano, S. Enhancement of hydrolysis through the formation of mixed hetero-metal species. *Talanta* **2005**, *65*, 229–238. [CrossRef] [PubMed]
37. Crea, P.; De Stefano, C.; Milea, D.; Sammartano, S. Formation and stability of mixed Mg^{2+}/Ca^{2+}/phytate species in seawater media. Consequences on ligand speciation. *Mar. Chem.* **2008**, *112*, 142–148. [CrossRef]
38. De Stefano, C.; Lando, G.; Milea, D.; Pettignano, A.; Sammartano, S. Formation and Stability of Cadmium(II)/Phytate Complexes by Different Electrochemical Techniques. Critical Analysis of Results. *J. Solut. Chem.* **2010**, *39*, 179–195. [CrossRef]
39. Crea, F.; De Stefano, C.; Milea, D.; Sammartano, S. Phytate–molybdate(VI) interactions in NaCl(aq) at different ionic strengths: Unusual behaviour of the protonated species. *New J. Chem.* **2018**, *42*, 7671–7679. [CrossRef]
40. Brønsted, J.N. Studies on solubility. IV. The principle of the specific interaction of ions. *J. Am. Chem. Soc.* **1922**, *44*, 877–898. [CrossRef]
41. Guggenheim, E.A.; Turgeon, J.C. Specific interaction of ions. *Trans. Faraday Soc.* **1955**, *51*, 747–761. [CrossRef]
42. Pitzer, K.S. Thermodynamics of Electrolytes. I. Theoretical Basis and General Equations. *J. Phys. Chem.* **1973**, *77*, 268–277. [CrossRef]
43. Pitzer, K.S.; Mayorga, G. Thermodynamics of Electrolytes. II. Activity and Osmotic Coefficients for Strong Electrolytes with on or Both Ions Univalent. *J. Phys. Chem.* **1973**, *77*, 2300–2308. [CrossRef]
44. Ciavatta, L. The Specific Interaction Theory in Evaluating Ionic Equilibria. *Ann. Chim. (Rome)* **1980**, *70*, 551–567.
45. Pitzer, K.S. *Activity Coefficients in Electrolyte Solutions*, 2nd ed.; CRC Press: Boca Raton, FL, USA, 1991.
46. Grenthe, I.; Puigdomenech, I. *Modelling in Aquatic Chemistry*; OECD: Paris, France, 1997.
47. Cigala, R.M.; Crea, F.; Lando, G.; Milea, D.; Sammartano, S. Solubility and acid-base properties of concentrated phytate in self-medium and in NaCl$_{(aq)}$ at T = 298.15 K. *J. Chem.* **2010**, *42*, 1393–1399.
48. Crea, F.; Cucinotta, D.; De Stefano, C.; Milea, D.; Sammartano, S.; Vianelli, G. Modeling solubility, acid-base properties and activity coefficients of amoxicillin, ampicillin and (+)6-aminopenicillanic acid, in NaCl$_{(aq)}$ at different ionic strengths and temperatures. *Eur. J. Pharm. Sci.* **2012**, *47*, 661–677. [CrossRef] [PubMed]
49. De Robertis, A.; Foti, C.; Patanè, G.; Sammartano, S. Hydrolysis of $(CH_3)Hg^+$ in Different Ionic Media: Salt Effects and Complex Formation. *J. Chem. Eng. Data* **1998**, *43*, 957–960. [CrossRef]
50. De Stefano, C.; Foti, C.; Gianguzza, A.; Martino, M.; Pellerito, L.; Sammartano, S. Hydrolysis of $(CH_3)_2Sn^{2+}$ in Different Ionic Media: Salt Effects and Complex Formation. *J. Chem. Eng. Data* **1996**, *41*, 511–515. [CrossRef]
51. Gianguzza, A.; Milea, D.; Millero, F.J.; Sammartano, S. Hydrolysis and chemical speciation of dioxouranium(VI) in aqueous media simulating the major ion composition of seawater. *Mar. Chem.* **2004**, *85*, 103–124. [CrossRef]

52. Hoellein, L.; Holzgrabe, U. Ficts and facts of epinephrine and norepinephrine stability in injectable solutions. *Int. J. Pharm.* **2012**, *434*, 468–480. [CrossRef]
53. Pettit, L.D.; Powell, K.J. IUPAC Stability Constants Database. Available online: http://publications.iupac.org/projects/posters01/pettit01.pdf (accessed on 22 January 2020).
54. Aydin, R. Study on the interaction of Yttrium(III) with adrenaline, noradrenaline, and dopamine. *J. Chem. Eng. Data* **2007**, *52*, 2400–2404. [CrossRef]
55. Crea, F.; De Robertis, A.; Sammartano, S. Dioxouranium carboxylate complexes. Formation and stability of acetate species at different ionic strengths in NaCl$_{aq}$. *Ann. Chim. (Rome)* **2003**, *93*, 1027–1035.
56. Smith, R.M.; Martell, A.E.; Chen, Y. Critical-Evaluation of Stability-Constants for Nucleotide Complexes with Protons and Metal-Ions and the Accompanying Enthalpy Changes. *Pure Appl. Chem.* **1991**, *63*, 1015–1080. [CrossRef]
57. Crea, F.; De Stefano, C.; Pettignano, A.; Sammartano, S. Hydrolysis of Dioxouranium(VI): A Calorimetric Study in NaCl(aq) and NaClO4(aq), at 25 °C. *Acta* **2004**, *414*, 185–189.
58. Crea, F.; Stefano, C.D.; Gianguzza, A.; Piazzese, D.; Sammartano, S. Protonation of carbonate in aqueous tetraalkylammonium salts at 25 degrees C. *Talanta* **2006**, *68*, 1102–1112. [CrossRef] [PubMed]
59. Bretti, C.; Cigala, R.M.; Crea, F.; Lando, G.; Sammartano, S. Thermodynamics of proton binding and weak (Cl−, Na+ and K+) species formation, and activity coefficients of 1, 2-dimethyl-3-hydroxypyridin-4-one (deferiprone). *J. Chem. Thermodyn.* **2014**, *77*, 98–106. [CrossRef]
60. Cardiano, P.; Cigala, R.M.; Crea, F.; De Stefano, C.; Milea, D.; Sammartano, S. Characterization of the thermodynamic properties of some benzenepolycarboxylic acids: Acid-base properties, weak complexes, total and neutral species solubility, solubility products in NaCl$_{aq}$, (CH3)4NCl$_{aq}$ and Synthetic Sea Water (SSW). *Fluid Phase Equilibria* **2019**, *480*, 41–52. [CrossRef]
61. Bretti, C.; Foti, C.; Porcino, N.; Sammartano, S. SIT parameters for 1:1 electrolytes and correlation with Pitzer coefficients. *J. Solut. Chem.* **2006**, *35*, 1401–1415. [CrossRef]
62. Setschenow, J.Z. Uber Die Konstitution Der Salzlosungenauf Grund Ihres Verhaltens Zu Kohlensaure. *Z. Phys. Chem.* **1889**, *4*, 117–125. [CrossRef]
63. Battaglia, G.; Cigala, R.M.; Crea, F.; Sammartano, S. Solubility and Acid-Base Properties of Ethylenediaminetetraacetic Acid in Aqueous NaCl Solution at 0 <I <6 mol kg$^{−1}$ and T = 298.15 K. *J. Chem. Eng. Data* **2008**, *53*, 363–367.
64. Crea, F.; De Stefano, C.; Irto, A.; Milea, D.; Pettignano, A.; Sammartano, S. Modeling the Acid-Base Properties of Molybdate(VI) in Different Ionic Media, Ionic Strengths and Temperatures, by EDH, SIT and Pitzer Equations. *J. Mol. Liq.* **2017**, *229*, 15–26. [CrossRef]
65. Jameson, R.F.; Neillie, W.F.S. Complexes formed by adrenaline and related compounds with transition-metal ions—III. *J. Inorg. Nucl. Chem.* **1966**, *28*, 2667–2675. [CrossRef]
66. Jameson, R.F.; Neillie, W.F.S. Complexes formed by adrenaline and related compounds with transition-metal ions—II complexes with copper(II). *J. Inorg. Nucl. Chem.* **1965**, *27*, 2623–2634. [CrossRef]
67. Aydin, R.; Inci, D. Potentiometric and Spectrophotometric Studies of the Complexation of Lanthanum(III) with Adrenaline, Noradrenaline, and Dopamine. *J. Chem. Eng. Data* **2012**, *57*, 967–973. [CrossRef]
68. Gao, F.; Han, J.F.; Wu, Z.J.; Wang, Y.; Yang, K.Y.; Niu, C.J.; Ni, J.Z. Studies on the coordination of Pr(III) with adrenaline by potentiometry and absorption spectroscopy. *Chin. Chem. Lett.* **1999**, *10*, 677–678.
69. Jameson, R.F.; Neillie, W.F. Complexes Formed by Adrenaline and Related Compounds with Transition-Metal Ions. I. Acid Dissociation Constants of the Ligands. *J. Chem. Soc.* **1965**, *65*, 2391–2395. [CrossRef] [PubMed]
70. Marzotto, A.; Mazzucco, E.; Galzigna, L. Spectral changes following the epinephrine-dioxouranium(VI) interaction. *Inorg. Nucl. Chem. Lett.* **1980**, *16*, 331–336. [CrossRef]
71. Moustafa, M.H. Studies on the binary and ternary comlexes of mercury(II) with gallic acid and adrenaline. *Ass. Univ. Bull. Environ. Res.* **2010**, *13*, 77–89.
72. De Stefano, C.; Foti, C.; Giuffrè, O.; Sammartano, S. Dependence on ionic strength of protonation enthalpies of polycarboxylic anions in NaCl aqueous solution. *J. Chem. Eng. Data* **2001**, *46*, 1417–1424. [CrossRef]
73. De Stefano, C.; Sammartano, S.; Mineo, P.; Rigano, C. Computer Tools for the Speciation of Natural Fluids. In *Marine Chemistry—An Environmental Analytical Chemistry Approach*; Gianguzza, A., Pelizzetti, E., Sammartano, S., Eds.; Kluwer Academic Publishers: Amsterdam, The Netherlands, 1997; pp. 71–83.
74. Gans, P. Hyperquad. Available online: http://www.hyperquad.co.uk/ (accessed on 20 May 2019).

75. De Stefano, C.; Princi, P.; Rigano, C.; Sammartano, S. The Calculation of Equilibrium Concentrations. ES4EC1: A Fortran Program for Computing Distribution Diagrams and Titration Curves. *Comput. Chem.* **1989**, *13*, 343–359. [CrossRef]
76. De Robertis, A.; De Stefano, C.; Rigano, C. Computer Analysis of Equilibrium Data in Solution. ES5CM Fortran and Basic Programs for Computing Formation Enthalpies from Calorimetric Measurements. *Acta* **1989**, *138*, 141–146.
77. Crea, F.; De Stefano, C.; Giuffrè, O.; Sammartano, S. Ionic strength dependence of protonation constants of N-Alkylsubstituted open chain diamines in $NaCl_{(aq)}$. *J. Chem. Eng. Data* **2004**, *49*, 109–115. [CrossRef]
78. Bretti, C.; Giacalone, A.; Gianguzza, A.; Milea, D.; Sammartano, S. Modeling S-carboxymethyl-L-cysteine protonation and activity coefficients in sodium and tetramethylammonium chloride aqueous solutions by SIT and Pitzer equations. *Fluid Phase Equilib.* **2007**, *252*, 119–129. [CrossRef]
79. Crea, P.; De Robertis, A.; De Stefano, C.; Milea, D.; Sammartano, S. Modelling the dependence on medium and ionic strength of glutathione acid-base behavior in $LiCl_{aq}$, $NaCl_{aq}$, KCl_{aq}, $CaCl_{aq}$, $(CH_3)_4NCl_{aq}$ and $(C_2H_5)_4NI_{aq}$. *J. Chem. Eng. Data* **2007**, *52*, 1028–1036. [CrossRef]
80. Cigala, R.M.; Cordaro, M.; Crea, F.; De Stefano, C.; Fracassetti, V.; Marchesi, M.; Milea, D.; Sammartano, S. Acid–Base Properties and Alkali and Alkaline Earth Metal Complex Formation in Aqueous Solution of Diethylenetriamine-N,N,N',N'',N''-pentakis(methylenephosphonic acid) Obtained by an Efficient Synthetic Procedure. *Ind. Eng. Chem. Res.* **2014**, *53*, 9544–9553. [CrossRef]
81. Bretti, C.; Cigala, R.M.; Lando, G.; Milea, D.; Sammartano, S. Some Thermodynamic Properties of Aqueous 2-Mercaptopyridine-N-Oxide (Pyrithione) Solutions. *J. Solut. Chem.* **2014**, *43*, 1093–1109. [CrossRef]
82. Cataldo, S.; Crea, F.; Gianguzza, A.; Pettignano, A.; Piazzese, D. Solubility and acid-base properties and activity coefficients of chitosan in different ionic media and at different ionic strengths, at T = 25 °C. *J. Mol. Liq.* **2009**, *148*, 120–126. [CrossRef]
83. Foti, C.; Gianguzza, A.; Milea, D.; Sammartano, S. Hydrolysis and chemical speciation of $(C_2H_5)_2Sn^{2+}$, $(C_2H_5)_3Sn^+$ and $(C_3H_7)_3Sn^+$ in aqueous media simulating the major composition of natural waters. *Appl. Organomet. Chem.* **2002**, *16*, 34–43. [CrossRef]

Sample Availability: Samples of the compounds are not available from the authors.

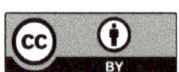

© 2020 by the authors. Licensee MDPI, Basel, Switzerland. This article is an open access article distributed under the terms and conditions of the Creative Commons Attribution (CC BY) license (http://creativecommons.org/licenses/by/4.0/).

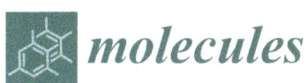

Article

Speciation Studies of Bifunctional 3-Hydroxy-4-Pyridinone Ligands in the Presence of Zn^{2+} at Different Ionic Strengths and Temperatures

Anna Irto [1], Paola Cardiano [1], Salvatore Cataldo [2], Karam Chand [3], Rosalia Maria Cigala [1], Francesco Crea [1], Concetta De Stefano [1], Giuseppe Gattuso [1], Nicola Muratore [2], Alberto Pettignano [2], Silvio Sammartano [1,*] and M. Amélia Santos [3,*]

1. Dipartimento di Scienze Chimiche, Biologiche, Farmaceutiche e Ambientali, Università di Messina, Viale F. Stagno d'Alcontres 31, 98166 Messina, Italy; airto@unime.it (A.I.); pcardiano@unime.it (P.C.); rmcigala@unime.it (R.M.C.); fcrea@unime.it (F.C.); cdestefano@unime.it (C.D.S.); ggattuso@unime.it (G.G.)
2. Dipartimento di Fisica e Chimica Emilio Segrè, ed. 17, Università di Palermo, Viale delle Scienze, I-90128 Palermo, Italy; salvatore.cataldo@unipa.it (S.C.); nicola.muratore@unipa.it (N.M.); alberto.pettignano@unipa.it (A.P.)
3. Centro de Química Estrutural, Instituto Superior Técnico, Universidade de Lisboa, Av. Rovísco Pais 1, 1049-001 Lisboa, Portugal; kc4chemistry@gmail.com
* Correspondence: ssammartano@unime.it (S.S.); masantos@tecnico.ulisboa.pt (M.A.S.); Tel.: +39-0906765749 (S.S.); +351-218419273 (M.A.S.)

Academic Editors: Francesco Crea and Alberto Pettignano
Received: 11 October 2019; Accepted: 6 November 2019; Published: 12 November 2019

Abstract: The acid–base properties of two bifunctional 3-hydroxy-4-pyridinone ligands and their chelating capacity towards Zn^{2+}, an essential bio-metal cation, were investigated in NaCl aqueous solutions by potentiometric, UV-Vis spectrophotometric, and ^1H NMR spectroscopic titrations, carried out at $0.15 \leq I/mol^{-1} \leq 1.00$ and $288.15 \leq T/K \leq 310.15$. A study at $I = 0.15$ mol L^{-1} and $T = 298.15$ K was also performed for other three Zn^{2+}/L^{z-} systems, with ligands belonging to the same family of compounds. The processing of experimental data allowed the determination of protonation and stability constants, which showed accordance with the data obtained from the different analytical techniques used, and with those reported in the literature for the same class of compounds. ESI-MS spectrometric measurements provided support for the formation of the different Zn^{2+}/ligand species, while computational molecular simulations allowed information to be gained on the metal–ligand coordination. The dependence on ionic strength and the temperature of equilibrium constants were investigated by means of the extended Debye–Hückel model, the classical specific ion interaction theory, and the van't Hoff equations, respectively.

Keywords: 3-hydroxy-4-pyridinone; speciation; acid–base properties; extended Debye–Hückel; Zn-complexation; specific ion interaction theory; van't Hoff equation; sequestering ability

1. Introduction

The 3-hydroxy-4-pyridinones (3,4-HPs) are a family of compounds that are derivatives of deferiprone (DFP), which have been extensively developed as possible strong chelators and metal-related pharmaceutical drugs, due to their important roles in pharmaceutical and bioenvironmental processes, in the sequestration or release of specific metal cations (M^{n+}) from or into the human body, and as metal carriers for therapeutics or imaging purposes [1,2]. These compounds feature a 6-membered N-heterocyclic aromatoid ring with hydroxyl and ketone groups in the ortho position, conferring them a significant binding ability towards hard divalent and trivalent metal cations (M^{2+}, M^{3+}) [3]. In the last two decades, their development has been considerably spreading, since several studies [1,3,4] have demonstrated that the 3-hydroxy-4-pyridinones may strongly sequester metal cations (Fe^{3+}, Al^{3+}, etc.), resulting in the formation of species with a higher thermodynamic stability with respect to the precursor deferiprone [5,6]. At the same time, they can be considered good alternatives to deferoxamine (DFO or Desferal®) [7] as iron chelators, because the use of 3,4-HPs does not involve serious drawbacks, such as high toxicity and costs, oral activity, or other possible undesired side effects. As already reported in previous papers [8,9], the 3-hydroxy-4-pyridinones can also be extra-functionalized to improve their lipophilic–hydrophilic balance and increase their affinity towards cells biological membranes.

The present paper investigates the acid–base properties of two bifunctional 3,4-HPs, ligands (L2: (S)-2-amino-4-((2-(3-hydroxy-2-methyl-4-oxopyridin-1(4H)-yl)ethyl)amino)-4-oxobutanoic acid and L5: 1-(3-aminopropyl)-3-hydroxy-2-methylpyridin-4(1H)-one, Figure 1), at different ionic strength and temperature conditions ($0.15 \leq I/\text{mol L}^{-1} \leq 1.00$, $288.15 \leq T/K \leq 310.15$) in $NaCl_{(aq)}$. This ionic medium was selected because it is the principal inorganic component of many natural and biological fluids [10–12]. Therefore, performing studies under the experimental conditions of these fluids, namely at $I \sim 0.01$–0.10 mol L^{-1} and 0.70 mol L^{-1} for fresh and marine waters, or $I \sim 0.16$ mol L^{-1} for blood plasma, allows simulation and possibly predictions of the behaviour of real systems [13,14]. Moreover, although these 3,4-HPs metal chelators have already proven to have an inherently high affinity towards *hard* metal cations, such as Al^{3+} [8], it is interesting to study their interaction with biologically relevant M^{2+}, in order to assure that along with their sequestering role of *hard* M^{3+}, they do not lead to a significant depletion of important divalent bio-metal cations, in particular Zn^{2+}. In fact, Zn^{2+} is an essential trace mineral required for the metabolism of several enzymes, cell division processes, DNA, and protein synthesis [15]. Furthermore, it has an important role in the proper growth and development of the human body, helps to protect the skin and muscles from premature aging, and has antioxidant functions against free radicals [16]. Zinc also participates in regulation of immune functions through the activation of T lymphocytes (T cells), which help the body to control and regulate the immune responses and to attack infected or cancerous cells [17]. Therefore, the binding ability of the cited 3,4-HPs towards Zn^{2+} was investigated, as well as for three other ligands (L1: 4-(3-hydroxy-2-methyl-4-oxopyridin-1(4H)-yl)butanoic acid, L3: (S)-2-amino-4-((3-(3-hydroxy-2-methyl-4-oxopyridin-1(4H)-yl)propyl)amino)-4-oxobutanoic acid, and L4: (S)-2-amino-5-(3-hydroxy-2-methyl-4-oxopyridin-1(4H)-yl)pentanoic acid; Figure 1), all of which belong to the same class of compounds. From an experimental point of view, potentiometric measurements, using specific electrodes for H^+ ion activity (ISE-H^+), and ultraviolet-visible (UV-Vis) spectrophotometric measurements were carried out at $I = 0.15$ mol L^{-1} in $NaCl_{(aq)}$ and $T = 298.15$ K, and in the case of L2 and L5 3-hydroxy-4-pyridinones, also at $0.15 \leq I/\text{mol L}^{-1} \leq 1.00$, $288.15 \leq T/K \leq 310.15$. Electrospray mass (ESI-MS) spectrometric measurements were performed to investigate the possible formation of Zn^{2+}/ligand species with different stoichiometry at $I = 0.15$, 1.00 mol L^{-1} in $NaCl_{(aq)}$ and in the absence of ionic medium, at $T = 298.15$ K. Proton nuclear magnetic resonance (^{1}H NMR) spectroscopic titrations and computational studies were also carried out to gain information on the Zn^{2+}–ligand coordination mode. The protonation and stability data, determined for the different experimental conditions, were used to model the dependence of thermodynamic parameters on ionic strength by means of the extended Debye–Hückel (EDH) equation and the specific ion interaction theory (SIT), while the effect of temperature was determined using the van't Hoff equation. Finally, the sequestering ability of the 3-hydroxy-4-pyridinones towards the metal cation under study was investigated by calculating the empirical parameter $pL_{0.5}$, already proposed in [18], at different pH, ionic strength, and temperature conditions.

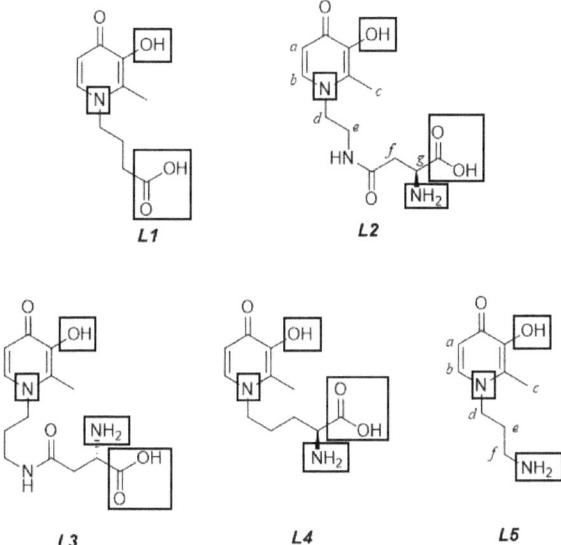

Figure 1. Structures of the 3-hydroxy-4-pyridinones under study, with protonable groups highlighted with rectangles. The letters represent for the proton nuclear magnetic resonance (^{1}H NMR) titration peak assignment.

2. Results and Discussion

2.1. Equilibria and Thermodynamic Models

The acid–base properties of the ligands (L^{z-}) were investigated, taking into account the following stepwise ($\log K_r^H$; Equation (1)) and overall ($\log \beta_r^H$; Equation (2)) equilibria, respectively:

$$H^+ + H_{(r-1)}L^{-(z-(r-1))} = H_rL^{-(z-r)} \qquad \log K_r^H \qquad (1)$$

and

$$rH^+ + L^{z-} = H_rL^{-(z-r)} \qquad \log \beta_r^H \qquad (2)$$

where r is the rth protonation step; z is the charge of the completely deprotonated 3-hydroxy-4-pyridinones.

The metal hydrolytic behavior is described by the equilibrium:

$$pZn^{2+} + rH_2O = Zn_p(OH)_r^{(2p-r)} + rH^+ \qquad \log \beta_r^{OH} \qquad (3)$$

The stepwise and overall stability constants of the Zn^{2+}-ligands species are given as follows:

$$pZn^{2+} + H_rL_q^{-(zq-(r-1))} = Zn_pL_qH_r^{(2p+r-qz)} + H^+ \qquad \log K_{pqr} \qquad (4)$$

$$pZn^{2+} + qL^{z-} + rH^+ = Zn_pL_qH_r^{(2p+r-qz)} \qquad \log \beta_{pqr} \qquad (5)$$

If ternary metal–ligand hydrolytic species are formed, equilibria refer to:

$$pZn^{2+} + qL^{z-} + rH_2O = Zn_pL_q(OH)_r^{(2p-r-zq)} + rH^+ \qquad \log \beta_{pq\text{-}r} \qquad (6)$$

The protonation and stability of formation constants, concentrations, and ionic strengths are expressed in the molar (c, mol L^{-1}) or molal (m, mol (kg H$_2$O)$^{-1}$) scales. Molar to molal conversions were performed by means of appropriate density values.

The dependence on ionic strength (*I*) of the thermodynamic parameters was studied using an extended Debye–Hückel-type equation [19]:

$$\log K = \log K^0 - z^* \cdot DH + C \cdot I \qquad (7)$$

where $\log K^0$ is the equilibrium constant atinfinite dilution; z^* is the Σ (charge)^2_reactants − Σ (charge)^2_products; DH is the $0.51 \cdot (I^{1/2}/(1 + 1.5 I^{1/2}))$, Debye–Hückel term; C is the empirical parameter for the dependence of the equilibrium constants on the ionic strength.

If the equilibrium constants are expressed in the molal concentration scale, Equation (7) can be modified to obtain the classical specific ion interaction theory (SIT) [20–22], where C parameter is replaced by $\Delta \varepsilon$:

$$\Delta \varepsilon_{ij} = \sum_i \varepsilon(i, j) \qquad (8)$$

where $\varepsilon(i, j)$ is the interaction coefficient for an ith species with a jth component of opposite charge.

Furthermore, protonation and formation constants determined at different temperatures were used to calculate the enthalpy values by applying the van't Hoff equation, assuming that the contribution of ΔC_p in a small temperature range, in our case 288.15–310.15 K, is negligible:

$$\log K_T = \log K_\theta + (\Delta H_\theta / 2.303 R)(1/\theta - 1/T) \qquad (9)$$

where θ is the reference temperature (298.15 K); T is temperature in Kelvin; ΔH_θ is enthalpy change at reference temperature; R is 8.314 J K^{-1} mol^{-1} and is the universal gas constant.

To complete the thermodynamic picture of the Zn^{2+}/ligand system behavior in NaCl aqueous solution, the Gibbs free energy was calculated from the equilibrium constants, as reported by Equation (10):

$$\Delta G = -RT \ln K \qquad (10)$$

From the knowledge of the enthalpy changes and the Gibbs free energy, the $T\Delta S$ values, as known, were detemined at the same experimental conditions:

$$T\Delta S = \Delta H - \Delta G \qquad (11)$$

2.2. Protonation Constants of the Ligands

The protonation constants of the ligands (Figure 1) have already been published at $I = 0.15$ mol L^{-1} in NaCl$_{(aq)}$ and T = 298.15 K and 310.15 K (Table S1) [8]. As a continuation of this study, the research group undertook a complete investigation on the acid–base properties of two 3-hydroxy-4-pyridinones, namely L2 and L5, in NaCl$_{(aq)}$ at $0.15 \le I$/mol L$^{-1} \le 1.00$ and $288.15 \le T$/K ≤ 310.15.

Both the ligands were synthesized in the H$_r$(L)^0 neutral species form; the possible protonable sites, as shown in Figure 1, can be assigned to:

1. the hydroxyl group of the aromatoid ring;
2. the –NH$_2$ and –COOH groups, potentially present in the alkyl moiety;
3. the pyridinone nitrogen in the N-heterocyclic ring, with the proton supplied by excess of inorganic acid [8].

2.2.1. L2 Behavior in Aqueous Solution

L2 ligand is an aspartic acid 3-hydroxy-4-pyridinone hybrid featuring all of the abovementioned protonable groups; its acid–base properties were investigated by means of UV-Vis spectrophotometric measurements, carried out at different ionic strengths and temperatures in NaCl aqueous solution.

Analysis of the experimental data led, in all cases, to the determination of four protonation constants, namely $\log K_1^H$ (9.88–10.99), $\log K_2^H$ (6.03–9.32), $\log K_3^H$ (3.97–4.93), and $\log K_4^H$ (3.06–3.73), as reported in Table 1 and Table S2 (in molar and molal concentration scales, respectively). These were already attributed, by means of ^{1}H NMR titrations, to –OH, –NH$_2$, –COOH, and the pyridinone nitrogen atom, respectively. Table S3 shows the average chemical shift values calculated for each protonated species at I = 0.15 mol L^{-1} in NaCl$_{(aq)}$ and T = 298.15 K [8].

Table 1. Experimental overall [1] and stepwise [2] protonation constants of L2 and L5 ligands at different temperatures and ionic strengths in NaCl$_{(aq)}$.

Ligand	I/mol L^{-1}	T/K	logβ_r^H [1] (logK_r^H) [2]			
			HL$^{(1-z)}$	H$_2$L$^{(2-z)}$	H$_3$L$^{(3-z)}$	H$_4$L$^{(4-z)}$
L2 [3]	0.149	288.15	10.28 ± 0.01 [4]	19.56 ± 0.01 [4] (9.28)	24.29 ± 0.08 [4] (4.73)	27.46 ± 0.08 [4] (3.17)
	0.506	298.15	9.962 ± 0.005	17.63 ± 0.03 (7.668)	22.52 ± 0.02 (4.89)	25.62 ± 0.02 (3.10)
	0.744	298.15	9.882 ± 0.008	17.25 ± 0.07 (7.365)	22.18 ± 0.10 (4.93)	25.41 ± 0.10 (3.23)
	1.012	298.15	10.059 ± 0.001	16.78 ± 0.02 (6.721)	21.18 ± 0.03 (4.40)	24.91 ± 0.12 (3.73)
L5 [5]	0.166	288.15	10.53 ± 0.03 [4]	19.92 ± 0.02 [4] (9.39)	23.58 ± 0.03 [4] (3.66)	-
	0.165	298.15	10.82 ± 0.07	20.44 ± 0.06 (9.62)	24.02 ± 0.07 (3.58)	-
	0.140	298.15	11.20 [6] ± 0.02	20.466 [6] ± 0.006 (9.266)	23.679 [6] ± 0.007 (3.213)	-
	0.473	298.15	9.99 ± 0.01	19.17 ± 0.01 (9.18)	22.46 ± 0.01 (3.29)	-
	0.723	298.15	9.79 ± 0.03	18.86 ± 0.03 (9.07)	22.02 ± 0.04 (3.16)	-
	1.008	298.15	10.31 ± 0.02	19.32 ± 0.03 (9.01)	23.38 ± 0.06 (4.06)	-

Note: [1] logβ_r^H refers to Equation (2); [2] logK_r^H refers to Equation (1); [3] data obtained by means of ultraviolet-visible (UV-Vis) spectrophotometric measurements; [4] standard deviation; [5,6] protonation constants determined by potentiometric and ^{1}H NMR titrations, respectively.

As examples of the ionic strength effect on the acid–base properties of the ligand, the protonation constant trends vs. I are shown in Figure 2, clearly indicating that the behavior of each protonable site is different than the others. With the exception of –NH$_2$ group, whose logK_2^H values constantly decrease with increasing ionic strength, the remaining sites undergo a tendency inversion at I = 0.75–1.00 mol L^{-1} in NaCl$_{(aq)}$.

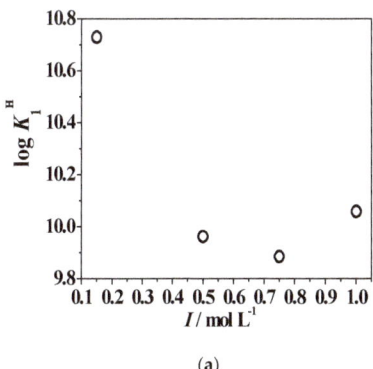

(a)

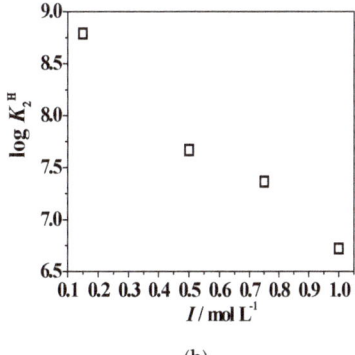

(b)

Figure 2. *Cont.*

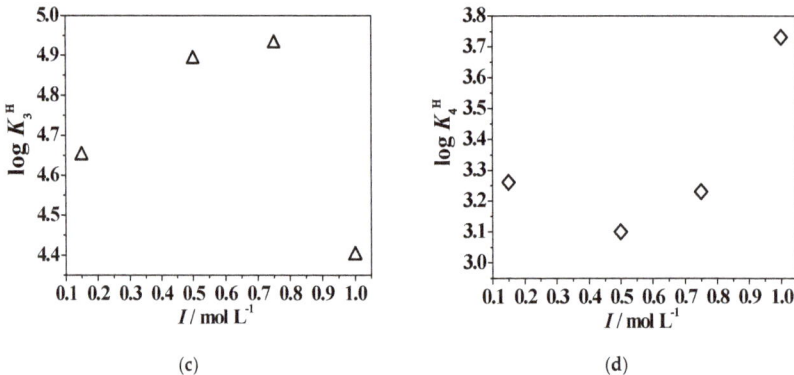

Figure 2. Trend of $\log K_1^H$ (a), $\log K_2^H$ (b), $\log K_3^H$ (c), and $\log K_4^H$ (d) L2 protonation constants vs. the ionic strength (in mol L^{-1}) in NaCl$_{(aq)}$ and T = 298.15 K.

Furthermore, a comparison between protonated species distribution at T = 298.15 K, I = 0.506 mol L^{-1}, and 1.012 mol L^{-1} is reported in Figure 3A. The H$_4$(L2)$^{2+}$ species is present at pH ~ 2.0, with percentages higher than 90% at both experimental conditions, while the H$_3$(L2)$^+$ reaches the 80% and 51% of formation at pH ~ 4.0 with increasing ionic strength. The bis-protonated H$_2$(L2)^0$_{(aq)}$ species is characterized by an opposite trend, achieving its maximum (88%) at lower pH (pH ~ 5.5) and with I = 1.012 mol L^{-1} than with I = 0.506 mol L^{-1} (pH ~ 6.3, 93%). The H(L2)$^-$ starts to form at pH ~ 4.2 and reaches 87% and 96% of formation at pH ~ 8.9 and 8.4, with the variable increasing. At last, the completely deprotonated species (L2)$^{2-}$ reaches about 90% at both ionic strength conditions. The effect of this variable can be further examined by the analysis of Figure 3B, where a comparison between the UV-Vis titration curves is reported, recorded at the same experimental conditions as those used to draw the distribution diagram.

The absorbance spectra vary with pH increase due to the different behaviours of the protonated species. In all cases, as already found at I = 0.15 mol L^{-1} in NaCl$_{(aq)}$ and T = 298.15 K [8], an absorption band at λ_{max} = 278 nm and pH ~ 2.0 was recorded, featuring an increase of intensity at pH ~ 4.5 and 4.9 at I = 0.506 mol L^{-1} and 1.012 mol L^{-1}, respectively. A batochromic shift and the formation of different isosbestic points were noticed. Furthermore, a general intensity increase of each UV-Vis absorbance maximum with increasing ionic strength was observed across the pH range investigated, probably due to a noteworthy contribution of the ionic medium to the ligand speciation in aqueous solution.

The deconvolution of the UV-Vis spectrophotometric data allowed us to calculate the molar absorbivities (ε/mol^{-1} L cm^{-1}) of each species; as an example, the ε variation with pH is reported in Figure S1 at T = 298.15 K and I = 0.506 mol L^{-1} and 1.012 mol L^{-1} in NaCl$_{(aq)}$. The values of the molar absorbivities in these conditions are:

- ε_{max}(H$_4$(L2)$^{2+}$) = 5221 and 5742 at λ_{max} = 278 nm with increasing ionic increasing;
- ε_{max}(H$_3$(L2)$^+$) = 8756 and 9400 at λ_{max} = 291 nm, I = 0.506 mol L^{-1} and 1.012 mol L^{-1}, respectively;
- ε_{max}(H$_2$(L2)^0$_{(aq)}$) = 7468 and 9681 at λ_{max} = 284 nm and 281 nm, respectively;
- ε_{max}(H(L2)$^-$) = 5016 at λ_{max} = 296 nm and both the variable conditions;
- ε_{max}((L2)$^{2-}$) = 7913 and 8276 at λ_{max} = 311 nm, with increasing ionic strength.

To investigate the effect of temperature on the speciation of the ligands in NaCl aqueous solution, UV-Vis spectrophotometric measurements were performed at I = 0.15 mol L^{-1} and T = 288.15 K, which together with the data already published in the literature at T = 298.15 K and 310.15 K [8] showed a trend for protonation constants with the considered variables. Analyzing the data reported in Table 1 and Table S1 (in molar and molal concentration scales, respectively), a different tendency was found for the hydroxyl group than for the others (carboxylic, amino, and pyridinone nitrogen groups); $\log K_1^H$

values increased with temperature, while for the other protonation constants an opposite trend can be observed. In particular, the significant variation of $\log K_2^H$ for $T = 288.15$ K–298.15 K and $T = 310.15$ K could probably be explained by the literature data, which reported a compound similar to L2, mimosine. It was observed that the contribution of the ligand structure to the resonance hybrid leading to a partial positive charge on the pyridinone nitrogen ring [23], together with the possible temperature effect, could cause a noteworthy decrease of protonation constants, attributed to the $-NH_2$ group, in comparison with the typical values usually obtained for this protonable site ($\log K^H \sim 9.0$–9.5) [24].

In Figure S2, a comparison between the distribution diagrams of the ligand at $I = 0.15$ mol L^{-1} in NaCl$_{(aq)}$, $T = 288.15$ K, and $T = 310.15$ K showed that the species formation percentages decrease with temperature increase. In physiological conditions, they are shifted towards lower pH values, with the exception of the H(L2)$^-$ species, which, as already evidenced, displays different behavior than the other ones compared with the considered variable.

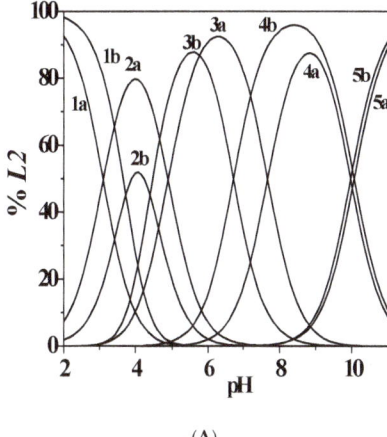 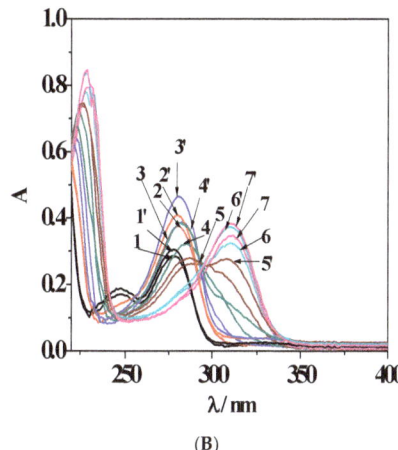

(A) (B)

Figure 3. (A) Distribution diagram of L2 ($c_L = 5.3 \cdot 10^{-5}$ mol L^{-1}) species at $T = 298.15$ K and $I = 0.506$ (a) and 1.012 (b) mol L^{-1} in NaCl$_{(aq)}$. Species: (1) H$_4$(L2)$^{2+}$; (2) H$_3$(L2)$^+$; (3) H$_2$(L2)$^0_{(aq)}$; (4) H(L2)$^-$; (5) (L2)$^{2-}$. (B) UV-Vis spectrophotometric titration curves of L2 under the same experimental conditions as for the distribution diagram and at different pH values. At $I = 0.506$ mol L^{-1}: (1) pH = 2.01, λ_{max} = 278 nm; (2) pH = 3.62, λ_{max} = 275 nm; (3) pH = 4.90, λ_{max} = 283 nm; (4) pH = 7.39, λ_{max} = 285 nm; (5) pH = 9.68, λ_{max} = 290 nm; (6) pH = 10.56, λ_{max} = 310 nm; (7) pH = 11.00, λ_{max} = 310 nm. At $I = 1.012$ mol L^{-1}: (1') pH = 2.00, λ_{max} = 278 nm; (2') pH = 3.59, λ_{max} = 279 nm; (3') pH = 4.50, λ_{max} = 280 nm; (4') pH = 8.40, λ_{max} = 283 nm; (5') pH = 9.84, λ_{max} = 296 nm; (6') pH = 10.60, λ_{max} = 310 nm; (7') pH = 10.99, λ_{max} = 311 nm.

2.2.2. L5 Ligand Protonation

The second 3-hydroxy-4-pyridinone under study, L5, shown in Figure 1, features three protonable moieties, namely the hydroxyl group, the pyridinone nitrogen atom, and the terminal amine group of the alkylic chain.

^{1}H NMR measurements were carried out at $I = 0.15$ mol L^{-1} in NaCl$_{(aq)}$ and $T = 298.15$ K to further analyze L5 acid–base behavior, which was previously investigated using UV-Vis spectrophotometric and spectrofluorimetric techniques [8]. The protonation constants (Table 1), refined using the HypNMR computer program, were in good agreement with those previously reported [8]. The collected spectra show a single set of signals shifted upfield with pH increase. As expected, all the resonances of protons closer to the pyridinone nitrogen of the aromatoid ring are more or less shielded in the pH range 2–4.5, thus confirming that this is the first group to be deprotonated, as already observed in similar ligands [8]. In detail, the *a* and *b* signals are characterized by a comparable upfield shift (0.48 and

0.33 ppm, respectively) in the cited pH range, whereas they do not change to a great extent from pH 4.5 to 7.5 and start to decrease again at alkaline pH. A less significant upfield shift can also be observed for *c* and *d* protons at pH < 4.5, and once again, the chemical shifts follow the behavior already discussed for the pyridinone protons. The other two signals, namely *e* and *f*, show an opposite trend with pH increase, since they start to considerably change from neutral pH and greater, confirming the deprotonation sequence already reported.

From the speciation data it is known that at pH ~ 2.0 the $H_3(L5)^{2+}$ species should be present in solution with a percentage of ca. 95%, whilst between 5.2 and 6.4 the most abundant species should be the $H_2(L5)^+$, reaching 99.8%; the spectra recorded in these conditions were compared with the calculated chemical shifts obtained by HypNMR for the same species. The calculated δ values for $H_3(L5)^{2+}$ and $H_2(L5)^+$, listed in Table S3, are in excellent agreement with the ones observed in the spectra recorded at the pH level where these species reach the maxima. In addition, Figure S3 shows the almost total overlap between observed and calculated chemical shifts for some selected nuclei.

The acid–base properties of *L5* were also studied by potentiometric measurements performed under different ionic strength and temperature conditions in $NaCl_{(aq)}$. The treatment of the experimental data allowed the determination of three protonation constants (Table 1 and Table S1): $\log K_1^H$ (9.79–11.20), $\log K_2^H$ (5.96–6.92), and $\log K_3^H$ (3.00–4.06).

The effect of the ionic strength on the protonation of the *L5* ligand can be observed in Figure 4 and Figure S4. In the first case, the trend of $\log K_r^H$ vs. *I* is reported, showing for this ligand a behavior similar to that found for analogous functional groups in *L2*. Therefore, the absence of the amidic moiety or the carboxyl group in the *L5* ligand structure, with respect to the first ligand, would not seem to influence the effect of the ionic strength increasing on the acid–base properties of the 3-hydroxy-4-pyridinone.

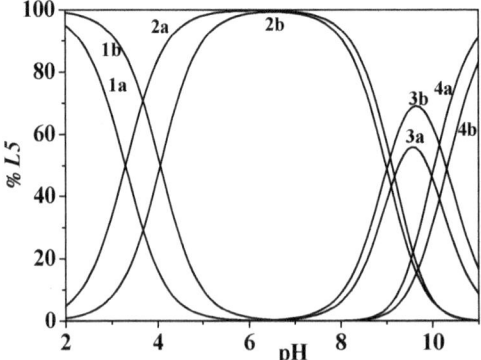

Figure 4. Distribution diagram of *L5* ($c_L = 1.0 \cdot 10^{-3}$ mol L^{-1}) species at T = 298.15 K, I = 0.473 (a) and I = 1.008 (b) mol L^{-1} in $NaCl_{(aq)}$. Species: (1) $H_3(L5)^{2+}$; (2) $H_2(L5)^+$; (3) $H(L5)^0_{(aq)}$; (4) $(L5)^-$.

In Figure 4, the ligand speciation diagrams, drawn at T = 298.15 K, I = 0.473 mol L^{-1}, and I = 1.008 mol L^{-1} in $NaCl_{(aq)}$, show that all the species are uniformly distributed along the pH range investigated. The $H_3(L5)^{2+}$ species is present in solution at pH ~ 2.0, reaching more than 90% in both the experimental conditions. This species achieves the maximum formation percentage at pH ~ 6.4; at pH ~ 9.6, $H(L5)^0_{(aq)}$ reaches 56% and 70% and $(L5)^-$ reaches 91% and 83% at I = 0.473 mol L^{-1} and I = 1.008 mol L^{-1}, respectively. Therefore, this figure shows a trend of protonations occurring at slightly higher pH values with ionic strength increasing.

Regarding the temperature effect, potentiometric data determined at I = 0.15 mol L^{-1} in $NaCl_{(aq)}$ and T = 288.15 K allowed us to obtain a trend for protonation constants, together with the values already determined at T = 298.15 K and in physiological conditions [8]. Table 1 and Table S1 show that $\log K_1^H$ values increase from the lowest temperature to $T = 298.15$ K, followed by an inversion of tendency at $T = 310.15$ K. For $\log K_2^H$, the variation of some logarithmic units on the protonation constant at physiological temperature was already discussed in the previous subparagraph (L2 behavior in aqueous solution) [23]. $\log K_3^H$, attributed to the pyridinone nitrogen atom, similar to the same moiety in L2, is characterized by a decrease with variable increase. To better observe the temperature effect on the speciation of the ligand in NaCl aqueous solution, in Figure S5 a comparison between the distribution diagrams of L5 at $I = 0.15$ mol L^{-1} in NaCl$_{(aq)}$, $T = 288.15$ K, and $T = 310.15$ K is depicted. The figure clearly indicates that the formation of protonated species occurs at higher pH values with temperature increasing.

2.3. Hydrolysis of the Metal Cation

The acid–base properties of Zn^{2+} in NaCl$_{(aq)}$ were already known and have been reported in the literature under different ionic strength and temperature conditions (Table S4) [6,25,26].

2.4. Binding Ability Towards Zn^{2+}

The investigation on the Zn^{2+} interactions with the bifunctional 3-hydroxy-4-pyridinones (L1–L5) led to the determination of species with different stoichiometry ($Zn_pL_qH_r^{(2p+r-qz)}$). The best possible speciation schemes were selected considering different criteria, such as:

- simplicity and probability of the model;
- formation percentages of the species across the pH range under investigation;
- statistical parameters (standard deviation on $\log \beta_{pqr}$ values and on the fitting values of the systems);
- values of corresponding ratios with single variances in comparison with those from the accepted model.

The high number of experiments performed (and of experimental points collected) showed the differences in variance between the accepted model and other models to be significant.

In Table 2, the stability constants of all of the Zn^{2+}/3-hydroxy-4-pyridinones complex species are reported at $I = 0.15$ mol L^{-1} in NaCl$_{(aq)}$ and $T = 298.15$ K. The experimental data, whenever possible, were determined by means of potentiometry (1st column), UV–Vis spectrophotometry (2nd column), and ^{1}H NMR spectroscopy (3rd column); the average (4th column) of the obtained values was also calculated. The measurements were carried out in the pH ranges of 2.0–10.5 for potentiometric and UV–Vis investigations, and 2.0–8.1 for ^{1}H NMR ones.

As can be inferred from the analysis in Table 2, for the mentioned experimental conditions, a trend of stability of the species can be observed due to a common complex, namely $ZnL^{(2-z)}$:

$$L4 > L3 > L5 > L2 > L1$$

This trend could be explained by assuming that the stability of the Zn^{2+}/L^{z-} systems may be favored by the simultaneous presence on the ligand molecules of carboxylic and amino groups or even different alkyl chains; in fact, there is a decrease with decreasing alkyl chain length (L2) and with the absence of an amino group (L1). In the case of L2 and L5, experiments at $0.15 \leq I/\text{mol L}^{-1} \leq 1.00$ and $288.15 \leq T/(K \leq 310.15$ were also carried out to give a more complete thermodynamic picture of the Zn^{2+}/ligand systems.

Table 2. Overall [1], stepwise [2] experimental, and average [3] stability constants of Zn^{2+}/3-hydroxy-4-pyridinone species obtained by potentiometric [4], UV-Vis spectrophotometric [5], and ^{1}H NMR [6] spectroscopic measurements at $I = 0.15$ mol L^{-1} in NaCl$_{(aq)}$ and $T = 298.15$ K.

	$\log\beta_{pqr}$ [1] $(\log K_{pqr})$ [2]			$\log\beta_{pqr}$ [1] $(\log K_{pqr})$ [2]			$\log\beta_{pqr}$ [1] $(\log K_{pqr})$ [2]
I/mol L^{-1}	0.146	0.147	0.150	0.145	0.150		0.148
Species	L1			L2			L3
ZnLH$^{(3-z)}$	-	15.50 [4] ± 0.06 [7] (4.77)	15.51 [5] ± 0.08 [7](4.78)	15.79 [6] ± 0.31 [7] (5.05)	15.56 [3] ± 0.08 [8] (4.83)		17.06 [4] ± 0.09 [6] (6.10)
ZnL$^{(2-z)}$	7.27 [4] ± 0.03 [7]	8.12 ± 0.06	8.11 ± 0.04	8.54 ± 0.48	8.20 ± 0.10		9.52 ± 0.06
ZnL(OH)$^{(1-z)}$	0.25 ± 0.07 (9.45) [9]	−0.72 ± 0.09 (8.48) [9]	−0.55 ± 0.04 (8.64) [9]	−0.72 ± 0.09 (8.64) [9]	−0.68 ± 0.06 (8.56) [9]		0.70 ± 0.08 (9.90) [9]
	$\log\beta_{pqr}$ [1] $(\log K_{pqr})$ [2]				$\log\beta_{pqr}$ [1] $(\log K_{pqr})$ [2]		
I/mol L^{-1}	0.145	0.150	0.147	0.149	0.150	0.145	0.150
Species	L4				L5		
ZnLH$^{(3-z)}$	16.69 [4] ± 0.05 [7] (5.59)	16.68 [5] ± 0.20 [7] (5.58)	16.68 [3] ± 0.02 [8] (5.58)	17.21 [4] ± 0.06 [7] (6.13)	17.41 [5] ± 0.07 [7] (6.33)	17.64 [6] ± 0.08 [7] (6.56)	17.46 [3] ± 0.09 [8] (6.38)
ZnL$^{(2-z)}$	9.68 ± 0.04	9.68 ± 0.10	9.68 ± 0.08	9.89 ± 0.08	9.08 ± 0.02	9.04 ± 0.04	9.22 ± 0.20
ZnL(OH)$^{(1-z)}$	0.60 ± 0.09 (9.80) [9]	0.33 ± 0.20 (9.53) [9]	0.46 ± 0.08 (9.66) [9]	-	-	-	-

Note: [1] $\log\beta_{pqr}$ refers to Equation (5); [2] $\log K_{pqr}$ refers to Equation (4); [3] values obtained by averaging potentiometric, UV-Vis spectrophotometric, and ^{1}H NMR spectroscopic data; [4,5,6] $\log\beta_{pqr}$ determined by potentiometry, UV-Vis spectrophotometry, and ^{1}H NMR spectroscopy, respectively; [7] standard deviation; [8] errors on weighed data; [9] $\log K_{11-1}$ refers to equilibrium: $Zn(OH)^+ + L^{z-} = ZnL(OH)^{(1-z)}$.

2.4.1. Zn^{2+}/L1, L3 and L4 Systems

The study on Zn^{2+}/L1 complexation allowed the determination of a model characterized by two species: $Zn(L1)^0{}_{(aq)}$ and $Zn(L1)OH^-$. The distribution diagram reported in Figure 5a, drawn at $I = 0.146$ mol L^{-1} in NaCl$_{(aq)}$ and $T = 298.15$ K, shows that the metal–ligand interaction starts at pH ~ 3.9 with the formation of $Zn(L1)^0{}_{(aq)}$ species reaching the 68% of formation at pH ~ 6.3, while the mixed hydroxo complex achieves its maximum formation percentage at pH ~ 10.5.

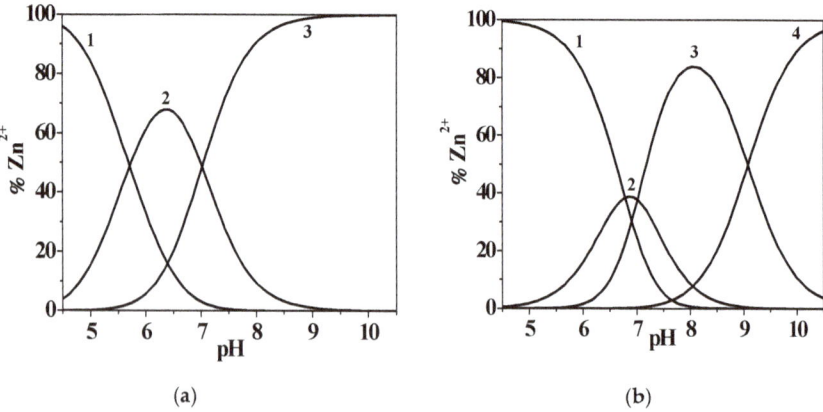

Figure 5. Distribution diagrams of Zn^{2+}/L1 (a) and L4 (b) ($c_{Zn}{}^{2+} = 4.3 \cdot 10^{-4}$ mol L^{-1}, $c_L = 1.2 \cdot 10^{-3}$ mol L^{-1}) species at $I = 0.150$ mol L^{-1} in NaCl$_{(aq)}$, $T = 298.15$ K. (a) Species: (1) free Zn^{2+}; 2. $Zn(L1)^0{}_{(aq)}$; (3) $Zn(L1)OH^-$. (b) Species: (1) free Zn^{2+}; 2. $Zn(L4)H^+$; (3) $Zn(L4)^0{}_{(aq)}$; (4) $Zn(L4)OH^-$.

L3 and L4 ligands, as shown in Figure 1, feature another protonable site, namely the –NH$_2$ group, with respect to L1; L3 is also characterized by an amidic moiety close to the amino and carboxylic groups.

The speciation schemes obtained for these Zn^{2+}/3,4-HPs systems are characterized by the formation of $ZnL^0_{(aq)}$, $ZnLOH^-$, and $ZnLH^+$ species. As listed in Table 2, the stability constants determined for Zn^{2+}/L3 and L5 ligands are higher than the ones obtained for L1, indicating that a possible involvement of the $-NH_2$ and amidic moieties could not be excluded in the metal–ligand interaction (for further details, see Section 2.4.2. Zn^{2+}/L2 system section); furthermore, in the case of the Zn^{2+}/L4 system, the formationconstant values at $I = 0.15$ mol L^{-1} in $NaCl_{(aq)}$ and $T = 298.15$ K are in good agreement among the different analytical techniques used. Figure 5b shows a distribution diagram drawn at $I = 0.147$ mol L^{-1} in $NaCl_{(aq)}$ and $T = 298.15$ K for the Zn^{2+}/L4 system.

With respect to the previous diagram, in this case the metal–ligand complexation starts at a higher pH value (pH ~ 4.7), in correspondence with the $Zn(L4)H^+$ species, which reaches 39% formation at pH ~ 6.9, while the simple 1:1 stoichiometry and the mixed-hydroxo complexes achieve 84% and 95% formation at pH ~ 8.0 and 10.5, respectively. The Zn^{2+}/L3 system displays a similar distribution, as observable in Figure S6.

2.4.2. Zn^{2+}/L2 Investigation

The solution study of the L2 ligand in the presence of Zn^{2+} was performed by means of potentiometric, UV-Vis spectrophotometric, and ^{1}H NMR investigation at $I = 0.15$ mol L^{-1} in $NaCl_{(aq)}$ and $T = 298.15$ K. The determined speciation model is characterized by three species, namely $Zn(L2)H^+$, $Zn(L2)^0_{(aq)}$, and $Zn(L2)OH^-$. In Table 2, the stability constants, determined with quite good accordance among the different analytical techniques, are reported together with the average of the obtained results. These last data are called "suggested values", which are useful for describing the system behavior in a more complete way by taking into account different component concentrations, namely high concentrations ($c_L \sim 10^{-2}$–10^{-3} mol L^{-1}) in potentiometric and ^{1}H NMR measurements, and low concentrations ($c_L \sim 10^{-5}$ mol L^{-1}) in UV-Vis spectrophotometric measurements.

The acid–base properties of L2 have already been studied by ^{1}H NMR spectroscopy and reported elsewhere [8]; conversely, the titrations performed in the presence of Zn^{2+} are herein commented on for the first time. The measurements were stopped at about pH ~ 8.1 due to the formation of sparingly soluble species. All the collected spectra showed only a single set of peaks, thus proving that the species formed in the solution present fast exchange on the NMR time scale, as observed for similar systems [4,27]. From the comparison of the data collected from the Zn^{2+}/L2 system with that of free L2, it can be argued that the presence of the metal cation leaves the signals referred to as *a*, *b*, *c*, and *d* almost unchanged below pH 4.5–5 (i.e., the protons closer to the hydroxo-oxo moiety). In detail, *a*, *c*, and *d* peaks show a common behavior, being slightly deshielded with respect to the corresponding signals of the free ligand, starting from approximately pH 5.0. At the same time, the resonance due to *b* undergoes a downfield shift compared to the L2 system from pH 4.5 onwards. The non-equivalent *f* protons, here reported as f_1 and f_2, display an opposite trend due to the presence of Zn^{2+}, with one being shielded and the other deshielded, starting from a more acidic pH than before (i.e., approximately 3.2). The *e* methylene as well as *g* methyne protons seem to be unaffected by the presence of the metal along the investigated pH range. It is worth remembering that each observed shift resulting from fast-exchanging species corresponds to an averaged shift, so that apparently some signals may not change upon pH increase or in the presence of metal as a result of mutual exchange. In this case, the calculation of the single resonances for each nucleus of the species present in equilibrium is required according to the selected speciation model, to gain deeper insight into the system in solution. Accordingly, by comparing the chemical shifts of the expected species calculated by means of HypNMR (Table S5) with the free ligand ones, it appears that for $Zn(L2)H^+$ the peaks more affected by the presence of the metal cation are *a*, *b*, f_1, f_2, and *g*, suggesting that the interactions occur both *via* hydroxo-oxo as well as amide part of the ligand. In the case of the other expected species, namely $Zn(L2)^0_{(aq)}$, the shifts, although less pronounced, involve the same protons, so that similar conclusions may be drawn. On these bases, it appears that for both species all the coordination sites of L2 allow the formation of the complexes, even though we do not feel confident enough to claim that clear indications have been obtained from NMR investigations for this system. Regardless, once again NMR studies provide useful information about the reliability of the system speciation profile. Further evidence of the structural features of the complexes was gathered by computer modeling. Preliminary attempts to calculate the preferred conformation of Zn(L2)H$^+$ and Zn(L2)^0$_{(aq)}$ in vacuo at the functional density level of theory did not produce reliable minima. It was, therefore, envisaged that placement of the ligand L2 and the Zn^{2+} cation within a cluster of 100 explicit water molecules would provide a more accurate description of the zinc–ligand interaction [28]. PM6 (Parameterization Method 6) semiempirical calculations yielded minimum energy geometries for the Zn(L2)H$^+$ and Zn(L2)^0$_{(aq)}$ complexes, both featuring the zinc cation in close proximity to the carboxylate moiety (Figure 6). Interestingly, the pyridinone oxygen atoms are not involved in complexation, regardless of their protonation state, although they are strongly solvated (water molecules not shown). Likewise, the amide moiety is seensolvated, but the zinc cation is too far away to interact with the carbonyl oxygen. The involvement of the carboxylate group is in line with the data obtained by ^{1}H NMR, with special reference to the diastereotopic hydrogen atoms f_1 and f_2. The increased chemical shift difference between the two resonances upon the addition of Zn^{2+} may be the result of the hampered rotational freedom of the aminoacidic moiety due to the interaction of the carboxylate with the metal. In agreement with this, the methyne proton g also undergoes a significant shift, and the modest shift of the e protons confirms the passive role played by the amide group.

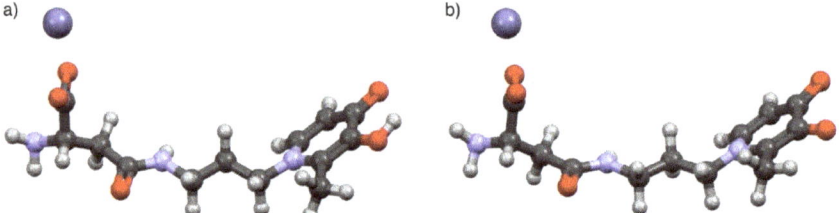

Figure 6. Ball-and-stick views of the PM3-optimized geometry (calculated within a cluster of 100 explicit water molecules) of the Zn^{2+}/L2 species: (**a**) Zn(L2)H$^+$ and (**b**) Zn(L2)^0$_{(aq)}$. Oxygen = red; carbon = grey; hydrogen = white, nitrogen = blue; zinc = dark blue.

UV-Vis spectrophotometric titrations were also carried out at $0.15 \leq I/\text{mol L}^{-1} \leq 1.00$ and $288.15 \leq T/\text{K} \leq 310.15$ to evaluate the effect of ionic strength and temperature on the speciation. The model obtained at $I = 0.15$ mol L^{-1} in NaCl$_{(aq)}$ and $T = 298.15$ K was confirmed atthe other experimental conditions and the Zn^{2+}/ligand complex formation constants are reported in Table 3.

The stepwise formation constants of Zn(L2)H$^+$ and Zn(L2)^0$_{(aq)}$ increase with I and decrease with T, as observable in Figure 7 for the metal–ligand 1:1 stoichiometry species. Concerning the hydrolytic mixed species, the stability decreases with ionic strength, but with an inversion of tendency at $I = 0.75$–1.00 mol L^{-1}, whilst the effect of temperature is opposite to that of the other two species. The influence of ionic strength on the speciation can be further examined by the analysis of Figure S7, in which a comparison between the UV-Vis titration curves is reported, recorded at $I = 0.501$ mol L^{-1} and 1.005 mol L^{-1} and $T = 298.15$ K. Analogous to the spectra reported in Figure 3B, for both ionic strength conditions, the intensity of the usual band at $\lambda_{max} = 278$ nm increases up to pH ~ 4.1, as already observed for the protonation reaction. Above pH ~ 5.2, a decrease of absorbance with a bathochromic shift and a further raise of signal with respect to the protonated species occur. An increase of the UV-Vis titration curve intensity with the variable increase was also noticed for the complexes along all pH ranges investigated.

Table 3. Overall [1] and stepwise [2] experimental stability constants of $Zn^{2+}/L2$ and $L5$ species determined at different ionic strengths and temperatures in $NaCl_{(aq)}$.

System	I/mol L^{-1}	T/K	$\log\beta_{111}$ [1] ($\log K_{111}$) [2]	$\log\beta_{110}$ [1,2]	$\log\beta_{11-1}$ [1] ($\log K_{11-1}$) [3]
$Zn^{2+}/L2$	0.147	288.15	15.90 [1] ± 0.03 [4] (5.62)	8.79[1] ± 0.10[4]	−1.50 [1] ± 0.12 [4] (8.18)[3]
	0.501	298.15	14.95 ± 0.05 (4.99)	8.34 ± 0.03	−1.26 ± 0.05 (7.82)
	0.759	298.15	14.97 ± 0.10 (5.085)	8.839 ± 0.009	−1.055 ± 0.009 (8.067)
	1.005	298.15	15.47 ± 0.08 (5.44)	9.26 ± 0.01	−0.804 ± 0.003 (8.357)
	0.152	310.15	15.50 ± 0.04 (4.51)	7.93 ± 0.16	0.47 ± 0.04 (9.25)
$Zn^{2+}/L5$	0.161	288.15	17.51 [1] ± 0.10 [4] (6.97)	9.67[1] ± 0.10[4]	-
	0.472	298.15	16.45 ± 0.02 (6.46)	9.03 ± 0.04	-
	0.725	298.15	16.09 ± 0.04 (6.29)	8.91 ± 0.06	-
	0.951	298.15	16.75 ± 0.09 (6.44)	8.49 ± 0.11	-
	0.155	310.15	16.65 ± 0.10 (6.08)	8.08 ± 0.11	-

Note: [1] $\log\beta_{pqr}$ refers to Equation (4); [2] $\log K_{pqr}$ refers to Equation (5); [3] $\log K_{11-1}$ refers to equilibrium: $Zn(OH)^+ + L^{2-} = ZnL(OH)^-$; [4] standard deviation.

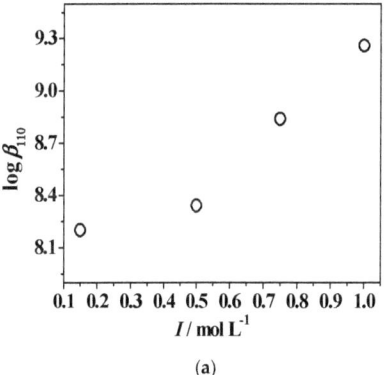 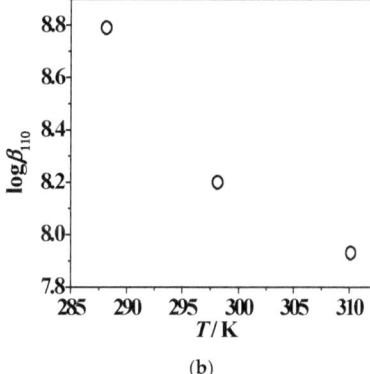

(a)   (b)

Figure 7. Trends of $Zn^{2+}/L2$ suggested $\log\beta_{110}$ values vs. the ionic strength (mol L^{-1}) in $NaCl_{(aq)}$ and T = 298.15 K (**a**) and vs. the temperature at I = 0.15 mol L^{-1} (**b**).

In Figure S8a, the distribution diagram of $Zn^{2+}/L2$ species, drawn at the same experimental conditions employed for the UV-Vis titration curves described previously, shows that all the species reach percentages higher than 20%, and in particular, at I = 1.005 mol L^{-1} the formation of $Zn(L2)H^+$ and $Zn(L2)^0_{(aq)}$ is shifted towards more acidic pH values than at I = 0.501 mol L^{-1}. In Figure S8b, the effect of temperature on the speciation is highlighted: the beginning of metal complexation is favored at higher temperature, starting from pH ~3.5 and 5.0 at T = 310.15 K and 288.15 K, respectively. The

Zn(L2)H$^+$ and Zn(L2)OH$^-$ complex formations reach higher percentages at high temperature, while Zn(L2)$^0_{(aq)}$ is characterized by an opposite trend. Low (<5%) formation percentages of the hydrolytic Zn(OH)$_2{}^0_{(aq)}$ species are observed in both T conditions; at T = 310.15 K, these start to form at pH ~ 6.8, whereas at lower temperature values this occurs at pH > 9.0.

2.4.3. Zn^{2+}/L5 System

The same analytical techniques employed for the previous system were used for the investigation of Zn^{2+}/L5 complexation at I = 0.15 mol L^{-1} in NaCl$_{(aq)}$ and T = 298.15 K. The speciation model, considered the best possible match with the already cited criteria, is characterized by two complex species, namely Zn(L5)H^{2+} and Zn(L5)$^+$. The stability constants are in good agreement among the different techniques, and the suggested values are reported in Table 2.

All ^{1}H NMR investigations carried out in Zn^{2+}/L5-containing solutions by varying the metal/ligand ratio and the relative concentrations, show comparable spectra in the same pH conditions, as well as a single set of resonances, indicating that although complex species may be present in solution, all of them are involved in a fast mutual exchange. By comparing the spectra collected for L5 acid–base properties with the ones recorded for the titrations on the Zn^{2+}-containing solutions, it appears that up to about pH 5.0 the chemical shifts due to the protons indicated as a, b, c, and d (i.e., the ones closer to pyridinone nitrogen on the aromatoid part of L5), are not influenced by the presence of the metal in the solution. Conversely, upon pH increasing, a and b signal results, as well as to a lesser extent c and d, shifted with respect to the corresponding free ligand peaks. In addition, the presence of the metal in the solution does not result in any shifting of e and f signals up to pH ~8.0; it is worth mentioning that the titrations stopped at approximately pH 9.0 due to the formation of sparingly soluble species. All of this experimental evidences suggest that at neutral pH only the hydroxo-oxo part of the ligand is involved in the formation of the expected species in these conditions, namely Zn(L5)H^{2+}, whereas at higher pH the whole L5 structure is involved in the Zn(L5)$^+$ formation. As usual, the theoretical chemical shifts, due to the nuclei belonging to each single complex species, were calculated by means of HypNMR (Table S5); once known, they were employed to recalculate the weight average chemical shifts, which should be closer to the observed ones if the proposed speciation model is reliable. From Figure 8, the almost total overlap of the experimental and the calculated average chemical shifts can be clearly observed, shown here for a, c, d, and f nuclei of L5 in the Zn^{2+}/L5 system, thus confirming the model employed for the rationalization of the data coming from potentiometric and spectrophotometric investigations.

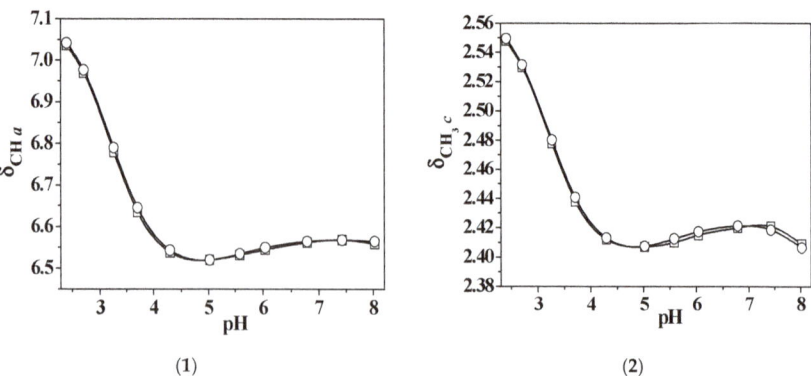

Figure 8. *Cont.*

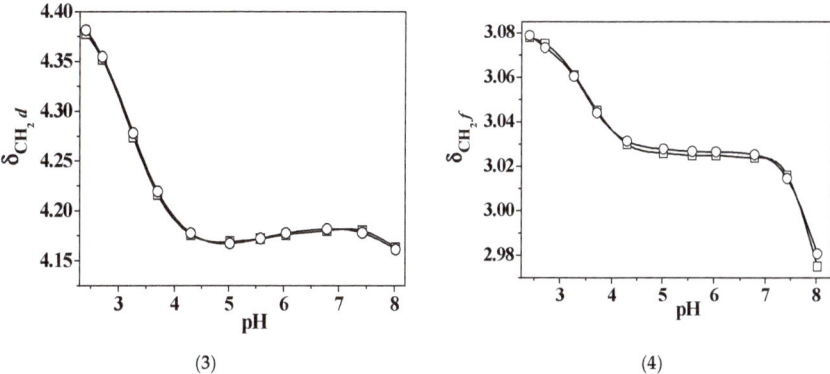

Figure 8. Observed (□) and calculated (○) values of chemical shifts of: *a* (**1**), *c* (**2**), *d* (**3**), and *f* (**4**) nuclei of L5 in Zn^{2+}/L5 system vs. pH at c_{Zn2+} = 3.3·10^{-2} mol L^{-1}, c_L = 1.0·10^{-2} mol L^{-1}, and I = 0.15 mol L^{-1} in NaCl$_{(aq)}$ and T = 298.15 K.

The geometry of the Zn(L5)H^{2+} and Zn(L5)$^+$ species was obtained by performing a preliminary equilibrium conformer search with a molecular modelling force field (MMFF). The minimum energy conformers were refined by the PM6 (Parameterization Method 6) semiempirical method, and the resulting structures were used as inputs for a geometry optimization at the DFT level of theory (B3LYP/6-31G(d)) [29]. Both complexes returned a similar arrangement (Figure 9), with the Zn^{2+} cation interacting with both the oxygen atoms of the pyridinone ring, again confirming the conclusions drawn by the ^{1}H NMR experiments. The only significant difference between the two complexes was in the oxygen–metal distances, which were found to be longer in Zn(L5)H^{2+} (=O···Zn^{2+}···OH of 1.85 and 2.04 Å, respectively) than in Zn(L5)$^+$ (=O···Zn^{2+}···O$^-$ of 1.85 and 1.84 Å, respectively), probably owing to the additional electrostatic attraction in the latter species.

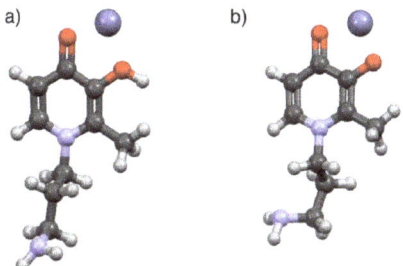

Figure 9. Ball-and-stick views of the DFT-optimized geometry (B3LYP/6-31G(d)) of the Zn^{2+}/L5 species: (**a**) Zn(L5)H^{2+} and (**b**) Zn(L5)$^+$. Oxygen = red; carbon = grey; hydrogen = white, nitrogen = blue; zinc = dark blue.

Potentiometric studies were also performed at different ionic strengths (0.15 ≤ I/mol L^{-1} ≤ 1.00) and temperatures (288.15 ≤ T/K ≤ 310.15) to check the influence of these variables on the speciation. In Table 3, the formation constants determined at the different experimental conditions are reported.

As also observable in Figure S9I, the logβ_{110} values decrease with I and T increasing. The same behavior characterizes the logK_{110} trend with temperature increase, while its stability decreases with ionic strength increasing, and it shows an inversion tendency at I = 1.00 mol L^{-1}. The variables effect can also be increased, as seen by the distribution diagrams in Figure S9II, drawn for two conditions: ionic strength increase, namely I = 0.161, 0.472, 0.951 mol L^{-1}, T = 298.15 K; and temperature increase, I = 0.15 mol L^{-1}, T = 288.15 K, and T = 310.15 K. In the first case, the Zn^{2+}/3-hydroxypyridinone complexation starts at pH ~ 3.0 and the percentages of Zn(L5)H^{2+} species increase with ionic strength, reaching values of 67%, 81%, and 92% in the pH range of 6.6–6.9. The metal–ligand 1:1 stoichiometry species formation, instead, is shifted at more alkaline pH conditions with I increase. In the second case, similarly to the previous system, metal complexation is favored at high temperature, beginning at pH < 2.0. The main species at physiological pH levels is Zn(L5)H^{2+}, where the formation of hydrolytic Zn(OH)$_2{}^0{}_{(aq)}$ and Zn(OH)$_3{}^-$ species occur, which does not happen at lower temperatures.

Confirmation of Zn^{2+}/L5 Species Formation by ESI-MS

In the literature, Clarke et al. [30] reported the results of a potentiometric and UV-Vis spectrophotometric studies on the speciation of deferiprone, a 1,2-dimethyl-3-hydroxy-4-pyridinone ligand, in the presence of trivalent and divalent metal cations, including Zn^{2+} at I = 0.15 mol L^{-1} in KCl$_{(aq)}$ and T = 298.15 K. In the case of zinc, two complexes were obtained, namely a 1:1 and a 1:2 stoichiometry metal–ligand species. On the contrary, Grgas-Kužnar's group [31] reported the results of an investigation on a Zn^{2+}/dopamine system at I = 0.50 mol L^{-1} in NaNO$_{3(aq)}$ and T = 303.15 K, determining only the Zn(Dop)H$^+$ species. Dopamine is characterized by a similar structure to L5, namely by an aromatic ring with two –OH substituents in the ortho position and an ethylamine group. As already discussed, the study presented in this paper on Zn^{2+}/3-hydroxy-pyridinone systems, did not lead to the determination of the 1:2 stoichiometry metal–ligand species, at the experimental conditions of the measurements, performed with different analytical techniques.

In light of these considerations, amongthe Zn^{2+}/(3-hydroxy-4-pyridinone) systems, the Zn^{2+}/L5 system was selected for further studies. Therefore, with the aim of confirming the Zn(L5)$^+$ complex formation and further verifying the possible determination of a Zn(L5)$_2{}^0{}_{(aq)}$ species, ESI-MS (Electrospray mass) measurements were performed on samples at different ionic strength conditions, such as I = 0.15 and 1.00 mol L^{-1} in NaCl$_{(aq)}$ at pH ~ 10.5. This pH value was chosen because it represents a condition under which only the 1:1 stoichiometry metal–ligand species is present in solution (see Figure 9), taking into account the speciation model already reported. The focus on this pH is also significant because the formation of the 1:2 stoichiometry metal–ligand species may occur in approximately the same pH range. Some measurements were also carried out in the absence of ionic medium to make comparisons among the possible species formed for NaCl-containing systems.

Prior to investigating the metal–ligand complexation, the spectra of ligand and metal cation were studied separately at the already cited experimental conditions. As observable in the distribution diagrams for L5 reported in Figure S5, and in accordance with the data already reported by this research group [8], the monoprotonated ligand species is present in solution at pH ~ 10.5, together with the fully deprotonated one. From the analysis of ESI-MS spectra recorded at all selected experimental conditions, the formation of three main ligand species was noticed, with m/z = 183.1, 205.1, and 221.1 (Table 4), attributable to the [H(L5) + H]$^+$ species and to the [H(L5) + Na]$^+$ and [H(L5) + K]$^+$ adducts, respectively.

Table 4. ESI-MS signals obtained for L5, Zn^{2+}, and Zn^{2+}/L5 systems.

Species	Theoretical m/z	Experimental m/z	Formula
[H(L5) + H]$^+$	183.11	183.1	C$_9$H$_{15}$N$_2$O$_2$
[H(L5) + Na]$^+$	205.10	205.1	C$_9$H$_{14}$N$_2$NaO$_2$
[H(L5) + K]$^+$	221.07	221.1	C$_9$H$_{14}$N$_2$KO$_2$
[Zn(H$_2$O)$_3$]$^{2+}$	58.98	59.0	ZnH$_6$O$_3$
[Zn + NaCl]$^{2+}$	60.94	61.0	ZnClNa
[Zn(H$_2$O)$_5$]$^{2+}$	76.99	76.9	ZnH$_{10}$O$_5$
[Zn(OH)]$^+$	80.93	81.0	ZnHO
[Zn(OH)(H$_2$O)]$^+$	98.94	98.9	ZnH$_3$O$_2$
[Zn(H$_2$O)$_6$(L5) + H + NaCl]$^{2+}$	206.03	206.0	ZnC$_9$H$_{26}$N$_2$ClNaO$_8$

The observation of the sodium and potassium adducts is very common in ESI-MS spectra, possible due to background impurities and to the considerable presence, in some cases, of ionic medium NaCl in solution [32]. Furthermore, an intensity decrease of the $[H(L5) + H]^+$ peak with ionic strength increase was noticed, in particular at $I = 1.00$ mol L^{-1}, due to a signal suppression attributable to the ionic medium effect, leading to a significant salt-adducted species formation [33–35].

Regarding the metal behavior, firstly it was investigated at pH ~ 10.5, but under all experimental conditions ($I = 0.15$, 1.00 mol L^{-1} in NaCl$_{(aq)}$, absence of ionic medium) the formation of a white, sparingly soluble species, probably attributable to Zn(OH)$_2{}^0{}_{(s)}$, made this investigation difficult. For these reasons, we decided to carry out some measurements at similar experimental conditions to the literature ones in the pH range of 6.0–7.5, in order to gain information on the ESI-MS Zn^{2+} behavior in aqueous solution and make comparisons with some data already present in the literature. ZnI$_2$ ($c_{Zn2+} = 0.002$ mol L^{-1}) was used instead of ZnCl$_2$ as a source of zinc and in the absence of ionic medium, however formation of the sparingly soluble species was not observed. At this pH range, as observable in Figure S10, the distribution diagram of Zn^{2+} in the absence of ionic medium, drawn using literature hydrolytic constants [6,25,26], shows that the metal cation is almost totally present in the free form, together with low percentages (<10%) of Zn(OH)$^+$ species. In accordance with the literature data [36], from the analysis of ESI-MS Zn^{2+} spectra, peaks related to the formation of $[Zn(H_2O)_n]^{2+}$ and $[Zn(OH)(H_2O)_n]^+$ clusters were noticed, as well as those attributable to chloride and sodium adducts, as reported in Table 4.

Concerning the Zn^{2+}/L5 complexation, the analysis of ESI-MS spectra, recorded at $I = 0.15$ and 1.00 mol L^{-1} in NaCl$_{(aq)}$, and in the absence of ionic medium, showed the presence of peaks related to L5 in all cases (i.e., $[H(L5) + H]^+$, $[H(L5) + Na]^+$, and $[H(L5) + K]^+$ adducts). In addition, the formation of the 1:1 stoichiometry metal–ligand complex was detected in the form of an adduct cluster with water molecules, Na$^+$, and Cl$^-$ ions, caused either by the background or the ionic medium effect (Table 4). Similar to the investigation of L5 spectra, also in this case the effect of NaCl was significant, and a signal suppression of peaks with ionic strength increasing characterized the complex under study. Moreover, regarding the possible formation of the 1:2 stoichiometry metal–ligand species, a small peak with a value of $m/z = 448.9$ was noticed only in the spectra in the absence of ionic medium, and was not present in any of those recorded at $I = 0.15$ and 1.00 mol L^{-1}. This signal, perhaps, could be attributable to a possible adduct $[Zn(L5)_2 + Na]^+$ with a theoretical value of $m/z = 449.11$, but the difference between the theoretical and the experimental values seems excessive for the type of instrument used.

Actually, on light of this consideration, and taking into account that all the results reported in the present paper were obtained from measurements in the presence of NaCl, we feel confident to state that under the used experimental conditions, the 1:2 stoichiometry metal–ligand species does not form, but we cannot exclude its formation under other conditions.

2.5. Dependence on Ionic Strength and Temperature

The dependence on ionic strength and temperature of L2 and L5 protonation and stability constants towards Zn^{2+} in NaCl$_{(aq)}$ was modeled using Equations (7)–(9). The thermodynamic parameters (equilibrium constants atinfinite dilution, C and $\Delta\varepsilon$ empirical parameters, ΔH values), determined by taking into account the values obtained from UV-Vis spectrophotometric, spectrofluorimetric [8], potentiometric, and ^{1}H NMR measurements, are reported in Table 5, together with the overall and stepwise free energy (ΔG) and the entropy changes ($T\Delta S$). The assessment of thermodynamic parameters provides a complete picture of the systems, whose equilibrium constants can be predicted for any experimental conditions.

Table 5. Thermodynamic parameters for the dependence on ionic strength and temperature of L2 and L5 protonation, and Zn^{2+} complex formation in $NaCl_{(aq)}$ at $T = 298.15$ K.

Species	$\log^T\beta_{pqr}$ [1] ($\log^T K_{pqr}$) [2]	C [3]	$\Delta\varepsilon$ [4]	ΔH [5,6] (Stepwise ΔH)	ΔG [5,6] (Stepwise ΔG)	$T\Delta S$ [5,6] (Stepwise $T\Delta S$)
$H(L2)^-$	11.32 ± 0.08 [7]	−0.71 ± 0.10 [7]	−0.69 ± 0.15 [7]	55 ± 12 [7]	−61.2 ± 0.2 [7]	116 ± 4 [7]
$H_2(L2)^0_{(aq)}$	20.54 ± 0.02 (9.22)	−2.72 ± 0.07	−2.74 ± 0.15	−200 ± 3 (−255)	−111.4 ± 0.5 (−50.2)	−88 ± 3 (−204)
$H_3(L2)^+$	25.35 ± 0.03 (4.81)	−2.94 ± 0.02	−2.88 ± 0.07	−260 ± 4 (−60)	−137.9 ± 0.5 (−26.5)	−122 ± 6 (−34)
$H_4(L2)^{2+}$	28.34 ± 0.04 (2.99)	−2.88 ± 0.02	−2.86 ± 0.10	−269 ± 14 (−9)	−156.5 ± 0.5 (−18.6)	−112 ± 6 (10)
$Zn(L2)H^+$	16.26 ± 0.12 (4.94)	0.59 ± 0.10	0.64 ± 0.07	−27 ± 9 (−80)	−88.5 ± 0.2 (−27.4)	61 ± 8 (−53)
$Zn(L2)^0_{(aq)}$	8.77 ± 0.05	2.12 ± 0.06	2.01 ± 0.01	−62 ± 1	−46.3 ± 0.2	−16 ± 1
$Zn(L2)OH^-$	−0.10 ± 0.01 (8.86)	0.25 ± 0.10	0.37 ± 0.05	153 ± 3 (96)	3.0 ± 0.2 (−49.4)	150 ± 3 (146)
$H(L5)^0_{(aq)}$	11.12 ± 0.10 [7]	−0.83 ± 0.10 [7]	−0.80 ± 0.19 [7]	1 ± 4 [7]	−63 ± 0.4 [7]	64 ± 4 [7]
$H_2(L5)^+$	20.54 ± 0.10 (9.42)	−1.26 ± 0.20	−1.24 ± 0.20	−271 ± 2 (−272)	−112.6 ± 1.1 (−49.6)	−158 ± 7 (−222)
$H_3(L5)^{2+}$	23.86 ± 0.08 (3.32)	−1.42 ± 0.20	−1.50 ± 0.32	−322 ± 12 (−51)	−135.1 ± 1.1 (−22.5)	−187 ± 12 (−29)
$Zn(L5)H^{2+}$	17.33 ± 0.18 (6.00)	−0.60 ± 0.09	−0.49 ± 0.14	−65 ± 8 (−66)	−97.7 ± 0.3 (−34.7)	33 ± 8 (−31)
$Zn(L5)^+$	10.57 ± 0.10	−1.24 ± 0.11	−1.38 ± 0.10	−127 ± 15	−52.1 ± 0.8	−75 ± 15

Note: [1,2] $\log^T\beta_{pqr}$ and $\log^T K_{pqr}$ refer to Equations (1) and (2), and (4)–(6), respectively, and are calculated under infinite dilution; in the molal concentration scale, their values are very similar to the results reported in molar one, with maximum differences of 0.002 logarithmic units; [3] parameter determined using Equation (7); [4] parameter calculated using Equation (8); [5] in kJ mol^{-1}; [6] at $I = 0.15$ mol kg^{-1}; [7] standard deviation.

The stepwise protonation enthalpy changes calculated at $I = 0.15$ mol L^{-1} and $T = 298.15$ K resulted in good agreement among the protonable groups belonging to both the ligands under investigation, and in all cases the reactions were spontaneous ($\Delta G < 0$). The protonation of –OH groups resulted an endothermic process, with positive ΔH values and a consequent heat absorbance from the system environment, while the entropic contribution was the driving force for the formation of protonated species. On the contrary, the protonation of the remaining sites is exothermic in nature, with negative ΔH values and a resulting heat transfer from the system environment. The comparison with the calculated $T\Delta S$ values allowed us to assert that for –NH$_2$, –COOH, and pyridinone nitrogen atoms, the enthalpic factor provided the driving force for the formation of protonated species. In the case of Zn^{2+}/3-hydroxy-pyridinone interactions, as listed in Table 5, for both ligands the enthalpic contribution is the main driving force for the complex formation of ZnLH$^{(3-z)}$ and ZnL$^{(2-z)}$ species, which is exothermic in nature; Zn(L2)OH$^-$ is instead characterized by an opposite tendency.

2.6. Literature Data Comparison

2.6.1. Protonation of the Ligands

The acid–base properties of L2 and L5, reported in this paper in NaCl$_{(aq)}$ at different ionic strength and temperature conditions, can be compared with data published in the literature by our research group on the same two ligands at $I = 0.15$ mol L^{-1} in NaCl$_{(aq)}$ and at $T = 298.15$ K and 310.15 K [8], and also by other authors for products (see Figure S11) characterized by similar structures and functional groups. In particular, it is possible to make the comparison of the two ligands' protonation constants at $I = 0.15$ mol L^{-1} in NaCl$_{(aq)}$ and $T = 298.15$ K (Table 1), with data from Clevette and coworkers [5], Crisponi's group [37–39], and Clarke et al. [30] (listed in Table 6). The first author worked at the same experimental conditions reported above, while the second and the third groups worked at conditions of $I = 0.15$ mol L^{-1} in KCl$_{(aq)}$ and $T = 298.15$ K. Bretti et al. [40] published a complete study on deferiprone

(DFP) behaviour in NaCl aqueous solution, studied by means of potentiometric measurements carried out at $0.10 \leq I/\text{mol L}^{-1} \leq 4.92$ and $283.15 \leq T/K \leq 318.15$.

Table 6. Literature protonation constants reported at different temperatures, ionic strengths, and ionic media in molar concentration scale.

Ligand	I/molL^{-1}	T/K	Ionic Medium	$\log K_1^H$	$\log K_2^H$	$\log K_3^H$	$\log K_4^H$	Ref.
DFP	0.099	283.15	NaCl	10.00	3.80	-	-	[40]
	0.152	298.15	NaCl	9.82	3.67	-	-	[40]
	0.150		NaCl	9.86	3.70	-	-	[5]
	0.495		NaCl	9.70	3.74	-	-	[40]
	1.005		NaCl	9.66	3.83	-	-	[40]
	0.100	310.15	NaCl	9.70	3.60	-	-	[40]
	0.100	298.15	KCl	9.82	3.66	-	-	[39]
	0.150		KCl	9.82	3.66	-	-	[37,38]
	0.150		KCl	9.77	3.68	-	-	[30]
	0.500		KCl	9.78	3.75	-	-	[39]
	1.000		KCl	9.75	3.80	-	-	[39]
	0.100	310.15	KCl	9.70	3.57	-	-	[39]
Pyridine	0.294	283.15	NaCl	5.50	-	-	-	[41]
	0.197	298.15	NaCl	5.28	-	-	-	[41]
	0.480		NaCl	5.37	-	-	-	[41]
	0.960		NaCl	5.52	-	-	-	[41]
	2.018	310.15	NaCl	5.66	-	-	-	[41]
Dopamine	0.147	288.15	NaCl	10.61	9.41	-	-	[24]
	0.162	298.15	NaCl	10.59	9.18	-	-	[24]
	0.504		NaCl	10.44	9.07	-	-	[24]
	0.737		NaCl	10.278	8.99	-	-	[24]
	0.982		NaCl	10.25	8.85	-	-	[24]
	0.165	310.15	NaCl	10.02	8.69	-	-	[24]
	0.500	303.15	NaNO$_3$	12.05	10.60	9.06	-	[31]
Aspartic acid	0.100	298.15	Na$^+$	9.66	3.71	1.95	-	[6]
	0.500		Na$^+$	9.58	3.68	1.98	-	[6]
	1.000		NaCl	9.61	3.64	2.00	-	[6]
	0.150	310.15	Na$^+$	9.33	3.64	1.94	-	[6]
Mimosine	0.150	310.15	KNO$_3$	8.86	7.00	2.62	1.10	[23]

The DFP protonation constants (Table 6), refined by the author at quite similar I and T conditions to those used in the present work, are in good agreement with the values obtained here for H(L2)$^-$, H$_4$(L2)$^{2+}$, H(L5)^0$_{(aq)}$, and H$_3$(L5)$^{2+}$ species, as reported in Table 1. As already mentioned in the literature [8] and in the section detailing L5 ligand acid–base properties, H(L2)$^-$ and H(L5)^0$_{(aq)}$ protonation constants are related to the –OH groups, while the H$_4$(L2)$^{2+}$ and H$_3$(L5)$^{2+}$ ones are related to the pyridinone nitrogen atom protonation.

The same research group [41] also reported the results of a potentiometric investigation carried out on pyridine in NaCl$_{(aq)}$, $0.29 \leq I/\text{mol L}^{-1} \leq 3.60$, and at $288.15 \leq T/K \leq 310.15$. In this case, the constant related to the nitrogen atom protonation showed similar ionic strength trends to those obtained for both the studied L2 and L5 ligands, but at similar experimental conditions to those reported here, the values reported by the author were higher than the ones we found. This difference may be due to a different electronic charge delocalization and to the absence on the pyridine ring structure of substituents and alkylic chains, which could influence the acid–base properties of the ligand. This research group [24] also investigated dopamine (Figure S11) behaviour in NaCl aqueous medium by means of potentiometric, UV-Vis spectrophotometric, and spectrofluorimetric measurements performed at $0.15 \leq I/\text{mol L}^{-1} \leq 1.02$ and $288.15 \leq T/K \leq 318.15$, where two protonable groups were determined, possibly related to the substituent groups, namely –OH in the aromatic ring and –NH$_2$ on the alkyl chain, which were present on the molecules. The affinity between dopamine data (Table 6) and L2 and L5 protonation constants (Table 1) at the different experimental conditions could be explained by the similarity of some dopamine moieties with respect to the ligand structures under investigation. Analogous data were obtained by Grgas-Kužnar's group [31], using a potentiometric study performed at $I = 0.50$ mol L^{-1} in NaNO$_{3(aq)}$ and $T = 303.15$ K. In this case, the only difference was the protonation constant value related to the other –OH group present on the molecule structure, which was detectable only by carrying out measurements at alkaline pH conditions.

L2 acid–base properties at different ionic strengths and temperatures can be compared with aspartic acid behavior, from which it is derived, reported by Martell et al. [6] at $0.10 \leq I$/mol L$^{-1} \leq 1.00$ in Na$^+$ ionic medium and $T = 298.15$ K and 310.15 K. The L2 protonation constants reported in this paper in Table 1 for the –NH$_2$ and –COOH groups are in good agreement with the literature data (Table 6), also providing a logK^H value for a second carboxylic group, which is not present in our structure.

Lastly, as already mentioned in the sections detailing L2 and L5 behavior in aqueous solution, there was a good accordance among the –NH$_2$ groups' protonation constants at $I = 0.15$ mol L^{-1} in NaCl$_{(aq)}$ and $T = 310.15$ K [9], along with the corresponding value for mimosine [23] (Table 6, Figure S11), studied at the same temperature and ionic strength but in KNO$_{3(aq)}$.

2.6.2. Zn^{2+}/Ligands Systems

Comparisons can be performed among the data for ZnL$^{(2-z)}$ species reported in the literature (Table 7) for similar ligand structures and functional groups as the investigated 3-hydroxy-4-pyridinones.

Clarke et al. [30] published a value of log$K_{110} = 7.19$ at $I = 0.15$ mol L^{-1} in KCl$_{(aq)}$ and $T = 298.15$ K, which is similar to the corresponding one here obtained for the Zn^{2+}/L1 system at $I = 0.15$ mol L^{-1} in NaCl$_{(aq)}$ and $T = 298.15$ K. The authors also determined the formation of a Zn(DFP)$^0{}_{2(aq)}$ species, while a hydrolytic mixed species was obtained here with L1.

Analogous to the acid–base properties, comparison can also be made between results and Zn^{2+}/pyridine (L = Py) complexation data present in the literature. In particular, Desai et al. [42] and Kapinos and coworkers [43] reported the results of potentiometric studies carried out at $I = 0.10$ mol L^{-1} in NaClO$_{4(aq)}$ and $I = 0.50$ mol L^{-1} in NaNO$_{3(aq)}$ and $T = 298.15$ K, respectively, with stability constants values of about 7–8 orders of magnitude lower than those we obtained for the ZnL$^{(2-z)}$ species, as could be expected due to the absence of functional groups that may participate in the metal coordination. The first author reported a speciation model characterized by protonated, simple 1:1 (Zn(Py)$^{2+}$), 1:2 (Zn(Py)$_2{}^{2+}$), and 1:3 (Zn(Py)$_3{}^{2+}$) metal–ligand stoichiometry species, while the second one only reported the formation of the Zn(Py)$^{2+}$ complex.

Table 7. Literature stability constants of Zn^{2+}/ligands species reported for different temperatures, ionic strengths, and ionic media in molar concentration scale.

Ligand	I/mol L^{-1}	T/K	Ionic Medium	logK_{111}	logK_{110}	logK_{120}	logK_{130}	Ref.
DFP	0.100	298.15	KCl	-	7.19	6.34	-	[30]
Pyridine	0.100	298.15	NaClO$_4$	5.50	1.10	0.60	0.38	[44]
	0.500	298.15	NaNO$_3$	-	1.15	-	-	[43]
Dopamine	0.500	293.15	NaNO$_3$	7.28	-	-	-	[31]
Aspartic acid	0.100	298.15	NaNO$_3$	-	5.35	-	-	[45]
	0.100		Na$^+$	-	5.87	-	-	[6]
	0.500		Na$^+$	-	5.60	9.93	-	[6]
	1.000		Na$^+$	-	5.64	-	-	[6]
	0.100	303.15	Na$^+$	-	-	10.16	-	[6]
	0.150	310.15	Na$^+$	1.55	5.82	10.13	-	[6]

Grgas-Kužnar's group [31], as mentioned above, reported the results of a potentiometric investigation carried out on the Zn^{2+}/dopamine (L = Dop) system at I = 0.50 mol L^{-1} in NaNO$_{3(aq)}$ and T = 303.15 K. The obtained speciation model was characterized only by the Zn(Dop)H$^+$ species, confirming the formation of the monoprotonated complex, as we also obtained for all the metal/–NH$_2$-containing ligand group (L2–L5) systems, which were studied at I = 0.15 mol L^{-1} in NaCl$_{(aq)}$ and T = 298.15 K. The stability constants found in the literature (Table 7) are ~1–2 orders of magnitude higher than the values presented here, probably because the stability of the formed Zn^{2+}/3,4-HPs species can be influenced by the absence of a hydroxyl group and the presence, in some cases, of carboxylic and amidic moieties.

Sajadi and coworkers [45] published the results of a potentiometric speciation study of Zn^{2+} in the presence of aspartic acid (Asp), of which L2 and L3 ligands are derivatives, carried out at I = 0.10 mol L^{-1} in NaNO$_{3(aq)}$ and T = 298.15 K, while Martell et al. [6] reported data from investigations in Na$^+$ ionic medium at different experimental conditions, such as $0.10 \leq I$/mol L$^{-1} \leq 1.00$ at T = 298.15 K, I = 0.10 mol L^{-1} at T = 303.15 K, and I = 0.15 at 310.15 K. In almost all cases, the authors obtained the Zn(Asp)$^0_{(aq)}$ species, with values 3.5–3.8 orders of magnitude higher than the ones reported here; the formation of Zn(Asp)H$^+$ and Zn(Asp)$_2^{2-}$ species also occurred only at some experimental conditions.

2.7. Sequestering Ability

The sequestering ability of a ligand towards a metal cation can be evaluated by the determination of an empirical parameter, pL$_{0.5}$. It has already been proposed by the research group and represents the total concentration of ligand that is required to sequester 50% of a metal cation present in trace concentration in solution. This parameter is described by the following sigmoidal-type Boltzmann equation (Equation (12)):

$$x_M = \frac{1}{1 + 10^{(pL - pL_{0.5})}} \tag{12}$$

where x_M is the mole fraction of the metal cation complexed by the ligand, pL = $-\log c_L$, and pL$_{0.5}$ = $-\log c_L$, if x_M = 0.5. A detailed description of pL$_{0.5}$ calculation, importance, and applications is reported in the literature [18].

An investigation on the sequestering ability of the five 3-hydroxy-4-pyridinone ligands towards Zn^{2+} was carried out at I = 0.15 mol L^{-1} in NaCl$_{(aq)}$ and T = 298.15 K, and in the case of L2 and L5, also at different ionic strengths ($0.15 \leq I$/mol L$^{-1} \leq 1.00$) and temperatures ($288.15 \leq T$/K ≤ 310.15).

From the data reported in Table 8 and the graphs in Figure 10, it can be argued that for all the systems the sequestering ability assumes significant values starting from pH ~ 3.0–4.0, due to the beginning of metal complexation with pH increasing up to pH ~ 9.0, where the possible formation of Zn^{2+} hydrolytic or mixed-hydrolytic species may influence the systems. At physiological pH level (pH ~ 7.4), I = 0.15 mol L^{-1} in NaCl$_{(aq)}$, and T = 298.15 K, the sequestering ability is influenced, as expected, by the different acid–base properties of the ligands, and it decreases with alkyl chain length; the trend is: L1 > L5 > L4 > L3 > L2. Concerning the ionic strength effect, as already stated for L2 protonation behaviour, the presence of sodium chloride would seem to stabilize the system, which may be the reason why, as shown in Table 8 and Figure 10, the sequestering ability increases with increasing I, while in the case of Zn^{2+}/L5 species, it reaches its maximum value at T = 310.15 K.

Table 8. The $pL_{0.5}$ [1] values of Zn^{2+}/ligand systems with different pH, ionic strengths, and temperatures in $NaCl_{(aq)}$.

System	pH	$pL_{0.5}$	I/mol L^{-1}	T/K	System	pH	$pL_{0.5}$	I/mol L^{-1}	T/K
Zn^{2+}/L1	2.5	<1.0	0.15	298.15	Zn^{2+}/L2	7.4	6.3	0.75	298.15
	3.0	<1.0	0.15	298.15		7.4	6.8	1.00	298.15
	4.0	1.0	0.15	298.15		7.4	5.2	0.15	310.15
	5.0	2.5	0.15	298.15	Zn^{2+}/L3	7.4	4.2	0.15	298.15
	6.0	3.6	0.15	298.15	Zn^{2+}/L4	7.4	4.4	0.15	298.15
	7.4	5.5	0.15	298.15	Zn^{2+}/L5	7.4	5.4	0.15	288.15
	8.1	6.7	0.15	298.15		2.5	<1.0	0.15	298.15
	9.0	7.6	0.15	298.15		3.0	<1.0	0.15	298.15
	10.0	7.3	0.15	298.15		4.0	<1.0	0.15	298.15
Zn^{2+}/L2	7.4	6.3	0.15	288.15		5.0	2.0	0.15	298.15
	2.5	<1.0	0.15	298.15		6.0	3.0	0.15	298.15
	3.0	<1.0	0.15	298.15		7.4	4.7	0.15	298.15
	4.0	<1.0	0.15	298.15		8.1	5.8	0.15	298.15
	5.0	1.0	0.15	298.15		9.0	6.6	0.15	298.15
	6.0	2.0	0.15	298.15		10.0	4.7	0.15	298.15
	7.4	3.8	0.15	298.15		7.4	5.2	0.50	298.15
	8.1	5.0	0.15	298.15		7.4	5.3	0.75	298.15
	9.0	5.7	0.15	298.15		7.4	5.1	1.00	298.15
	10.0	5.5	0.15	298.15		7.4	6.3	0.15	310.15
	7.4	5.6	0.50	298.15					

[1] Values calculated using Equation (12).

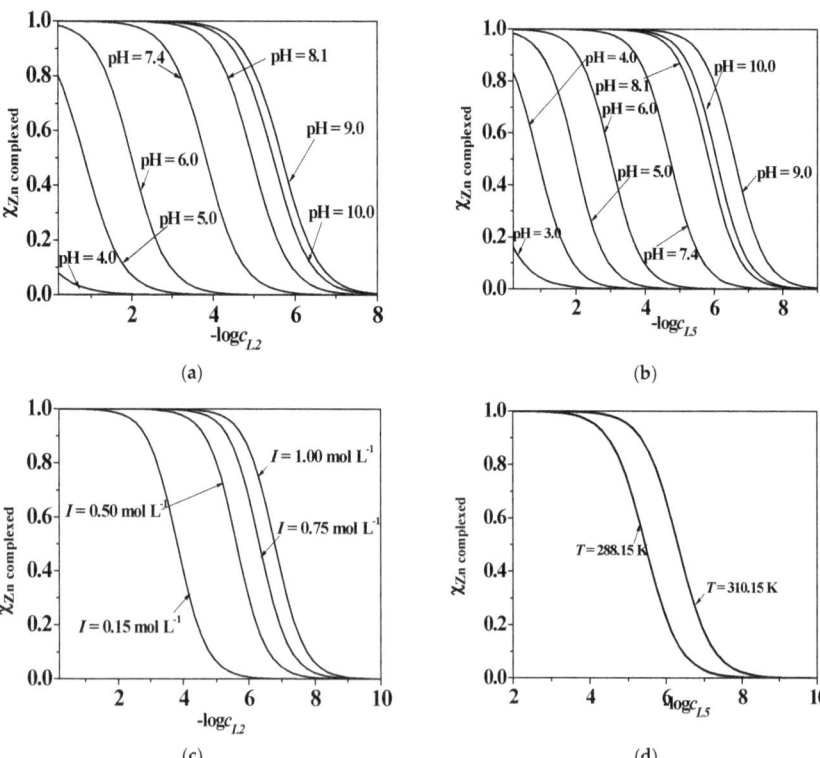

Figure 10. Sequestration diagrams of Zn^{2+}/L2 and L5 species with different pH (**a**,**b**), ionic strength (**c**), and temperature (**d**) values.

2.8. Zn^{2+} Depletion vs. Al^{3+} Sequestration

A comparison of this paper's data can be performed with those already reported in the literature by this research group for the Al^{3+} complexation by the same bifunctional ligands [8], at $I = 0.15$ mol L^{-1} in $NaCl_{(aq)}$ and $T = 298.15$ K. The main purpose of this paper, as already mentioned, was to verify, from a thermodynamic point of view, if there could be a significant depletion of an important divalent bio-metal such as Zn^{2+}, along with the strong sequestering activity towards the trivalent metal cations. In particular, the determined stability constants related to the $ZnL^{(2-z)}$ species (Table 2) and the corresponding values reported in Table S6 at the same experimental conditions for the $AlL^{(3-z)}$ complex can be compared, observing that for all the bifunctional ligands the stability of the simple Al 1:1 stoichiometry species is much higher than those obtained with Zn^{2+}. Moreover, a comparison among the physiological $pL_{0.5}$ values calculated for all the ligands towards both the metal cations (Table 8 and Table S6) can be carried out, showing that the sequestering ability of 3-hydroxy-4-pyridinones is stronger towards Al^{3+} than Zn^{2+} for *L1*, *L2*, *L3*, and *L4* ligands, with values of $\Delta pL_{0.5} = 0.8, 3.9, 2.2$, and 3.0, respectively. Only in the case of *L5* is the tendency is opposite, due to the absence of the –COOH group in the ligand structure (Figure 1), which, as already pointed in the literature, should allow the formation of the sparingly soluble $Al(OH)_3{}^0{}_{(s)}$ species under acidic pH values (pH ~ 5.0), influencing in a noteworthy way the sequestering ability of the ligand towards Al^{3+} [46].

In light of these considerations, it is possible to claim, from a thermodynamic point of view, that no competition between Zn^{2+}/Al^{3+} should occur since the ligands promote the removal of *hard* metal cations from the human body, while avoiding the possibility of bio-metal depletion.

3. Materials and Methods

3.1. Chemicals

HCl and NaOH standard solutions were prepared for dilution of Riedel–deHäen concentrated ampoules and were standardized against sodium carbonate and potassium hydrogen phthalate, respectively. Sodium hydroxide solutions were preserved from atmospheric CO_2 using soda lime traps. The NaCl ionic medium aqueous solutions were prepared by weighing the pure salt purchased from Fluka, which was previously dried in an oven at $T = 383.15$ K for at least 2 h. The reagents used for all investigations were of the highest available purity and the solutions were prepared with analytical grade water (R = 18 MΩ cm^{-1}), using grade A glassware. The ligands under study, namely *L1–L5* (see Figure 1), were synthesized following procedures already reported in the literature [8]. The Zn^{2+} solutions were prepared by weighing $ZnCl_2$ Fluka salt without further purification, and standardized using EDTA (ethylenediaminetetraacetic acid) standard solutions; their purity was always ≥98% [47].

3.2. Analytical Equipment and Procedures

3.2.1. Potentiometric Tools and Procedure

A Metrohm Titrando (model 809) and a potentiometer with a combined glass electrode (Ross type 8102, from Thermo-Orion) coupled with an automatic burette were used for the potentiometric experiments. This apparatus was connected to a computer and automatic titrations were performed with MetrohmTiAMO 1.2 software, to control titrant delivery, data acquisition, and e.m.f. (electromotive force) stability. Estimated accuracy was ±0.15 mV and ±0.003 mL for e.m.f. and titrant volume readings, respectively. The titrations were carried out using 25 mL of thermostated solution under magnetic stirring. Purified presaturated nitrogen was bubbled into the solutions to keep out the presence of oxygen and carbon dioxide.

For each measurement, titrations of hydrochloride with standard sodium hydroxide solutions were performed, at the same ionic medium, ionic strength, and temperature conditions as those used for the investigated systems, to refine the electrode potential (E^0), the acidic junction potential ($Ej = j_a[H^+]$), and the ionic product of water (K_w) values. The pH scale used was the free scale and pH≡ −log[H$^+$], where [H$^+$] is the free proton concentration. Then, 80–100 data points were collected for each titration and the equilibrium state during the experiments was checked by adopting necessary precautions, such as checking the necessary time to reach equilibrium and performing back titrations.

The acid–base properties and binding ability of L5 (Figure 1, $5.0·10^{-4} \leq c_{L5}/\text{mol L}^{-1} \leq 1.5·10^{-3}$) towards Zn^{2+} ($3.9·10^{-4} \leq c_{Zn2+}/\text{mol L}^{-1} \leq 1.0·10^{-3}$) were investigated by means of potentiometric measurements at metal/ligand ratios between 1:4 and 1:1, $0.15 \leq I/\text{mol L}^{-1} \leq 1.00$ in NaCl$_{(aq)}$, $288.15 \leq T/K \leq 310.15$, and in the pH range of 2.0–10.5. Zn^{2+}/(L1–L4) complexation was studied by performing potentiometric measurements at $I = 0.15$ mol L^{-1} in NaCl$_{(aq)}$, $T = 298.15$ K, in the pH range of 2.0–10.5, and with the same concentrations of ligands and metal cations used for the Zn^{2+}/L5 system.

3.2.2. UV-Vis Spectrophotometric Equipment and Procedure

Spectrophotometric measurements were performed by means of an UV-Vis spectrophotometer (Varian Cary 50 model) equipped with an optic fiber probe, featuring a 1 cm fixed-path length. The instrument was linked to a computer and Varian Cary WinUV software was used to record the signal of absorbance (A) vs. wavelength (λ/nm). Simultaneously, potentiometric data were collected using a combined glass electrode (Thermo-Orion Ross type 8102) connected to a potentiometer. A Metrohm 665 automatic burette was used to deliver the sodium hydroxide titrant in 25 mL thermostated cells. A magnetic stirrer ensured the homogeneity of the solutions during the measurements. N$_{2(g)}$ was bubbled in the solutions for at least 5 min before starting the titrations, with the purpose of excluding the possible presence of atmospheric oxygen and carbon dioxide.

UV-Vis spectrophotometric titrations were carried out in NaCl$_{(aq)}$ at $0.15 \leq I/\text{mol L}^{-1} \leq 1.00$, $288.15 \leq T/K \leq 310.15$, and in the wavelength range of $200 \leq \lambda/\text{nm} \leq 800$, to study L2 ($4.0·10^{-5} \leq c_L/\text{mol L}^{-1} \leq 6.0·10^{-5}$) protonation and binding ability towards Zn^{2+} ($2.0·10^{-5} \leq c_{Zn2+}/\text{mol L}^{-1} \leq 6.0·10^{-5}$), with metal/ligand ratios between 1:4 and 1:1. The metal complexation by the other ligands (L1, L3–L5, Figure 1) was investigated by performing measurements at $I = 0.15$ mol L^{-1} in NaCl$_{(aq)}$, $T = 298.15$ K, $2.0 \leq pH \leq 10.5$. An analogous wavelength range and the concentrations of 3-hydroxy-4-pyridinones and Zn^{2+} used for the Zn^{2+}/L2 system were also selected for these metal–ligands investigations.

3.2.3. ^{1}H NMR Apparatus and Procedure

^{1}H NMR measurements were recorded using a Bruker AVANCE 300 operating at 300 MHz in 9:1 H$_2$O/D$_2$O solution. The chemical shifts were measured with respect to 1,4-dioxane and converted relative to tetramethylsilane (TMS), employing $\delta_{(dioxane)} = 3.70$ ppm. The acid–base properties of L2 have already been investigated and are reported elsewhere [8], whilst L5 behavior in aqueous solution was studied using ^{1}H NMR titrations in $1.0·10^{-2}$ mol L^{-1} ligand solutions, in the pH range of 2.0–11.0, with $I = 0.15$ mol L^{-1} in NaCl$_{(aq)}$ and $T = 298.15$ K. The spectra of the Zn^{2+}-containing solutions in the presence of L2 or L5 were recorded by adding known volumes of a sodium hydroxide solution to mixtures of the ligands ($5.0·10^{-3} \leq c_L/\text{mol L}^{-1} \leq 1.0·10^{-2}$) and the metal cation ($2.5·10^{-3} \leq c_{Zn2+}/\text{mol L}^{-1} \leq 1.0·10^{-2}$), in the same ionic medium and pH range already mentioned.

3.2.4. MS Spectroscopy Apparatus and Procedure

Electrospray mass (ESI-MS) spectrometric spectra were recorded on an Agilent LC/MS instrument in positive ion mode using a LC/QQQ 6420 series spectrometer equipped with an electrospray ionization source model G1948B. The instrument was used as simple ESI-MS equipment, thus the column was bypassed and 5 µL of the samples were introduced by flow injection analysis, with water as the solvent flow phase at a flow rate of 0.4 mL min^{-1}. Preliminary experiments were performed to establish optimal experimental settings for the ESI-MS conditions, which were capillary voltage 4 kV, fragmentor voltage 135 V, and source temperature 300 °C. Nitrogen was used as the nebulization and desolvation gas at 15 psi and 11 L min^{-1}. Spectra were obtained in MS2 scan mode with the Agilent software Masshunter B.06.00.

The mass spectra of L5, Zn^{2+}, and their mixtures were investigated at I = 0.15 and 1.00 mol L^{-1} in $NaCl_{(aq)}$ and in the absence of ionic medium. Ligand and metal concentrations were $1.0 \cdot 10^{-3} \leq c_L$/mol $L^{-1} \leq 5.4 \cdot 10^{-3}$ and $1.0 \cdot 10^{-3} \leq c_{Zn^{2+}}$/mol $L^{-1} \leq 5.0 \cdot 10^{-3}$, respectively. The pH of each measurement solution was adjusted using NaOH standard solutions.

3.3. Computer Programs

The determination of the acid–base titration parameters, such as E^0, pK_w, and j_a, and analytical concentration of reagents was carried out using the non-linear least squares ESAB2M [48] computer program. The potentiometric data were elaborated using the BSTAC [49] computer program and checks were performed by means of the HYPERQUAD 2008 software [50]. This last program was also used to analyze UV-Vis spectrophotometric data. Since for L5 protonation investigations, as well as for Zn^{2+}/L5 and Zn^{2+}/L2 ^{1}H-NMR titrations, protons were found to rapidly exchange on the NMR time scale, HypNMR was employed to calculate the individual chemical shifts of all the species present at equilibria, together with the protonation constants, as well as the stability constants [51]. The LIANA [52] computer program was used to refine the parameters for the dependence of thermodynamic parameters on ionic strength and temperature. HySS program [53] allowed the calculation of species formation percentages and the representation of distribution or speciation diagrams.

3.4. Computational Studies

The conformational analysis of the Zn^{2+}/L2 and Zn^{2+}/L5 systems was carried out with the molecular mechanics force field (MMFF) by using the Monte Carlo method to randomly sample the conformational space.

For the Zn^{2+}/L5 complexes, the equilibrium geometries were further refined using semi-empirical methods (PM6), and finally optimized at the density functional level of theory (DFT, B3LYP functional) using the 6-31G(d) basis set.

As for the Zn^{2+}/L2 complexes, the conformational analysis was carried out in a water cluster consisting of 100 explicit solvent (water) molecules with the molecular mechanics force field (MMFF), without constraints. The geometry obtained was further refined by semiempirical methods at the PM6 level. All quantum mechanical calculations were performed using Spartan'10 (Wavefunction, Inc., California) [54].

4. Conclusions

The acid–base behavior of two bifunctional 3-hydroxy-4-pyridinone ligands, namely L2 and L5, which are derivatives of deferiprone, was investigated by potentiometric, UV-Vis spectrophotometric, and ^{1}HNMR titrations at different temperatures and ionic strengths in $NaCl_{(aq)}$. Regarding the protonation of L2, the results of UV-Vis studies conducted at different I values showed a speciation model with a general trend of protonations occurring at slightly higher pH values with ionic strength, probably due to a noteworthy contribution of the ionic medium to the ligand speciation in aqueous solution. The speciation model obtained for L5 was confirmed by means of ^{1}H NMR spectroscopic titrations performed at I = 0.15 mol L^{-1} and T = 298.15 K. This analytical technique resulted an effective tool to possibly attribute the protonation constants to the corresponding functional groups. Furthermore, a speciation study of both 3-hydroxy-4-pyridinones in the presence of Zn^{2+} was performed under the same experimental conditions as the protonation study; an investigation at I = 0.15 mol L^{-1} and T = 298.15 K was also carried out for the other three Zn^{2+}/L^{z-} systems with ligands belonging to the same class of compounds. The elaboration of the experimental data allowed the determination of overall and stepwise stability constants and metal–ligand species with different stoichiometry ($Zn_pL_qH_r^{(2p+r-qz)}$). The obtained values were in accordance with the different analytical techniques and with the data already reported in the literature for ligands with analogous structures and protonable groups. ESI-MS spectrometric measurements performed under different experimental conditions confirmed the formation of 1:1 zinc–L5 species. Computational studies provided useful information on the geometry of metal–ligand coordination, showing that $L2$ binds with Zn^{2+} mainly by its carboxylate moiety, whereas $L5$, in all the pH ranges where zinc–ligand species are formed, takes advantage of the hydroxo-oxo moiety of the pyridinone ring.

The dependence on ionic strength of equilibrium constants was investigated by means of two commonly used models, the extended Debye–Hückel (EDH) model and the classical specific ion interaction theory (SIT). The study of temperature effect, using the van't Hoff equation, allowed the determination of protonation and formation enthalpy changes calculated at $I = 0.15$ mol L^{-1} and $T = 298.15$ K; the Gibbs free energy and the entropy change were also calculated. For both ligands, the protonation of –OH groups resulted an endothermic process, while an inverse behavior characterized the remaining sites, with reactions being exothermic in nature. Regarding Zn^{2+}/3-hydroxy-pyridinone interactions, the enthalpic contribution resulted in the main driving force for the complex formation of $ZnLH^{(3-z)}$ and $ZnL^{(2-z)}$ species, which was exothermic in nature; the formation of $Zn(L2)OH^-$ was instead characterized by an opposite tendency.

Furthermore, on the light of the comparison between the Zn^{2+} data reported in the present paper and those published in the literature for Al^{3+}/3,4-HP complexation, from a thermodynamic point of view it is possible to affirm that no competition between Zn^{2+}/Al^{3+} should occur, since the ligands are able to promote the removal of the *hard* metal cation from the human body, while avoiding the possibility of bio–metal (zinc) depletion. At physiological pH, $I = 0.15$ mol L^{-1} in $NaCl_{(aq)}$, and $T = 298.15$ K, the sequestering ability follows the trend: $L1 > L5 > L4 > L3 > L2$; in addition, it increases with I increasing, while for $Zn^{2+}/L5$ species, it reaches its maximum value at $T = 310.15$ K.

Supplementary Materials: The following are available online, Figures S1–S11, Tables S1–S5.

Author Contributions: Conceptualization, M.A.S., S.S., C.D.S., and A.I.; formal analysis, A.I., K.C., G.G., A.P., N.M., and S.C.; investigation, A.I., P.C., and N.M.; data curation, A.I., R.M.C., F.C., and P.C.; writing—original draft preparation, A.I., P.C., G.G., and N.M.; writing—review and editing, A.I., R.M.C., and F.C.; supervision, M.A.S., S.S., and C.D.S.; project administration, M.A.S., S.S., and C.D.S.; funding acquisition, M.A.S., S.S., and C.D.S.

Funding: The authors from the University of Messina and Palermo thank *Ministero dell'Istruzione, dell'Università e della Ricerca* (MIUR) for financial support (co-funded by the PRIN project with prot. 2015MP34H3). The authors from (IST) University of Lisbon thank the Portuguese *Fundação para a Ciência e Tecnologia* (FCT) for financial support for the projects UID/QUI/00100/2013 and PEst-C/SAU/LA0001/2011-2013, and the postdoctoral fellowship (K.C.). Acknowledgements are also due to the Portuguese NMR (IST-UL Center) and Mass Spectrometry Networks (Node IST-CTN) for providing access to their facilities.

Conflicts of Interest: The authors declare no conflict of interest.

References

1. Santos, M.A. Recent developments on 3-hydroxy-4-pyridinones with respect to their clinical applications: Mono and combined ligand approaches. *Coordin. Chem. Rev.* **2008**, *252*, 1213–1224. [CrossRef]
2. Santos, M.A.; Chaves, S. 3-hydroxypyridinone derivatives as metal sequestering agents for therapeutic use. *Future Med. Chem.* **2015**, *7*, 383–410. [CrossRef] [PubMed]
3. Queiros, C.; Amorim, M.J.; Leite, A.; Ferreira, M.; Gameiro, P.; de Castro, B.; Biernacki, K.; Magalhães, A.; Burgess, J.; Rangel, M. Nickel(II) and Cobalt(II) 3-Hydroxy-4-pyridinone Complexes: Synthesis, Characterization and Speciation Studies in Aqueous Solution. *Eur. J. Inorg. Chem. Wiley Online Libr.* **2011**, 131–140. [CrossRef]
4. Irto, A.; Cardiano, P.; Chand, K.; Cigala, R.M.; Crea, F.; De Stefano, C.; Gano, L.; Gattuso, G.; Sammartano, S.; Santos, M.A. New bis-(3-hydroxy-4-pyridinone)-NTA-derivative: Synthesis, binding ability towards Ca^{2+}, Cu^{2+}, Zn^{2+}, Al^{3+}, Fe^{3+} and biological assays. *J. Mol. Liq.* **2018**, *272*, 609–624. [CrossRef]
5. Clevette, D.J.; Nelson, W.O.; Nordin, A.; Orvig, C.; Sjoeberg, S. The complexation of aluminum with N-substituted 3-hydroxy-4-pyridinones. *Inorg. Chem.* **1989**, *28*, 2079–2081. [CrossRef]
6. Martell, A.E.; Smith, R.M.; Motekaitis, R.J. *NIST Critically Selected Stability Constants of Metal Complexes Database, 8.0*; National Institute of Standard and Technology: Garthersburg, MD, USA, 2004.
7. Neilands, J.B. Microbial Iron Compounds. *Annu. Rev. Biochem.* **1981**, *50*, 715–731. [CrossRef] [PubMed]

8. Irto, A.; Cardiano, P.; Chand, K.; Cigala, R.M.; Crea, F.; De Stefano, C.; Gano, L.; Sammartano, S.; Santos, M.A. Bifunctional 3-hydroxy-4-pyridinones as effective aluminium chelators: Synthesis, solution equilibrium studies and in vivo evaluation. *J. Inorg. Biochem.* **2018**, *186*, 116–129. [CrossRef] [PubMed]
9. Santos, M.A.; Gil, M.; Marques, S.; Gano, L.; Cantinho, G.; Chaves, S. N-Carboxyalkyl derivatives of 3-hydroxy-4-pyridinones: Synthesis, complexation with Fe(III), Al(III) and Ga(III) and in vivo evaluation. *J. Inorg. Biochem.* **2002**, *92*, 43–54. [CrossRef]
10. Buffle, J. *Complexation Reactions in Aquatic Systems: An Analytical Approach*; Ellis Horwood: Chichester, UK, 1988.
11. Lentner, C. *Geigy Scientific Tables*, 8th ed.; CIBA-Geigy: Basilea, Switzerland, 1981.
12. Millero, F.J. *Physical Chemistry of Natural Waters*; John Wiley & Sons, Inc.: New York, NY, USA, 2001.
13. Kot, A.; Namiesnik, J. The role of speciation in analytical chemistry. *Trends Analyt. Chem.* **2000**, *19*, 69–79. [CrossRef]
14. Templeton, D.M.; Ariese, F.; Cornelis, R.; Danielsson, L.G.; Muntau, H.; Van Leeuwen, H.P.; Łobinsky, R. Guidelines for terms related to chemical speciation and fractionation of elements. Definitions, structural aspects, and methological approaches. *Pure App. Chem.* **2000**, *72*, 1453–1470. [CrossRef]
15. Deshpande, J.D.; Joshi, M.M.; Giri, P.A. Zinc: The trace element of major importance in human nutrition and health. *Int. J. Med. Sci. Public Health* **2013**, *2*, 1–6. [CrossRef]
16. Powell, S.R. The antioxidant properties of zinc. *J. Nutr.* **2000**, *130*, 1447S–1454S. [CrossRef] [PubMed]
17. Kaltenberg, J.; Plum, L.M.; Ober-Blöbaum, J.L.; Hönscheid, A.; Rink, L.; Haase, H. Zinc signals promote IL-2-dependent proliferation of T cells. *Eur. J. Immunol.* **2010**, *40*, 1496–1503. [CrossRef] [PubMed]
18. Crea, F.; De Stefano, C.; Foti, C.; Milea, D.; Sammartano, S. Chelating agents for the sequestration of mercury(II) and monomethyl mercury(II). *Curr. Med. Chem.* **2014**, *21*, 3819–3836. [CrossRef] [PubMed]
19. Foti, C.; Sammartano, S. Ionic Strength Dependence of Protonation Constants of Carboxylate Ions in NaCl$_{aq}$ ($0 \leq I \leq 5.6$ mol·kg^{-1}) and KCl$_{aq}$ ($0 \leq I \leq 4.5$ mol·kg^{-1}): Specific Ion Interaction Theory and Pitzer Parameters and the Correlation between Them. *J. Chem. Eng. Data* **2010**, *55*, 904–911. [CrossRef]
20. Biederman, G. Ionic Media. In *Dahlem Workshop on the Nature of Seawater*; Dahlem Konferenzen: Berlin, Germany, 1975.
21. Biederman, G. Introduction to the specific interaction theory with emphasis on chemical equilibria. In *Metal Complexes in Solution*; Jenne, E.A., Rizzarelli, E., Romano, V., Sammartano, S., Eds.; Piccin: Padua, Italy, 1986; pp. 303–314.
22. Grenthe, I.; Puigdomenech, I. *Modelling in Aquatic Chemistry*; OECD: Paris, France, 1997.
23. Stunzi, H.; Perrin, D.D.; Teitei, T.; Harris, R.L.N. Stability Constants of Some Metal Complexes Formed by Mimosine and Related Compounds. *Aust. J. Chem.* **1979**, *32*, 21–30. [CrossRef]
24. Bretti, C.; Crea, F.; De Stefano, C.; Foti, C.; Materazzi, S.; Vianelli, G. Thermodynamic Properties of Dopamine in Aqueous Solution. Acid–Base Properties, Distribution, and Activity Coefficients in NaCl Aqueous Solutions at Different Ionic Strengths and Temperatures. *J. Chem. Eng. Data* **2013**, *58*, 2835–2847. [CrossRef]
25. Baes, C.F.; Mesmer, R.E. *The Hydrolysis of Cations*; John Wyley & Sons: New York, NY, USA, 1976.
26. Pettit, D.; Powell, K.K. *Stability Constants Database, Academic Software*; IUPAC: Otley, UK, 1997.
27. Irto, A.; Cardiano, P.; Chand, K.; Cigala, R.M.; Crea, F.; De Stefano, C.; Gano, L.; Gattuso, G.; Sammartano, S.; Santos, M.A. A new bis-(3-hydroxy-4-pyridinone)-DTPA-derivative: Synthesis, complexation of di-/tri-valent metal cations and in vivo M3+ sequestering ability. *J. Mol. Liq.* **2019**, *281*, 280–294. [CrossRef]
28. Manganaro, N.; Lando, G.; Pisagatti, I.; Notti, A.; Pappalardo, S.; Parisi, M.F.; Gattuso, G. Hydrophobic interactions in the formation of a complex between a polycationic water-soluble oxacalix [4] arene and a neutral aromatic guest. *Supramol. Chem.* **2016**, *28*, 493–498. [CrossRef]
29. Colombo, S.; Coluccini, C.; Caricato, M.; Gargiulli, C.; Gattuso, G.; Pasini, D. Shape selectivity in the synthesis of chiral macrocyclic amides. *Tetrahedron* **2010**, *66*, 4206–4211. [CrossRef]
30. Clarke, E.T.; Martell, A.E. Stabilities of 1,2-dimethyl-3-hydroxy-4-pyridinone chelates of divalent and trivalent metal ions. *Inorg. Chim. Acta* **1992**, *191*, 57–63. [CrossRef]
31. Grgas-Kužnar, B.; Simeon, V.; Weber, O.A. Complexes of adrenaline and related compounds with Ni^{2+}, Cu^{2+}, Zn^{2+}, Cd^{2+} and Pb^{2+}. *J. Inorg. Nucl. Chem.* **1974**, *36*, 2151–2154. [CrossRef]

32. Huang, N.; Siegel, M.M.; Kruppa, G.H.; Laukien, F.H. Automation of a Fourier transform ion cyclotron resonance mass spectrometer for acquisition, analysis, and e-mailing of high-resolution exact-mass electrospray ionization mass spectral data. *J. Am. Soc. Mass Spectrom.* **1999**, *10*, 1166–1173. [CrossRef]
33. Annesley, T.M. Ion Suppression in Mass Spectrometry. *Clin. Chem.* **2003**, *49*, 1041–1044. [CrossRef] [PubMed]
34. Constantopoulos, T.L.; Jackson, G.S.; Enke, C.G. Effects of salt concentration on analyte response using electrospray ionization mass spectrometry. *J. Am. Soc. Mass Spectrom.* **1999**, *10*, 625–634. [CrossRef]
35. Karki, S.; Shi, F.; Archer, J.J.; Sistani, H.; Levis, R.J. Direct Analysis of Proteins from Solutions with High Salt Concentration Using Laser Electrospray Mass Spectrometry. *J. Am. Soc. Mass Spectrom.* **2018**, *29*, 1002–1011. [CrossRef] [PubMed]
36. Cheng, Z.L.; Siu, K.W.M.; Guevremont, R.; Berman, S.S. Electrospray mass spectrometry: A study on some aqueous solutions of metal salts. *J. Am. Soc. Mass Spectrom.* **1992**, *3*, 281–288. [CrossRef]
37. Crisponi, G.; Nurchi, V.M.; Zoroddu, M.A. Iron chelating agents for iron overload diseases. *Thalass. Rep.* **2014**, *4*, 2046.
38. Crisponi, G.; Remelli, M. Iron chelating agents for the treatment of iron overload. *Coordin. Chem. Rev.* **2008**, *252*, 1225–1240. [CrossRef]
39. Nurchi, V.M.; Crisponi, G.; Pivetta, T.; Donatoni, M.; Remelli, M. Potentiometric, spectrophotometric and calorimetric study on iron(III) and copper(II) complexes with 1,2-dimethyl-3-hydroxy-4-pyridinone. *J. Inorg. Biochem.* **2008**, *102*, 684–692. [CrossRef] [PubMed]
40. Bretti, C.; Cigala, R.M.; Crea, F.; Lando, G.; Sammartano, S. Thermodynamics of proton binding and weak (Cl$^-$, Na$^+$ and K$^+$) species formation, and activity coefficients of 1,2-dimethyl-3-hydroxypyridin-4-one (deferiprone). *J. Chem. Thermodyn.* **2014**, *77*, 98–106. [CrossRef]
41. Bretti, C.; Cigala, R.M.; De Stefano, C.; Lando, G.; Sammartano, S. Thermodynamics for Proton Binding of Pyridine in Different Ionic Media at Different Temperatures. *J. Chem. Eng. Data* **2014**, *59*, 143–156. [CrossRef]
42. Desai, A.G.; Kabadi, M.B. Stepwise stability constants of complexes of pyridine and substituted pyridines with zinc (II). *J. Inorg. Nucl. Chem.* **1966**, *28*, 1279–1282. [CrossRef]
43. Kapinos, L.E.; Sigel, H. Acid–base and metal ion binding properties of pyridine-type ligands in aqueous solution.: Effect of ortho substituents and interrelation between complex stability and ligand basicity. *Inorg. Chim. Acta* **2002**, *337*, 131–142. [CrossRef]
44. Desai, A.G.; Kabadi, M.B. On the ratio of successive stepwise complex formation constants: Zinc and cadmium complexes of pyridine and substituted pyridines. *Recueil des Travaux Chimiques des Pays-Bas* **1965**, *84*, 1066–1070. [CrossRef]
45. Sajadi, S.A.A. Metal ion-binding properties of L-glutamic acid and L-aspartic acid, a comparative investigation. *Nat. Sci.* **2010**, *2*, 85–90. [CrossRef]
46. Öhman, L.O. Equilibrium Studies of Ternary Aluminium (III) Hydroxo Complexes with Ligands Related to Conditions in Natural Waters. Ph.D. Thesis, University of Umeà, Umeà, Sweden, 1983.
47. Flaschka, H.A. *EDTA Titration*; Pergamon Press: London, UK, 1959.
48. De Stefano, C.; Princi, P.; Rigano, C.; Sammartano, S. Computer Analysis of Equilibrium Data in Solution. ESAB2M: An Improved Version of the ESAB Program. *Ann. Chim. (Rome)* **1987**, *7*, 643–675.
49. De Stefano, C.; Foti, C.; Giuffrè, O.; Mineo, P.; Rigano, C.; Sammartano, S. Binding of Tripolyphosphate by Aliphatic Amines: Formation, Stability and Calculation Problems. *Ann. Chim. (Rome)* **1996**, *86*, 257–280.
50. Gans, P.; Sabatini, A.; Vacca, A. Investigation of equilibria in solution. Determination of equilibrium constants with the HYPERQUAD suite programs. *Talanta* **1996**, *43*, 1739–1753. [CrossRef]
51. Frassineti, C.; Ghelli, S.; Gans, P.; Sabatini, A.; Moruzzi, M.S.; Vacca, A. Nuclear Magnetic Resonance as a Tool for Determining Protonation Constants of Natural Polyprotic Bases in Solution. *Anal. Biochem.* **1995**, *231*, 374–382. [CrossRef] [PubMed]
52. De Stefano, C.; Sammartano, S.; Mineo, P.; Rigano, C. Computer Tools for the Speciation of Natural Fluids. In *Marine Chemistry—An Environmental Analytical Chemistry Approach*; Gianguzza, A., Pelizzetti, E., Sammartano, S., Eds.; Kluwer Academic Publishers: Amsterdam, The Netherlands, 1997; pp. 71–83.

53. Alderighi, L.; Gans, P.; Ienco, A.; Peters, D.; Sabatini, A.; Vacca, A. Hyperquad simulation and speciation (HySS): A utility program for the investigation of equilibria involving soluble and partially soluble species. *Coord. Chem. Rev.* **1999**, *184*, 311–318. [CrossRef]
54. Shao, Y.; Molnar, L.F.; Jung, Y.; Kussmann, J.; Ochsenfeld, C.; Brown, S.T.; Gilbert, A.T.B.; Slipchenko, L.V.; Levchenko, S.V.; O'Neill, D.P.; et al. Advances in methods and algorithms in a modern quantum chemistry program package. *Phys. Chem. Chem. Phys.* **2006**, *8*, 3172–3191. [CrossRef] [PubMed]

Sample Availability: Not available.

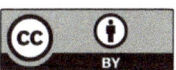

© 2019 by the authors. Licensee MDPI, Basel, Switzerland. This article is an open access article distributed under the terms and conditions of the Creative Commons Attribution (CC BY) license (http://creativecommons.org/licenses/by/4.0/).

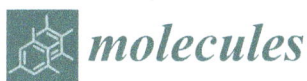

Article

Trends and Exceptions in the Interaction of Hydroxamic Acid Derivatives of Common Di- and Tripeptides with Some 3d and 4d Metal Ions in Aqueous Solution

András Ozsváth [1], Linda Bíró [1], Eszter Márta Nagy [1], Péter Buglyó [1], Daniele Sanna [2] and Etelka Farkas [1,*]

[1] Department of Inorganic and Analytical Chemistry, University of Debrecen, Egyetem tér 1, H-4032 Debrecen, Hungary; ozsvath.andras@science.unideb.hu (A.O.); linda.biro@science.unideb.hu (L.B.); neszma@hotmail.com (E.M.N.); buglyo@science.unideb.hu (P.B.)
[2] Istituto CNR di Chimica Biomolecolare, Trav. La Crucca 3, I-07040 Sassari, Italy; Daniele.Sanna@cnr.it
* Correspondence: efarkas@science.unideb.hu; Tel.: +36-52-512-900

Academic Editors: Francesco Crea and Alberto Pettignano
Received: 9 October 2019; Accepted: 30 October 2019; Published: 31 October 2019

Abstract: By using various techniques (pH-potentiometry, UV-Visible spectrophotometry, ^{1}H and ^{17}O-NMR, EPR, ESI-MS), first time in the literature, solution equilibrium study has been performed on complexes of dipeptide and tripeptide hydroxamic acids—AlaAlaNHOH, AlaAlaN(Me)OH, AlaGlyGlyNHOH, and AlaGlyGlyN(Me)OH—with 4d metals: the essential Mo(VI) and two half-sandwich type cations, [(η^6-p-cym)Ru(H$_2$O)$_3$]$^{2+}$ as well as [(η^5-Cp*)Rh(H$_2$O)$_3$]$^{2+}$, the latter two having potential importance in cancer therapy. The tripeptide derivatives have also been studied with some biologically important 3d metals, such as Fe(III), Ni(II), Cu(II), and Zn(II), in order to compare these new results with the corresponding previously obtained ones on dipeptide hydroxamic acids. Based on the outcomes, the effects of the type of metal ions, the coordination number, the number and types of donor atoms, and their relative positions to each other on the complexation have been evaluated in the present work. We hope that these collected results might be used when a new peptide-based hydroxamic acid molecule is planned with some purpose, e.g., to develop a potential metalloenzyme inhibitor.

Keywords: peptide hydroxamic acids; solution equilibrium; metal complexation; Ru(II)-, Rh(III)-based half-sandwich complexes; Mo(VI) complexes

1. Introduction

Hydroxamic acids containing one or more weak acidic function(s) -C(O)N(R)OH (R = H in primary, alkyl or aryl moiety in secondary derivatives) [1,2] are an important class of organic molecules with a huge number of biological activities, including the well-known, crucial role of the hydroxamate-based natural siderophores in the microbial iron uptake [3] or antifungal, antimalarial, metalloenzyme inhibitory effects [4,5]. Some derivatives may also behave as NO donors under certain conditions [6]. In some part, these diverse and important effects also depend on the significant H-bonding ability [7] or redox behaviour of this moiety [8,9], but predominantly, the rely on its strong chelating ability [1,2]. Consequently, investigation of complexation between metal ions and hydroxamic acids is permanently the focus of interest. The most typical coordination mode of a hydroxamate function involves chelation via deprotonated hydroxyl and carbonyl oxygen atoms providing a five-membered (O,O) chelate, which can be hydroxamato, if the function is mono-deprotonated, and hydroximato, if it is doubly-deprotonated. The latter type of chelate can only be formed with primary derivatives. A few examples have also been known for other modes of interactions [8,9]. Significantly increased versatility of the potential coordination modes exists in the presence of additional donors, such as amino or/and peptide groups in a hydroxamic derivative. This is clearly demonstrated by numerous results collected mostly on metal complexes of aminohydroxamic acids [10–16]. Significantly, increased interest toward the metal complexes of aminohydroxamic acids have been realised following the first publication on a pentanuclear β-alaninehydroxamate-based Cu(II)-containing metallacrown complex both in solution and in the solid state [14] and the discovery of numerous and diverse possibilities of applications of such compounds [15,16]. Peptide hydroxamic acids, however, despite the special interest in them e.g., to develop substrate-based metalloenzyme inhibitors [5], have very rarely been involved in solution studies [17–21]. Moreover, most of the results relate to complexes with $3d^{5-10}$ transition metal ions and only a few with 4d metals [21]. Following our solution equilibrium work done ca. thirty years ago on the complexation of ProLeuNHOH and ProLeuGlyNHOH with several 3d metals [17], we performed a detailed equilibrium study on complexation of a few simple dipeptide hydroxamic acids with Fe(III), Al(III), Ni(II), Cu(II), and Zn(II). The special interest in ProLeuGlyNHOH is due to the fact that human collagenase (a zinc(II)-containing metalloezyme) was isolated by means of an affinity column prepared with this tripeptide hydroxamic acid [22]. The obtained results showed the exclusive formation of (O,O) chelated hydroxamate species with the hard Fe(III) and Al(III) ions, while (O,O) and (NH$_2$,CO) chelated linkage isomers with Zn(II). These three metal ions were found not to induce deprotonation and parallel coordination of the peptide amide-N or primary hydroxamate-N, the processes of which, however, became deterministic with Cu(II) and especially with Ni(II) [19,20].

Out of the platinum group metals, only a recent publication from our lab discusses solution results on the rather complicated Pd(II)–AlaAlaNHOH, –AlaAlaN(Me)OH, –AlaGlyGlyNHOH, and –AlaGlyGlyN(Me)OH systems. In these systems, complexation and metal ion–induced hydrolytic and redox processes were found in a ligand-dependent extent [21]. No other metal from this group has previously been involved in investigations with peptide hydroxamic acids. The lack of interest came most probably from the high hydrolytic ability of these metals, as well as the inertness of their complexes. However, the intensive interest in relation to cancer therapy on numerous complexes with platinum group metals, together with the well-known fact that inertness of a complex is determined not only by the character of the metal ion but also by the mobility of the coordinated ligands, initiated studies in the past several years. For example, solution equilibrium measurements were successfully performed with half-sandwich type platinum group metal cations, including ruthenium and rhodium, in which an arene (benzene or its derivative such as 1-methyl-4-isopropylbenzene (p-cym)) or arenyl (pentamethyl-cyclopentadienyl (Cp*)) replaces three of the six solvent molecules, and complexation reactions can occur at the remaining three sites [23,24]. Recently, several types of hydroxamate-based ligands, including aminohydroxamic acids, have already been involved in solution equilibrium studies with these half-sandwich type cations [12,13], but only peptide hydroxamic acids are studied in the present work.

Likewise, according to the best of our knowledge, no publication can be found for complexes of peptide hydroxamic acids with molybdenum, despite the fact that this is an essential metal (the only one out of the 4d metals) and the biological activities of more than 50 enzymes are known to rely on it [25,26]. Again, the very high tendency of this metal for hydrolysis is one of the main reasons for the lack of investigations. Moreover, the stable form of Mo(VI) does not exist as an aqua-ion at all; only MoO_4^{2-} ion including various protonated forms of this oxido anion or its polymeric units exist [11].

As a continuation of our previous solution equilibrium work in this subject, in the present work, we have investigated the interaction of dipeptide and tripeptide hydroxamic acids, AlaAlaNHOH, AlaAlaN(Me)OH, AlaGlyGlyNHOH, and AlaGlyGlyN(Me)OH (see their structures in Scheme 1) with 4d metals, Mo(VI), and half-sandwich type cations of ruthenium(II), as well as rhodium(III), $[(\eta^6\text{-}p\text{-cym})Ru(H_2O)_3]^{2+}$, or $[(\eta^5\text{-Cp*})Rh(H_2O)_3]^{2+}$, respectively. To provide us with the possibility for a comparison between the results collected with 3d metals and 4d ones, investigation of the complexation with the (previously not studied) above tripeptide derivatives and metal ions as Fe(III), Ni(II), Cu(II), and Zn(II) was also performed.

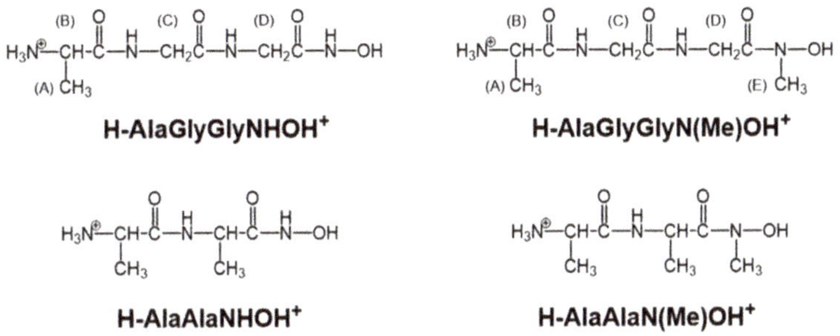

Scheme 1. Structures of the fully protonated ligands (H_2L^+).

H-AlaGlyGlyNHOH⁺

H-AlaGlyGlyN(Me)OH⁺

H-AlaAlaNHOH⁺

H-AlaAlaN(Me)OH⁺

2. Results

2.1. Protonation Equilibria of the Investigated Peptide Hydroxamic Acids

Each of the completely protonated form of the ligands have two deprotonation processes in the measurable pH-range; the calculated dissociation constants are presented in Table 1. Literature data could be found for the investigated dipeptide derivatives only in the presence of KCl, and those are in perfect agreement with the corresponding ones in Table 1 [19,20]. As can be seen in Table 1, there is practically no difference between the corresponding values of the di- and tripeptide derivatives determined either in the presence of KCl or KNO_3, but in accordance with earlier results, the dissociation constants for the secondary hydroxamic acids are 0.1–0.3 log unit smaller than those of the corresponding primary ones. This difference originates from the more enhanced delocalisation along the hydroxamate anions in the presence of an electron releasing alkyl group [20]. It is also known that the dissociation processes of the ammonium and hydroxamic groups considerably overlap each other [19]. Consequently, the values in Table 1 are macroconstants and cannot be ascribed unambiguously to the individual moieties. In one of our previous works, the dissociation microconstants were determined for the binding isomers of AlaAlaNHOH, and they supported the somewhat higher acidity of the ammonium group [19]. Since no significant difference can be assumed between the basicities of the investigated peptide hydroxamic acids, determination of dissociation microconstants for the additional ligands was beyond the scope of this work.

Table 1. Stepwise dissociation constants (pK) of the ligands at 25.0 °C, I = 0.20 M (KCl or KNO_3)*

Ligand	I = 0.20 M KCl		I = 0.20 M KNO_3	
	pK_1	pK_2	pK_1	pK_2
H-AlaAlaNHOH⁺	7.66 [1]	8.88 [1]	7.77(1)	8.89(1)
H-AlaAlaN(Me)OH⁺	7.74 [2]	8.74 [2]	7.77(1)	8.70(1)
H-AlaGlyGlyNHOH⁺	7.71(1)	8.82(1)	7.74(1)	8.82(1)
H-AlaGlyGlyN(Me)OH⁺	7.66(1)	8.63(1)	7.69(1)	8.57(1)

* 3σ standard deviations are in parentheses; [1] taken from [19]; [2] taken from [20].

2.2. Complexation of AlaGlyGlyNHOH and AlaGlyGlyN(Me)OH with Selected 3d Ions—Fe(III), Ni(II), Cu(II), and Zn(II)

Although the present solution equilibrium work has focused on the complexation of hydroxamic acid derivatives of common di- and tripeptides with the biologically important 4d metals Mo(VI), Ru(II), and Rh(III), a comparison between the results collected on complexes with the selected 3d and 4d metals has also been our aim.

Since detailed solution equilibrium results have been previously published only on the Fe(III), Ni(II), Cu(II), and Zn(II) complexes of the two dipeptide hydroxamic acids AlaAlaNHOH and

AlaAlaN(Me)OH [19,20], the present paper shortly discusses the results obtained for the two tripeptide hydroxamic acids AlaGlyGlyNHOH and AlaGlyGlyN(Me)OH.

The experimental results were collected on the Fe(III), Ni(II), Cu(II), and Zn(II) complexes of AlaGlyGlyNHOH and AlaGlyGlyN(Me)OH by the methods and under the conditions detailed in the Experimental section. The equilibrium models and logarithmic overall stability constants presented in Table 2 were determined by pH-potentiometry, except for the complexes with Fe(III), where combination of pH-metry and spectrophotometry provided the possibility for calculation of stability constants. The reason behind is the formation of complexes with [FeHL]$^{3+}$ stoichiometry below the pH-metrically measurable pH-range (far below pH 2). Their stability constants therefore were determined by fitting the spectra recorded on individual samples in the pH-range 0.7–1.6 (see Experimental part). These calculated constants were kept fixed when pH-metric titration curves, and UV-Visible spectra registered in the whole measured pH-range were fitted.

Table 2. Overall stability constants (logβ) for the Fe(III), Ni(II), Cu(II), and Zn(II) complexes formed with the investigated tripeptide hydroxamic acids at 25.0 °C, I = 0.20 M (KCl)*.

	AlaAlaNHOH [1]	AlaAlaN(Me)OH [2]	AlaGlyGlyNHOH	AlaGlyGlyN(Me)OH
[FeHL]$^{3+}$	17.62 [a]	18.08 [a]	17.74(1) [a]	17.64(1) [a]
[FeL]$^{2+}$	15.09	14.67	–	–
[FeH$_2$L$_2$]$^{3+}$	34.57	33.8	34.02(5)	33.70(7)
	34.00 [a]	34.71 [a]	34.00(2) [a]	33.76(1) [a]
[FeH$_3$L$_3$]$^{3+}$	49.40	50.01	48.7(2)	48.97(11)
	48.61 [a]	49.51 [a]	48.55(3) [a]	48.16(2) [a]
[NiHL]$^{2+}$	12.50	–	12.79(3)	11.6(2)
[NiL]$^{+}$	6.30	6.01	–	5.04(7)
[NiH$_{-1}$L]	−1.10	–	–	−3.3(1)
[NiH$_{-2}$L]$^{-}$	−9.57	–	−7.44(2)	−10.78(3)
[NiHL$_2$]$^{+}$	–	16.8	–	17.10(9)
[NiL$_2$]	–	9.13	–	–
[CuHL]$^{2+}$	14.70	15.02	14.45(7)	14.66(2)
[Cu$_2$L$_2$]$^{2+}$	23.20	–	–	–
[CuH$_{-1}$L]	4.43	3.04	–	3.52(2)
[CuH$_{-2}$L]$^{-}$	−5.24	−6.63	−5.38(5)	−5.28(2)
[CuH$_2$L$_2$]$^{2+}$	–	29.17	–	27.6(2)
[CuHL$_2$]$^{+}$	–	22.3	–	22.23(9)
[CuL$_2$]	–	14.8	–	14.8(1)
[CuH$_{-1}$L$_2$]$^{-}$	–	6.3	–	–
[Cu$_3$H$_{-4}$L$_2$]	5.89	–	–	–
[Cu$_3$H$_{-5}$L$_2$]$^{-}$	−3.56	–	–	–
[Cu$_3$H$_{-6}$L$_2$]$^{2-}$	−14.28	–	–	–
[ZnHL]$^{2+}$	12.35	12.00	12.47(2)	11.92(2)
[ZnL]$^{+}$	5.64	5.11	5.07(6)	4.55(2)
[ZnH$_{-1}$L]	−2.58	−3.23	−3.18(2)	−3.46(3)
[ZnHL$_2$]$^{+}$	17.52	17.12	–	–

* 3σ standard deviations are in parentheses; [a] Determined from UV-Vis data; [1] taken from reference [19]; [2] taken from reference [20].

For easier comparison, Table 2 also contains the previously published data for the complexes of dipeptide derivatives determined under the same conditions as used in the present study.

As shown in Table 2, there is a good agreement between both the equilibrium models and numerical values of the constants determined by pH-metry and spectrophotometry for the mono-, bis- and tris-complexes of primary and secondary di- and tripeptide derivatives with Fe(III). The only difference between the models is that the [FeL]$^{2+}$ complex—what was found with the dipeptide hydroxamic acids and was assumed to be a mixed hydroxido species—was not formed in measurable concentration with the two tripeptide derivatives. Based on the almost perfect agreement, the same coordination modes are assumed with the tripeptide derivatives as it was found with the dipeptide-based counterparts [19,20]:

coordination of the hydroxamate oxygens while the non-coordinating amino moiety is protonated. The UV-Visible spectra showing the well-known charge-transfer (C.T.) bands in both Fe(III)-tripeptide hydroxamic acid systems, clearly support this assumption. The registered spectra in the pH-range ca. 0.7–1.6 (where the [FeHL]$^{3+}$ is formed) are characteristic for an Fe(III)-monohydroxamato complex (λ_{max} = 510 nm). Upon increasing the pH, a decrease of the λ_{max} down to 460 nm in a second stepwise process by pH ca. 3–3.5 occurs (this process belongs to the formation of the bis-hydroxamato species [Fe(HL)$_2$]$^{3+}$), while as a result of a third process, the tris-hydroxamato species [Fe(HL)$_3$]$^{3+}$ is formed by ca. pH 6.5 with a characteristic λ_{max} = 420–425 nm. Above pH ca. 6.5, the formation of mixed hydroxido species was indicated to start by the spectra even at 1:5 metal to ligand ratio in both systems.

Zn(II) is the other metal ion, with which both the equilibrium models and stability constants are quite similar in all of the four systems. The only exception in the models is that bis-complex was found to form under our conditions with the dipeptide derivatives but not with the two tripeptide hydroxamic acids, most probably because of sterical reasons. All these findings suggest that Zn(II) behaves very similarly toward the two tripeptide-based ligands, as was previously supported by ^{1}H-NMR results for the complexes of AlaAlaNHOH [19] and AlaAlaN(Me)OH [20]. Consequently, AlaGlyGlyNHOH and AlaGlyGlyN(Me)OH are assumed to form moderate stability binding isomers with Zn(II), in which coordination occurs via either the five-membered (O,O)$_{hydr}$ chelate or the five-membered (NH$_2$,CO) chelate. Only one of these two possible chelates exists in [ZnHL]$^{2+}$ (which starts to form at pH ca. 4.8–5), while the other moiety is still in protonated, non-coordinated form. Upon increasing the pH, the formation of [ZnL]$^+$, followed by [ZnH$_{-1}$L], was found. They are most probably mixed hydroxido species and in the pH-range where the free ligand itself deprotonates (above pH 7) and the dissociation of the non-coordinating moiety also occurs. As in the case of Fe(III), there is no indication for the Zn(II)-induced deprotonation and coordination of peptide amide function in any of the investigated systems.

The situation is completely different with Ni(II) and Cu(II), in which metal ions accept N-donor ligands readily. At the same time, the different number and, in some part, type of the N-donors in the studied ligands results in different coordinating behaviour of them toward these metal ions: AlaAlaNHOH contains 3N (NH$_2$, N$_{amide}$, N$_{hydr.}$), AlaAlaN(Me)OH involves 2N (NH$_2$, N$_{amide}$) donor atoms, there are 4N donors in the tripeptide derivative AlaGlyGlyNHOH (NH$_2$, 2×N$_{amide}$, N$_{hydr.}$), while 3N in its secondary counterpart, AlaGlyGlyN(Me)OH (NH$_2$, 2×N$_{amide}$). The significant role of the amino-N, amide-N and for the primary hydroxamic derivatives, hydroxamate-N in the Ni(II)– and Cu(II)–AlaAlaNHOH and –AlaAlaN(Me)OH systems was discussed in our previous papers [19,20]. In the present work, both AlaGlyGlyNHOH and AlaGlyGlyN(Me)OH were found to react with Ni(II) above pH ca. 4. The first species, [NiHL], are formed in low extent below pH ca. 6, in which the ligands are assumed to coordinate in a similar manner as it was supported with the dipeptide derivative, either via five-membered (NH$_2$, CO) or (O,O)$_{hydr}$. The colour of the samples turned to yellow above pH ca. 6 with the primary derivative and above pH ca. 7 with its secondary counterpart. This latter pH is much lower than the value, where the color turned to yellow in the Ni(II)–AlaAlaN(Me)OH system, above pH 9 [20]. Above these pH values, the spectra registered in both systems are characteristic for square planar Ni(II) complexes (Figure 1a,b).

Although the most probable cooperative processes with the primary ligand were too slow to allow determination of stability constants for the stepwise equilibria, there is no doubt that four equivalents of base are consumed by the end of the titrations, up to pH ca. 11. The calculated stability constant for [NiH$_{-2}$L]$^-$ formed is shown in Table 2. The two dissociable protons of the ligand consume two equivalents of base, while the additional two react with the protons from the two peptide moieties. Consequently, [NiH$_{-2}$L]$^-$, which was found to be a mixed hydroxido complex with AlaAlaNHOH [19], is a 4N-coordinated complex with AlaGlyGlyNHOH, and the coordinating donor set is (NH$_2$,N$_{amide}$,N$_{amide}$,N$_{hydr}$). This assumption is further supported by the UV-Visible parameters (λ_{max} = 400 nm, ε ca. 200 M^{-1}cm^{-1}), which are similar to those obtained previously for the 4N-coordinated complex in the Ni(II)–ProLeuGlyNHOH system [17].

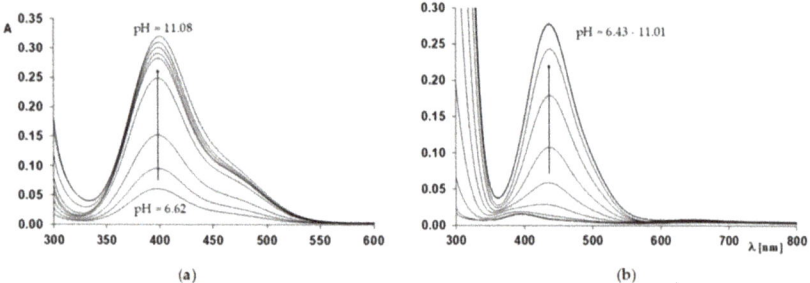

Figure 1. UV-Visible spectra recorded at different pH values for the (**a**) Ni(II)–AlaGlyGlyNHOH and (**b**) Ni(II)–AlaGlyGlyN(Me)OH systems at 1:1 ratio ($c_{Ni(II)}$ = 1.5 mM).

Like in the case of the primary counterpart, four equivalents of base were altogether consumed during the titration of Ni(II)–AlaGlyGlyN(Me)OH samples as well. There is no doubt that the final species, [NiH$_{-2}$L]$^-$, is a planar complex in this case, in which the metal ion is coordinated by the (NH$_2$, N$_{amide}$, N$_{amide}$, O$_{hydr}$) donor set. With this secondary tripeptide hydroxamic acid, however, the processes were fast enough to allow the calculation of stability constants for the intermediate species. At the same time, if the stepwise dissociation constants for the complexes using the corresponding overall stability constants in Table 2 are calculated, an irregular trend is found: pK$_{NiL}$ is higher than pK$_{NiH-1L}$, (5.04 − (−3.3) = 8.34 and −3.3 − (−10.78) = 7.48, respectively), showing cooperativity of the processes in this system, too. With AlaGlyGlyN(Me)OH, no hydrolysis, but bis-complex formation in a small extent and in a narrow pH-range (what was dominant with the secondary dipeptide, AlaAlaN(Me)OH [20]), was detected.

Between Cu(II) and the two tripeptide derivatives, complexation starts as low as pH ca. 2.5–3, where the competition between the proton and metal ion for the coordinating sites is very significant, as it was discussed previously [27]. An evaluation, based on this literature information allowed us to draw the conclusion that among the likely chelates (O,O)$_{hydr}$ has the highest conditional stability under the above acidic conditions. Consequently, the hydroxamate function behaves as anchor site for the Cu(II) ion. In fact, this coordination mode was unambiguously supported by both the characteristic charge transfer band at λ_{max} ca. 370–380 nm and the EPR results (g_{II} = 2.345 and 2.335, A_{II} = 160.5 × 10^{-4} and 159.8 × 10^{-4} cm^{-1} with AlaGlyGlyNHOH and AlaGlyGlyN(Me)OH, respectively) in the [CuHL]$^{2+}$ formed. Despite the fact that four equivalents of base were consumed with both of the ligands by pH ca. 11, several experimental findings collected above pH ca. 4.5 in the two systems differ from each other. Namely: (1) The primary derivative was capable of binding Cu(II) excess, the secondary not. (2) Bis-complexes were less favoured with the primary ligand but were present in low concentration also with this ligand. (3) The processes were very slow above pH 5 in the Cu(II)–AlaGlyGlyNHOH system, hindering the calculation of stability constants for some of the species formed, but those were significantly faster for the Cu(II)–AlaGlyGlyN(Me)OH system allowing calculations from the whole measured pH-range (see Table 2). Fortunately, EPR and UV-Visible measurements provided clear support for the different complexes formed in these two systems. For illustration, some EPR spectra recorded at various pH values for Cu(II)–AlaGlyGlyNHOH and Cu(II)-AlaGlyGlyN(Me)OH samples are shown in Figure S1 (a) and (b), respectively.

As Figure S1a reveals, with AlaGlyGlyNHOH in the pH-range ca. 6–7, the decreased intensity of the EPR signals supports the presence of a dinuclear species as major complex following [CuHL]$^{2+}$ with hydroxamate coordination. The existence of some EPR activity indicates that no spin-crossover but weak interaction exists between the two metal ions in the dinuclear complex. The calculated EPR parameters suggest that one of the Cu(II) is coordinated by two (O,O)$_{hydr}$ chelates (g_{II} = 2.283 and A_{II} = 181.7 × 10^{-4} cm^{-1}), while the other is coordinated by nitrogens. At pH = 9.2, the calculated parameters (g_{II} = 2.176 and A_{II} = 213.4 × 10^{-4} cm^{-1}) are in perfect agreement with those published for the 4N-coordinated complex in the Cu(II)–ProLeuGlyNHOH system (g_{II} = 2.181 and A_{II} = 208.5 × 10^{-4} cm^{-1}) [17]. This suggests an (NH$_2$,N$_{amide}$,N$_{amide}$,N$_{hydr}$)-type coordination mode in [CuH$_{-2}$L]$^-$, predominating at this pH. Additional support for the suggested coordination mode in this complex was provided by the λ_{max} = 500 nm of the d-d band in the UV-Visible spectrum.

Interestingly, the mononuclear bis-complex, [Cu(HL)$_2$]$^{2+}$ was found as a major species at ligand excess in the pH-range 4.7–6.5 with AlaGlyGlyN(Me)OH (see Figure S1b). The EPR parameters calculated for this complex show coordination of two hydroxamates (g_{II} = 2.283 and A_{II} = 181.7 × 10^{-4} cm^{-1}). In the pH-range 6.5–8.1 involvement of nitrogens in the coordination is clearly shown by the EPR spectra, but the presence of the C.T. band at λ_{max} = 380 nm in this pH range proves the involvement of the hydroxamate oxygens in the coordination too. Some cooperativity of the processes in this pH-range is indicated by the results and in [CuH$_{-1}$L], predominating at 1:1 metal ion to ligand ratio, highly distorted arrangement of the coordinated donors is shown by the appropriate EPR parameters (g_{II} = 2.172 and A_{II} = 124.3×10^{-4} cm^{-1}). Tentative binding modes for this species are shown in structures I and II in Scheme 2. The combination of g and A values suggests that the donor atoms involved in the metal coordination are strong donors (low g value) but the structure is very distorted (low A value); if also the g value was high we should think to a weak coordination [28,29]. Because we do not have a comparison with similar complexes having the same donor atoms coordinated but with a less distorted structure, we are not sure that the coordination is exactly the one that is reported as proposed structures I or II in Scheme 2. Upon increasing the pH further, [CuH$_{-2}$L]$^-$ becomes even more predominant with the (NH$_2$,N$_{amide}$,N$_{amide}$,O$_{hydr}$) donor set (structure III in Scheme 2).

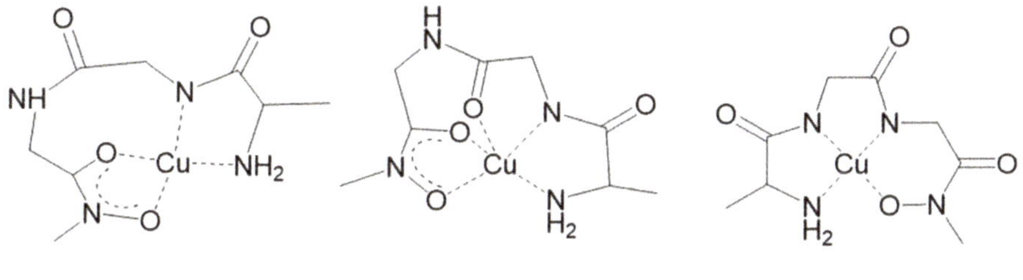

Scheme 2. Plausible binding modes in the complexes [CuH$_{-1}$L] (structures I and II) and the most possible mode in [CuH$_{-2}$L]$^-$ (structure III), L$^-$ = AlaGlyGlyN(Me)O$^-$.

2.3. Complexation of AlaAlaNHOH, AlaAlaN(Me)OH, AlaGlyGlyNHOH, and AlaGlyGlyN(Me)OH with the Essential 4d Ion Mo(VI)

The registered pH-potentiometric titration curves, similarly to the few previous results on Mo(VI)-monohydroxamic acid systems [30], indicated very strong interaction between the studied ligands and Mo(VI), but only under acidic conditions. No difference between the curves for the ligands or those registered in the Mo(VI)-containing samples was observed above pH ca. 7.5. To illustrate this, Figure 2 shows the titration curves registered for AlaAlaNHOH alone and for the Mo(VI)–AlaAlaNHOH system at various metal ion to ligand ratios.

All the titration curves can be fitted well (see fitting parameters in Table 3) for all the studied systems with the model involving the proton complexes of the ligands, hydroxido species of molybdenum(VI) (see the Experimental section), as well as the metal complexes [MoO$_2$(HL)$_2$]$^{2+}$ and [MoO$_3$(HL)]. The calculated overall stability constants of the species formed in equilibrium (1) are presented in Table 3. As an example, the inset in Figure 2 shows the concentration distribution curves of complexes formed in the Mo(VI)–AlaAlaNHOH system based on pH-metric results (similar curves were obtained for the Mo(VI)–AlaAlaN(Me)OH system).

$$MoO_4^{2-} + xL^- + 3xH^+ \rightleftharpoons [MoO_{4-x}(HL)_x]^{(x-1)+} + xH_2O \quad (1)$$

where x = 1 or 2.

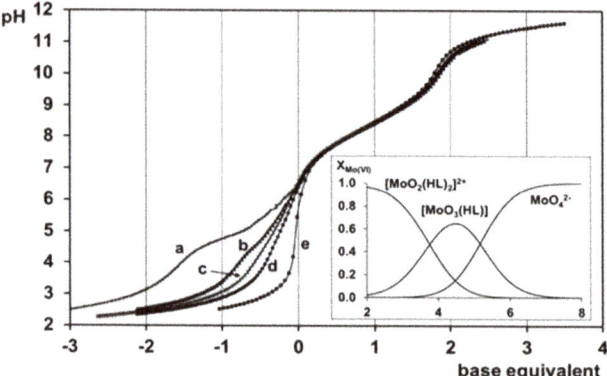

Figure 2. Titration curves of the Mo(VI)–AlaAlaNHOH system at (**a**) 1:1, (**b**) 1:2, (**c**) 1:3 and (**d**) 1:4 metal ion to ligand ratio with the titration curve of the (**e**) H$^+$–AlaAlaNHOH system (c_L = 6.00 mM) and in inset the calculated concentration distribution curves for the Mo(VI)–AlaAlaNHOH system at 1:4 metal ion to ligand ratio (c_L = 1.82 mM; negative base equivalents refer to an excess of acid in the samples).

Table 3. Overall stability constants (logβ) for the Mo(VI) complexes formed with the peptide hydroxamic acids at 25.0 °C, I = 0.20 M (KCl)*.

Species	AlaAlaNHOH	AlaAlaN(Me)OH	AlaGlyGlyNHOH	AlaGlyGlyN(Me)OH
[MoO$_2$(HL)$_2$]$^{2+}$	46.5(1)	47.78(7)	48.57(9)	46.44(2)
[MoO$_3$(HL)]	23.89(7)	24.52(5)	24.37(7)	23.92(2)
Fitting parameter (mL)^a	0.00317	0.00596	0.00662	0.00226
Number of fitted data	422	461	195	271

* 3σ standard deviations are in parentheses; ^{a} Fitting parameter is the average difference between the calculated and experimental titration curves expressed in the volume of the titrant.

Table 3 shows no significant differences between the stability constants determined in the four systems for the two types of complexes, [MoO$_2$(HL)$_2$]$^{2+}$ or [MoO$_3$(HL)], respectively. However, our previous results on the few Mo(VI)–monohydroxamic acid systems revealed that there were some processes that were not accompanied by pH-effect at all [30]. Consequently, pH-potentiometry alone could not detect all the solution equilibrium processes. Fortunately, additional information could be obtained using UV-Visible spectrophotometry, ^{1}H-NMR, and ^{17}O-NMR methods. Using these methods, the following results were obtained.

A high intensity C.T. band at λ_{max} ca. 290 nm could be detected in all the studied systems as low as pH 2, which started to decrease above pH 5. This band is known to refer to a molybdenum-dioxido-bis-hydroxamato species [30], so this finding, together with those based on ^{1}H-NMR measurements, clearly supports the predominance of hydroxamate coordinated species with all the four di- and tripeptide hydroxamic acids having the amino-moiety in non-coordinated, protonated form. Beside this very important similarity in the behaviour of the four ligands toward Mo(VI), the ^{1}H-NMR and especially ^{17}O-NMR spectra also indicated significant differences between the interactions with the primary and secondary derivatives. This is well demonstrated by the comparison of Figure 3a,b where ^{1}H-NMR spectra are presented, and Figure 4a,b where ^{17}O-NMR spectra recorded at various pH for the Mo(VI)–AlaAlaN(Me)OH and Mo(VI)–AlaAlaNHOH systems, respectively. (Similar experimental results were obtained for the corresponding tripeptide-based counterparts; those are not shown).

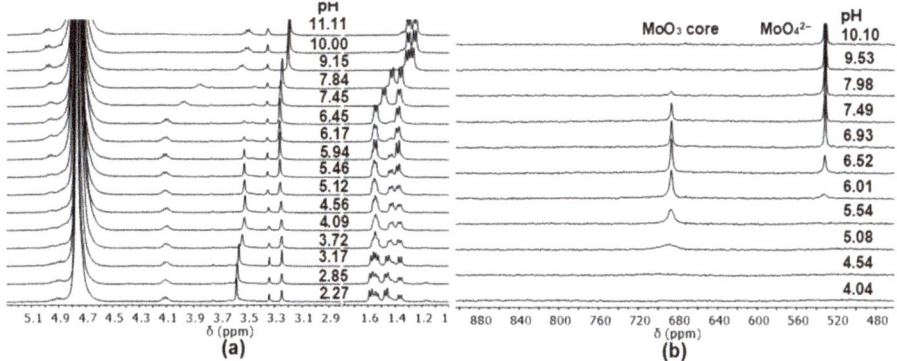

Figure 3. pH dependence of (**a**) ^{1}H-NMR (c_L = 0.015 M) and (**b**) ^{17}O-NMR (c_L = 0.15 M) spectra of the Mo(VI)–AlaAlaN(Me)OH system at 1:3 metal ion to ligand ratio. (^{1}H-NMR signal at 3.34 ppm refers to a few percent methanol impurity in the ligand).

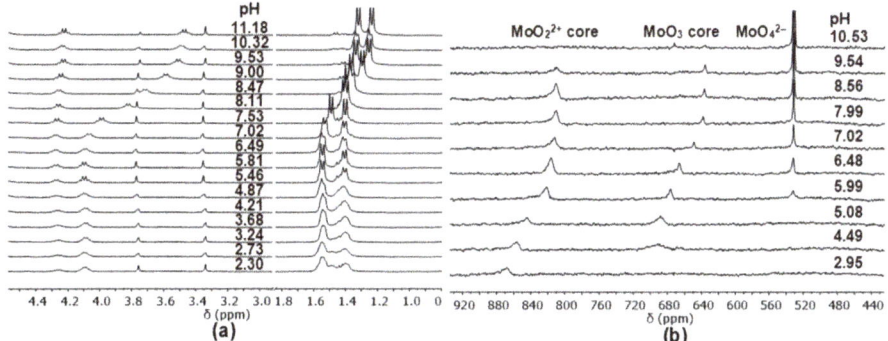

Figure 4. pH dependence of (**a**) ^{1}H-NMR (c_L = 0.015 M) and (**b**) ^{17}O-NMR (c_L = 0.15 M) spectra of the Mo(VI)–AlaAlaNHOH system at 1:3 metal ion to ligand ratio. (^{1}H-NMR signal at 3.34 ppm refers to few percent methanol impurity in the ligand).

As Figure 3a shows, complexation processes between Mo(VI) and the secondary derivative are slow enough on the NMR time scale to obtain individual signals for the non-dissociable protons locating close to the coordinating sites in the complexes compared to those for the free ligand. The fractions calculated from the relative intensities of these signals at pH 2 (ratio of the complexed and non-complexed ligand is 2:1) are in perfect agreement with the assumption that at this pH [MoO$_2$(HL)$_2$]$^{2+}$ exists exclusively in measurable concentration, while one third of the ligand remains in non-complexed form. Some broadening of the signals belonging to the complex is observable in the spectra above pH 4 and, parallel, small but measurable decrease in their chemical shift, either. This is the pH, where [MoO$_3$(HL)] is present in measurable concentration by the pH-metrically determined concentration distribution curves (see inset in Figure 2) and where the well-defined characteristic signal of the MoO$_3$-core at 680 ppm in the ^{17}O-NMR spectrum can already be detected in Figure 3. Various exchange processes might cause the disappearance of the characteristic signal of the MoO$_2^{2+}$ core [30]. The intensity of the ^{1}H and ^{17}O signals belonging to the MoO$_3$-containing species starts decreasing at pH ca. 6 and 7, respectively, and they disappear by pH ca. 7.5–8. Above this pH, only the existence of MoO$_4^{2-}$ ions and the free secondary ligand are supported by all the used methods. Consequently, these secondary peptide-based hydroxamic acids interact with Mo(VI) in the acidic and neutral pH-range, but they are not in the coordination sphere above neutral pH, where only MoO$_4^{2-}$ and the free ligand exist.

With primary derivatives, the situation is different. Although pH-potentiometry showed similar complexation behaviour with all the four studied ligands, ^{1}H and ^{17}O-NMR results indicate significant differences (*cf.* Figures 3 and 4). Very broad ^{1}H-NMR signals can be seen in Figure 4a for the Mo(VI)–AlaAlaNHOH system in the acidic region and sharpening of them at higher pH. Similar observation was made in the Mo(VI)–acetohydroxamic acid system, where, as a function of pH, various inter- and intramolecular exchange processes were suggested—faster ones in the acidic region, and formation of more inert species at higher pH [30].

^{17}O-NMR spectra of the Mo(VI)–AlaAlaNHOH system were recorded between pH ca. 3.0–10.5 at a metal ion to ligand ratio 1:3. The spectra in Figure 4b provide the following information.

1. Although the characteristic signal of MoO_4^{2-} appears at pH ca. 6 with this primary derivative (the same is seen in Figure 3b with the secondary counterpart), to some extent, the primary ligand remains in coordinative interaction with the MoO_2^{2+}-core up to pH ca. 10. Moreover, the pH-dependence of the chemical shift of the quite broad signals of the complexes with MoO_2^{2+}-core shows two inflexion points (two deprotonation processes). These experimental results support the formation of three different species with this core as a function of pH.
2. The very broad NMR signals of MoO_3 oxygens are clearly observable at ca. 688 ppm at pH 4.49, and their chemical shifts show one inflexion point as a function of pH (indicating one deprotonation step and two types of species with MoO_3 core). Furthermore, its intensity starts decreasing above pH 7 and almost disappears by pH 10.5.

Fitting the chemical shifts vs. pH curves by the computer program PSEQUAD provided the following dissociation constants (pK): pK_1 = 4.1(4), pK_2 = 5.7(1) for the MoO_2^{2+}-containing species and pK = 6.52(3) for the MoO_3-containing one. The corresponding values with the previously studied primary acetohydroxamic acid were pK_1 = 4.45, pK_2 = 6.74, and pK = 7.73, respectively [30]. There is no doubt that similar processes can be suggested with the primary peptide hydroxamic acids as were found with acetohydroxamic acid [30], in which two factors (strong hydrogen bonding character of a hydroxamate-NH and possibility of deprotonation of it resulting in the formation of a hydroximate chelate with very high stability) play a crucial role. The suggested two processes are shown in Equations (2) and (3) with MoO_2^{2+} core and in Equation (4) with MoO_3.

$$[MoO_2(HL)_2]^{2+} + 2H_2O \rightleftharpoons [MoO_2(HL)(OH)_2] + H_2L^+ + H^+ \tag{2}$$

$$[MoO_2(HL)(OH)_2] \rightleftharpoons [MoO_2(HLH_{-1})(OH)_2]^- + H^+ \tag{3}$$

$$[MoO_3(HL)(H_2O)] \rightleftharpoons [MoO_3(HLH_{-1})(H_2O)]^- + H^+ \tag{4}$$

where HL refers to the ligand coordinated via the hydroxamate chelate and the amino moiety is still protonated. HLH_{-1}^- symbolizes doubly deprotonated hydroximate function, with protonated amino end.

For the investigated Mo(VI)-primary peptide hydroxamic acid systems, the various most likely equilibrium processes are summarized in Scheme 3. Remarkable intramolecular exchange processes between the different species shown above (including water) result in significant broadening of the signals, as was detailed in our previous paper [30].

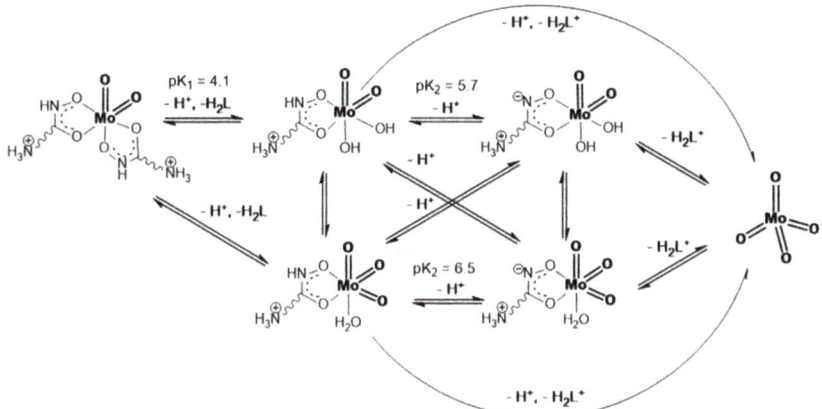

Scheme 3. The most likely equilibrium processes as a function of pH in Mo(VI)—primary peptide hydroxamic acid systems.

2.4. Complexation of AlaAlaNHOH or AlaAlaN(Me)OH with Two Half-Sandwich Type Cations—[(η^6-p-cym)Ru(H$_2$O)$_3$]$^{2+}$ or [(η^5-Cp*)Rh(H$_2$O)$_3$]$^{2+}$

The speciation profiles of the complexes formed in these systems were determined via a combined use of pH-potentiometry, ^{1}H-NMR, and ESI-MS. Fortunately the complex formation processes were fast enough in all of the systems to apply conventional pH-potentiometry; for details see the Materials and Methods section. Because the titration curves registered for the two systems containing the primary derivative, AlaAlaNHOH, were similar to each other. As a representative example, the curves registered for the [(η^5-Cp*)Rh(H$_2$O)$_3$]$^{2+}$-containing samples and the free ligand within the pH-range 2–11, together with the concentration distribution curves in inset, are depicted in Figure 5.

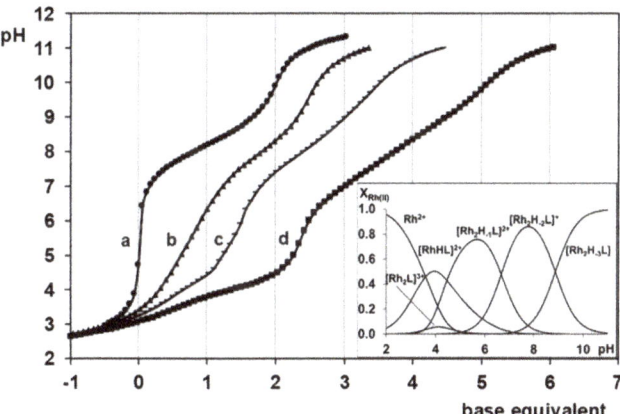

Figure 5. Titration curves of (**a**) the H$^+$-AlaAlaNHOH system and the [(η^5-Cp*)Rh(H$_2$O)$_3$]$^{2+}$-AlaAlaNHOH systems at (**b**) 1:2, (**c**) 1:1 and (**d**) 2:1 ratios (c_L = 1.62 mM) with the related concentration distribution curves in inset calculated at 1:1 metal ion to ligand ratio (c_L = 2.00 mM; negative base equivalent refers an excess of acid in the sample; "Rh" stands for [(η^5-Cp*)Rh(H$_2$O)$_3$]$^{2+}$).

The best fit of the titration curves was obtained with the model and stability constants collected in Table 4.

Table 4. Overall stability constants (logβ) for the [(η^6-p-cym)Ru(H$_2$O)$_3$]$^{2+}$ and [(η^5-Cp*)Rh(H$_2$O)$_3$]$^{2+}$ complexes formed with AlaAlaNHOH and AlaAlaN(Me)OH at 25.0 °C, I = 0.20 M (KNO$_3$)*.

Species	AlaAlaNHOH		AlaAlaN(Me)OH	
	[(η^6-p-cym)Ru]$^{2+}$	[(η^5-Cp*)Rh]$^{2+}$	[(η^6-p-cym)Ru]$^{2+}$	[(η^5-Cp*)Rh]$^{2+}$
[MHL]$^{2+}$	16.09(2)	15.54(1)	17.53(2)	15.89(1)
[ML]$^+$	–	–	11.61(3)	9.48(3)
[MH$_{-1}$L]	–	–	2.50(5)	2.62(2)
[M$_2$L]$^{3+}$	14.95(10)	13.57(8)	–	14.16(2)
[M$_2$H$_{-1}$L]$^{2+}$	11.16(5)	10.07(1)	–	–
[M$_2$H$_{-2}$L]$^+$	4.63(6)	3.40(3)	–	–
[M$_2$H$_{-3}$L]	–4.79(9)	–5.47(4)	–	–
Fitting parameter (mL)^a	0.00683	0.00417	0.00707	0.00575
Number of fitted data	302	183	201	244
pK_{MHL}	–	–	5.92	6.41
pK_{ML}	–	–	9.11	6.86

*3 σ standard deviations are in parentheses; ^{a} Fitting parameter is the average difference between the calculated and experimental titration curves expressed in the volume of the titrant.

As it is clearly seen in Table 4, identical equilibrium models were determined for the [(η^6-p-cym)Ru(H$_2$O)$_3$]$^{2+}$–AlaAlaNHOH and [(η^5-Cp*)Rh(H$_2$O)$_3$]$^{2+}$–AlaAlaNHOH systems. The only difference is that the stability constants are slightly higher for the complexes with the Ru-containing cation compared to Rh similarly as it was previously found with monohydroxamic acids and with aminohydroxamic acids [13,31]. Surprisingly, as Table 4 shows, apart from [MHL]$^{2+}$, only dinuclear complexes are formed in these systems, which predominate even at 1:1 metal ion to ligand ratio (see inset in Figure 5) and at ligand excess. The suggested coordination mode in the only mononuclear protonated complex is shown as structure IV in Scheme 4. (As an example, the binding modes are shown for the complexes formed with [(η^6-p-cym)Ru(H$_2$O)$_3$]$^{2+}$ but those are the same in the corresponding [(η^5-Cp*)Rh(H$_2$O)$_3$]$^{2+}$ containing complexes.)

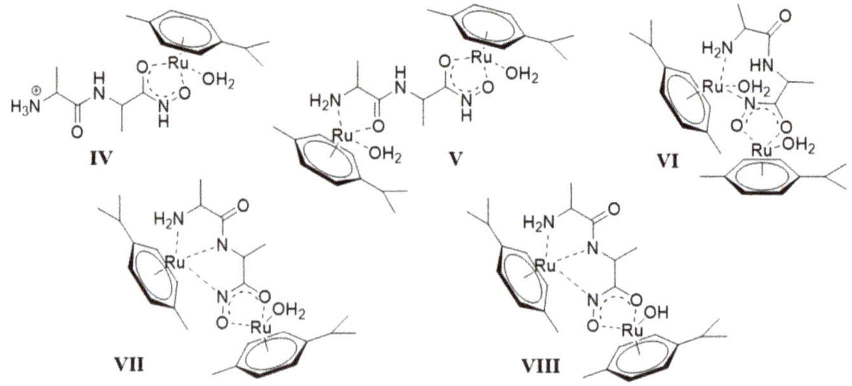

Scheme 4. Suggested structures for the complexes formed in [(η^6-p-cym)Ru(H$_2$O)$_3$]$^{2+}$–AlaAlaNHOH systems.

In IV, the hydroxamate chelate (having rather high conditional stability even under strongly acidic conditions with these metal ions [13]), together with a water molecule saturate the three coordination sites of a half-sandwich cation, while the amino group is protonated. The hydroxamate and, after deprotonation of the hydroxamate-NH, the hydroximate chelate is not displaced by other coordinating donors of this dipeptide-based primary hydroxamic acid remaining coordinated in the whole studied pH-range. That is the reason why the amino-N, the peptide moiety, and the hydroximate-N can only coordinate to another metal cation, forming dinuclear complexes in this way. The dominance of the dinuclear species might cause the high complexity of the ^{1}H-NMR spectra for the signals of the methyl groups of the Cp* ligand and especially that of the *p*-cymene aromatic protons above pH ca. 4. To illustrate this, pH-dependent chemical shifts of the *p*-cymene aromatic protons are shown in Figure S2. Additional support for the dominant formation of dinuclear complexes with AlaAlaNHOH in these systems was obtained by ESI-MS with the direct identification of $[M_2H_{-2}L]^+$ at and above pH = 8.01 (see Figure S3 for the measured and calculated spectra of this species).

The suggested binding modes in the dinuclear complexes $[M_2L]^{3+}$, $[M_2H_{-1}L]^{2+}$, $[M_2H_{-2}L]^+$, and $[M_2H_{-3}L]$ are shown as structures V, VI, VII and VIII, respectively, in Scheme 4.

Although the complexation processes with the secondary AlaAlaN(Me)OH were somewhat slower compared to those with the primary AlaAlaNHOH, they were still fast enough to perform direct pH-metric titrations. Because for AlaAlaN(Me)OH, the substitution of the hydrogen at the hydroxamic-nitrogen by a methyl moiety hinders the formation of either the hydroximate chelate with very high stability or the (NH$_2$,N$_{amide}$,N$_{hydr}$) tridentate coordination mode (both playing a very important role in the interaction between AlaAlaNHOH and the two studied metal ions, as seen in structures VI, VII and VIII), the significant differences between the equilibrium models obtained with the primary and secondary dipeptide hydroxamic acids (Table 4) are understandable. Apart from the minor species, $[M_2L]^{3+}$, with $[(\eta^5\text{-Cp*})Rh(H_2O)_3]^{2+}$ in an intermediate pH-range, only mononuclear complexes are seen in Table 4 with the secondary ligand. The model was also supported by the ESI-MS results. The existence of $[ML]^+$ and $[MH_{-1}L]$ were detected (the latter in its adduct with K$^+$) in both systems, while $[M_2L]^{3+}$ was detected only with $[(\eta^5\text{-Cp*})Rh(H_2O)_3]^{2+}$. The corresponding m/z values are shown in Table S1. Despite the almost identical equilibrium models, the binding modes cannot be the same in all of the suggested complexes with AlaAlaN(Me)OH and the two half-sandwich cations because the pH-metric titration curves indicate significant differences. This is demonstrated in Figure 6, where the titration curve of the ligand, and those registered at 1:1 metal ion to ligand ratio with the two cations are presented. In inset of Figure 6, the concentration distribution curves calculated using the pH-metric results are also shown.

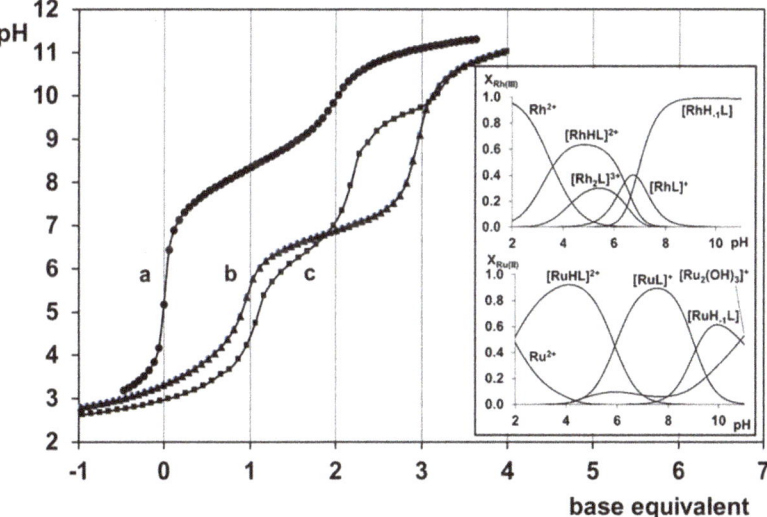

Figure 6. Representative titration curves for the (**a**) H$^+$–AlaAlaN(Me)OH, (**b**) $[(\eta^5\text{-Cp*})Rh(H_2O)_3]^{2+}$–AlaAlaN(Me)OH, and (**c**) $[(\eta^6\text{-}p\text{-cym})Ru(H_2O)_3]^{2+}$–AlaAlaN(Me)OH systems with their related concentration distribution curves in inset at 1:1 metal ion to ligand ratio. (c_L = 1.80 mM; negative base equivalent refers an excess of acid in the sample; "Rh" stands for $[(\eta^5\text{-Cp*})Rh(H_2O)_3]^{2+}$; "Ru" stands for $[(\eta^6\text{-}p\text{-cym})Ru(H_2O)_3]^{2+}$).

As can be seen in Table 4, the stability constants obtained for the [MHL]$^{2+}$ complexes are similar to the values of the corresponding ones with AlaAlaNHOH. This supports the same coordination mode (IV in Scheme 4) in [MHL]$^{2+}$ in all the studied systems. With the secondary ligand, however, this species is formed in a wider pH-range and higher extent than with the primary counterpart (cf. the corresponding speciation curves in Insets in Figures 5 and 6). The complex [M$_2$L]$^{3+}$, which was found only with the Rh(III)-containing cation, most probably has the binding mode shown in structure V in Scheme 4. Above pH ca. 5 [ML]$^+$ is formed in both systems, but predominates only in the [(η^6-p-cym)Ru(H$_2$O)$_3$]$^{2+}$-AlaAlaN(Me)OH system between pH ca. 6–8.5, while its amount is not significant at all with [(η^5-Cp*)Rh(H$_2$O)$_3$]$^{2+}$. Assuming that the terminal-NH$_3^+$ deprotonates in the [MHL]$^{2+}$ ⇌ [ML]$^+$ + H$^+$ equilibrium process, the pK values, that can be calculated using the corresponding stability constants in Table 4 (17.53 − 11.61 = 5.92 for the complex with [(η^6-p-cym)Ru(H$_2$O)$_3$]$^{2+}$, while 15.89 − 9.48 = 6.41 for the complex with [(η^5-Cp*)Rh(H$_2$O)$_3$]$^{2+}$) are significantly lower than the pK of the free ligand (see Table 1). This strongly suggests the coordination of the terminal amino-N in the [ML]$^+$ species. However, due to sterical reasons, the simultaneous coordination of the (O,O)$_{hydr}$ chelate and that of the amino-N are not possible at the three available sites of the same metal ion, and the stoichiometry of this species should be [M$_x$L$_x$]$^{x+}$. The suggested structure for [M$_2$L$_2$]$^{2+}$ is shown as structure IX in Scheme 5. Unfortunately, the methods applied could not provide direct information for the number of x, additional investigations are necessary to address this problem.

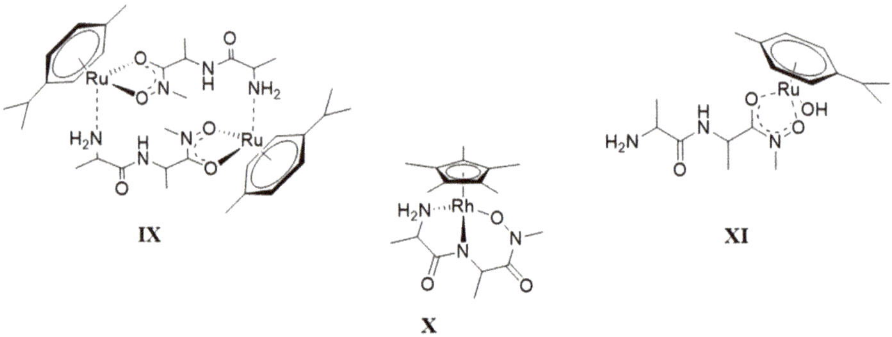

Scheme 5. Suggested binding modes for the complexes formed in half-sandwich metal ion–AlaAlaN(Me)OH systems.

On the contrary, rather large differences can be expected between the binding modes in [MH$_{-1}$L] formed with the two cations. As the comparison of curves b and c in Figure 6 reveals, the dissociation processes [MHL]$^{2+}$ ⇌ [ML]$^+$ + H$^+$ and [ML]$^+$ ⇌ [MH$_{-1}$L] + H$^+$ overlap with each other considerably in the [(η^5-Cp*)Rh(H$_2$O)$_3$]$^{2+}$-containing system (the corresponding pK values are 6.41 and 6.86 in Table 4), while those are completely separated from each other in the other system (the stepwise pK values are 5.92 and 9.11). The reason of this large difference originates from the rather different hydrolytic behaviour of the two half-sandwich cations, being the hydrolysis of the ruthenium-containing cation more pronounced [32]. As a consequence, [MH$_{-1}$L] can be formed with (NH$_2$,N$_{amide}$,O$_{hydr}$) tridentate coordination mode in the [(η^5-Cp*)Rh(H$_2$O)$_3$]$^{2+}$–AlaAlaN(Me)OH system only (structure X in Scheme 4), while the species with the same stoichiometry is a mixed hydroxido complex for the other metal ion (structure XI in Scheme 5).

2.5. Complexation of AlaGlyGlyNHOH or AlaGlyGlyN(Me)OH with the Two Half-Sandwich Type Cations—[(η^6-p-cym)Ru(H$_2$O)$_3$]$^{2+}$ or [(η^5-Cp*)Rh(H$_2$O)$_3$]$^{2+}$

Unfortunately, conventional pH-metric titrations could only be carried out below pH ca. 6 for the two systems containing one of the studied tripeptide hydroxamic acids and the [(η^6-p-cym)Ru(H$_2$O)$_3$]$^{2+}$ cation. Above this pH, the processes became too slow to reach pH equilibrium within maximum 30 min (see Materials and Methods section). As a consequence, calculations relating to the stoichiometry and stability constant of the complexes formed in these systems could only be carried out below pH 6. According to the pH-metric titration curves, however, the behaviour of the two ligands toward this half-sandwich cation is significantly different even in this narrow pH-range. For the primary derivative, two equivalents of base are consumed below pH 6 at 1:1 metal ion to ligand ratio, but only one with the secondary counterpart. There is no doubt that one equivalent base, in the pH-range ca. 2.5–4.5, is consumed for the neutralization of the proton released from the hydroxamic function and the (O,O)$_{hydr}$ chelate is formed. Direct proof for this assumption was obtained from the ^{1}H-NMR spectra, in which e.g., a new singlet of the C-terminal glycine-CH$_2$ protons (designated as "D" protons in the formula of AlaGlyGlyNHOH in Scheme 1) refers to the complex at 3.96 ppm, while the one for the non-complexed ligand is seen at 3.92 ppm. Indication is provided for the coordination of the amino-N in the pH-range of this second base-consuming process by the signal of the "B" protons in the ^{1}H-NMR spectra (the new signal belonging to the complex appears at 3.32 ppm). Most probably, due to sterical reasons this process was not observable with AlaGlyGlyN(Me)OH below pH 6 (spectra for this latter system are not presented here). The stoichiometries and the overall stability constants of the complexes yielding the best fit of the titration curves below pH 6 are as follows: [(η^6-p-cym)Ru(H$_2$O)$_3$]$^{2+}$-AlaGlyGlyNHOH: log$\beta_{[MHL]2+}$ = 17.19(2), log$\beta_{[ML]+}$ = 13.33(3); [(η^6-p-cym)Ru(H$_2$O)$_3$]$^{2+}$-AlaGlyGlyN(Me)OH: log$\beta_{[MHL]2+}$ = 17.14(2).

^{1}H-NMR measurements were also performed up to pH ca. 11 in these two systems, but detailed evaluation of them was not made because the spectra registered one hour after the preparation of the samples, as was often the case (see Materials and Methods section), which clearly did not refer to the equilibrium state in these samples above pH ca. 6. This was unambiguously supported by control measurements on a few samples where up to five days from the first registration the spectra were monitored again.

Fortunately, the processes were fast enough to perform pH-metric titrations in the [(η^5-Cp*)Rh(H$_2$O)$_3$]$^{2+}$–AlaGlyGlyN(Me)OH or –AlaGlyGlyNHOH systems, as demonstrated by Figure 7a,7b, respectively. The stoichiometry and overall stability constants of the complexes providing the best fit of the titration curves, together with the suggested binding modes of the complexes, are listed in Table 5. Concentration distribution curves calculated for the complexes formed in the above systems at 1:1 metal ion to ligand ratio using the corresponding stability constants are shown in Figure 7c,d, respectively.

Although some noticeable differences can be seen between the titration curves registered for the systems containing the primary and secondary ligands, Table 5 shows almost the same equilibrium models for the two systems (except the species [M$_2$_H$_2$L]$^+$, which was formed only with the primary derivative). A comparison of the two speciation profiles in Figure 7c,d however, indicated significant differences, especially in the intermediate pH-range (ca. 5–8). These differences are also supported by the ^{1}H-NMR spectra registered for the systems at 1:1 and 2:1 metal ion to ligand ratios. To illustrate this, Figure 8 shows the pH-dependence of the chemical shifts of the methyl (A) and (E) protons of AlaGlyGlyN(Me)OH as well as (A) protons of AlaGlyGlyNHOH in presence of equimolar amount of [(η^5-Cp*)Rh(H$_2$O)$_3$]$^{2+}$ in the pH-range ca. 2–11. Figure 8 reveals that individual signals belong to each of the complexes as well as to the free ligands in these systems. Consequently, the NMR results provided clear support to the speciation model and to the determination of the most likely binding modes in the complexes. (As an example, the registered spectra as a function of pH for the [(η^5-Cp*)Rh(H$_2$O)$_3$]$^{2+}$–AlaGlyGlyN(Me)OH system are shown in the Supplementary Figure S4.)

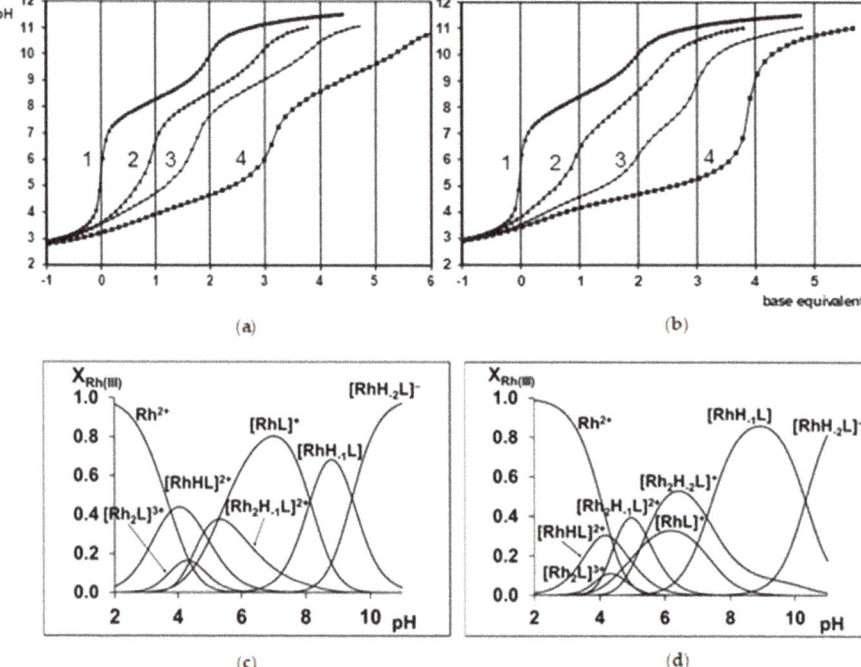

Figure 7. Titration curves with (**a**) AlaGlyGlyN(Me)OH and (**b**) AlaGlyGlyNHOH for (1) the H$^+$-ligand and the [(η^5-Cp*)Rh(H$_2$O)$_3$]$^{2+}$-ligand systems at (2) 1:2, (3) 1:1, and (4) 2:1 ratios (c_L = 1.62–1.82 mM, I = 0.20 M KNO$_3$); Calculated speciation curves for (**c**) the [(η^5-Cp*)Rh(H$_2$O)$_3$]$^{2+}$-AlaGlyGlyN(Me)OH (c_L = 1.82 mM) and (**d**) [(η^5-Cp*)Rh(H$_2$O)$_3$]$^{2+}$-AlaGlyGlyNHOH (c_L = 1.62 mM) systems at 1:1 ratio (negative base equivalent refers an excess of acid in the sample, "Rh" stands for [(η^5-Cp*)Rh(H$_2$O)$_3$]$^{2+}$).

Table 5. Overall stability constants (logβ) for the [(η^5-Cp*)Rh(H$_2$O$_3$)]$^{2+}$ complexes formed with tripeptide hydroxamic acids, together with their suggested binding modes at 25.0 °C, I = 0.20 M (KNO$_3$)*.

Species	AlaGlyGlyN(Me)OH		AlaGlyGlyNHOH	
	logβ	Coordinated Donor Atoms	logβ	Coordinated Donor Atoms
[MHL]$^{2+}$	15.53(4)	(O,O)$_{hydr}$	15.35(4)	(O,O)$_{hydr}$
[ML]$^+$	10.56(7)	(NH$_2$,N$_{amide}$)	10.42(6)	(NH$_2$,N$_{amide}$)
[MH$_{-1}$L]	2.42(6)	(NH$_2$,N$_{amide}$)	3.42(4)	(NH$_2$,N$_{amide}$, N$_{hydr}$)
[MH$_{-2}$L]$^-$	−7.02(7)	(NH$_2$,N$_{amide}$,N$_{amide}$)	−6.91(3)	(NH$_2$,N$_{amide}$,N$_{amide}$)
[M$_2$L]$^{3+}$	14.0(1)	(O,O)$_{hydr}$ + (NH$_2$,CO)	13.6(1)	(O,O)$_{hydr}$ + (NH$_2$,CO)
[M$_2$H$_{-1}$L]$^{2+}$	9.62(5)	(O,O)$_{hydr}$ + (NH$_2$,N$_{amide}$)	9.53(3)	(O,O)$_{hydr}$ + (NH$_2$,N$_{amide}$)
[M$_2$H$_{-2}$L]$^+$	-		4.12(3)	(O,O)$_{hydr}$ + (NH$_2$,N$_{amide}$,N$_{hydr}$)
Fitting parameter (mL)^a	0.0123		0.00599	
Number of fitted data	265		256	

*For the logβ values, 3σ standard deviations are in parentheses; ^{a} Fitting parameter is the average difference between the calculated and experimental titration curves expressed in the volume of the titrant; coordinated water molecules at the third coordination sites are omitted.

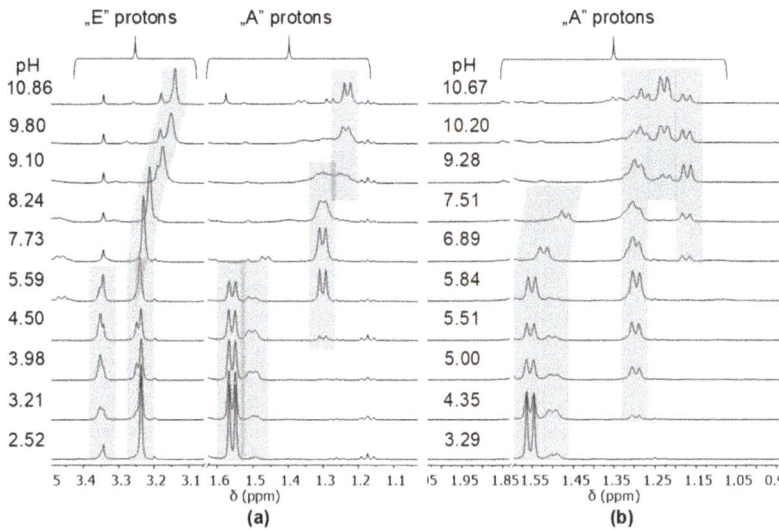

Figure 8. ^{1}H-NMR signals of E (singlets) and A (doublets) protons of the species formed in the (**a**) [(η^5-Cp*)Rh(H$_2$O)$_3$]$^{2+}$–AlaGlyGlyN(Me)OH and (**b**) [(η^5-Cp*)Rh(H$_2$O)$_3$]$^{2+}$–AlaGlyGlyNHOH systems at 1:1 metal ion to ligand ratio as a function of pH (c_L = 5.00 mM; ^{1}H-NMR signal at 3.34 ppm refers to methanol impurity in the ligand).

The conclusions, which can be drawn from a comparison of the equilibrium models/stability constants in Table 5, from the concentration distribution curves shown in Figure 7c,d and from the selected ^{1}H-NMR signals presented in Figure 8 are as follows: With the secondary derivative, the complexation starts above pH ca. 2 with the formation of [MHL]$^{2+}$, in which (O,O)$_{hydr}$ coordination mode is supported (a singlet in Figure 8a at 3.35 ppm belongs to the N-methyl (E) protons situating in the complexed ligand, while another one at 3.22 ppm to the protonated free ligand. The doublet at 1.55 ppm refers to the methyl protons of Ala (A)). Upon increasing the pH, first, the relative intensity of the singlet at 3.35 ppm increases up to pH ca. 4.5 and then starts to decrease and disappears by pH ca. 7. This suggests the displacement of the hydroxamate from the coordination sphere by pH 7, and, since the non-complexed hydroxamic function exists in its protonated form below and ca. pH 7, protonation of the displaced hydroxamate function occurs (a significant increase is seen in the intensity of the singlet at 3.22 ppm above pH 7). The appearance of a new doublet (1.55 ppm) at pH = 3.21 indicates the formation of a new species (this should be [M$_2$L]$^{2+}$), in which the hydroxamate chelate still exists, but the NH$_2$-function is also coordinated to another half-sandwich cation, most probably together with the neighbouring carbonyl-O. A new doublet at 1.30 ppm appears at pH ca. 4.5. Its relative intensity shows a sharp increase upon increasing the pH from 4.5 to 5.5, and some additional increase up to pH ca. 7.5 is observable, too. This signal starts to broaden, and its relative intensity decreases above pH ca. 8 but remains in the spectra up to as high as pH 9.8. Consumption of three equivalents of base and existence of three different species are shown in Figure 7a,c respectively, within the pH-range, where the doublet at 1.30 ppm exists. The three species, which are formed within the mentioned pH-range are the [M$_2$H$_{-1}$L]$^{2+}$, [ML]$^+$, and [MH$_{-1}$L]. As it is evident from the above NMR results, the coordination mode of the amino terminus of the tripeptide derivative in these three complexes is similar to each other and occurs, most probably, via (NH$_2$,N$_{amide}$,CO). The differences between the coordination modes of these complexes are due to the C-terminal end, where the hydroxamic function is situated. This latter function is deprotonated and coordinated to a second metal ion in [M$_2$H$_{-1}$L]$^{2+}$, it is non-coordinated and protonated in [ML]$^+$ (the formula of this species is in fact [MH(H$_{-1}$L)]$^+$), while it is non-coordinated and deprotonated in [MH$_{-1}$L]). (The deprotonation of the non-coordinated hydroxamic function is clearly seen in Figure 8a from the upfield shift of the resonance of the N-methyl singlet (E) from 3.22 ppm to 3.10 ppm between pH ca. 7–9.) The thermodynamically most stable complex, [MH₋₂L]⁻, in this system is present above pH 8 with the coordination mode of (NH₂,N$_{amide}$,N$_{amide}$), via two joined five-membered chelates.

Compared to the secondary derivative, the primary counterpart AlaGlyGlyNHOH has an additional and strong competitor donor, N$_{hydr}$ in its deprotonated form. Consequently, in this ligand, the number of the N-donors, which can be in chelatable position to each other, is four (NH₂, two N$_{amides}$, N$_{hydr}$), which is more than enough to saturate the three available coordination sites of [(η⁵-Cp*)Rh(H₂O)₃]²⁺. Although this results in higher variation of the binding modes with the primary ligand compared to the secondary one no difference can be seen between their coordination behaviour at the start of the interaction (pH ca. 2–3), where the (O,O)$_{hydr}$ dominates with both ligands and also the thermodynamically most stable complex, [MH₋₂L]⁻, has the same binding mode (NH₂, N$_{amide}$,N$_{amide}$) in both cases. The formation of [MH₋₂L]⁻ (cf. Figure 7c,d), however, is somewhat hindered with the primary derivative (its formation pH is above 9) compared to the secondary one (pH ~ 8). This difference clearly supports the importance of the N$_{hydr}$ coordination in the intermediate pH-range with AlaGlyGlyNHOH. The most important role of this donor is indicated by the NMR spectra (Figure 8b) in the pH-range ca. 7–10.5, where a new doublet at high field (1.18 ppm) exists. The pH-dependence of its intensity is very similar to the concentration profile of [MH₋₁L] (cf. Figures 7d and 8b) suggesting that this signal can be designated to the latter complex, in which, most probably, three nitrogens are coordinated to the metal cation (NH₂,N$_{amide}$,N$_{hydr}$). The differences between the binding modes in [MH₋₁L] formed with AlaGlyGlyN(Me)OH and AlaGlyGlyNHOH are well observable by the comparison of structures XII and XIII in Scheme 6.

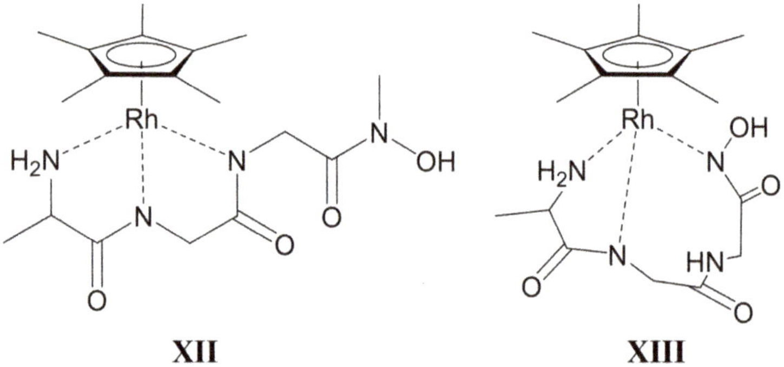

Scheme 6. Suggested binding modes for the [MH₋₁L] complexes formed in the [(η⁵-Cp*)Rh(H₂O)₃]²⁺–AlaGlyGlyN(Me)OH (structure **XII**) and [(η⁵-Cp*)Rh(H₂O)₃]²⁺–AlaGlyGlyNHOH (structure **XIII**) systems.

3. Discussion

Based on the solution equilibrium results and on the comparison of them, the following conclusions can be drawn regarding the complexes of primary and secondary hydroxamic derivatives of common di- and tripeptides, AlaAlaNHOH, AlaAlaN(Me)OH, AlaGlyGlyNHOH, and AlaGlyGlyN(Me)OH, with selected 3d metals, Fe(III), Ni(II), Cu(II), Zn(II), and 4d metals, tetraoxido anion of Mo(VI), half-sandwich type cations of Ru(II) and Rh(III), [(η⁶-p-cym)Ru(H₂O)₃]²⁺, and [(η⁵-Cp*)Rh(H₂O)₃]²⁺:

1. Due to its highest conditional stability out of the possible ones under highly acidic conditions, the hydroxamate-type chelate, (O,O)$_{hydr}$ is the anchor with all the studied metal ions, Mo(VI), Fe(III), Cu(II), Ru(II), and Rh(III), with which the interaction starts at pH ca. 3 or below. The situation is somewhat different with Ni(II) and Zn(II), where the interaction starts at pH ca. 4 or somewhat above. In these latter systems, binding isomers can exist because the coordination starts either via the five-membered (O,O)$_{hydr}$ or five-membered (NH₂,CO) chelate. For Zn(II),

these initial interactions were followed by hydrolytic processes resulting in the formation of mixed hydroxido complexes.

2. Exclusive hydroxamate-type coordination could be detected in the whole pH-range with Fe(III) and Mo(VI) (or also hydroximate-type one in the case of Mo(VI) with primary derivatives at higher pH). No role of the amino-N or peptide amide-N(s) was found in the complexation with these two metals. Consequently, there is no any significant difference between their complexation with the studied dipeptide and tripeptide derivatives. However, significant difference was found between the Mo(VI)-binding ability of the primary and secondary derivatives, the former being much more effective Mo(VI)-chelators. This is due to the significantly higher stability of the doubly deprotonated hydroximato chelate (which was detected in the Mo(VI)–primary derivative ligand systems up to pH ca. 10). On the contrary, the mono-deprotonated $(O,O)_{hydr}$ chelate cannot compete with the hydrolysis of the Mo(VI) above the neutral pH.

3. Out of the investigated metals, Ni(II) showed the highest preference towards the N-donors over the hydroxamate oxygens. This allows only a minor role of the $(O,O)_{hydr}$ at the beginning of the interaction. After that, Ni(II) forms with the primary AlaGlyGlyNHOH in slow cooperative processes a planar, 4N-coordinated $(NH_2, N_{amide}, N_{amide}, N_{hydr})$ 1:1 complex with very high stability, which exclusively exists above pH ca. 6. With the secondary counterpart, however, an $(NH_2, N_{amide}, N_{amide}, O_{hydr})$-coordinated planar complex is formed, with slightly lower stability and dominates only above pH ca. 7. The hydrolysis of the coordinated metal ion is hindered in both complexes, but, in the latter system, formation of bis-complexes in small extent can be observed in the presence of ligand excess. Nevertheless, even the secondary AlaGlyGlyN(Me)OH is a more effective ligand for Ni(II) (the situation is the same with Cu(II)) than the previously studied dipeptide derivatives [19,20].

4. Although the binding modes of the most stable Cu(II) complexes with AlaGlyGlyNHOH and with the secondary counterpart, the 4N-coordinated $(NH_2, N_{amide}, N_{amide}, N_{hydr})$ and $(NH_2, N_{amide}, N_{amide}, O_{hydr})$ planar 1:1 complexes, respectively, are the same as those with Ni(II); moreover their stability constants are significantly higher than those of the corresponding Ni(II) complexes (see Table 2), these species become predominant in the Cu(II)-containing systems in the higher pH-range only (above pH 8 and 9, respectively). This happens because the $(O,O)_{hydr}$ can play a crucial role in the interaction with Cu(II), and this is not the case for Ni(II). As a result of the measurable competition between the different types of potential donors even at neutral pH, the processes become very slow especially in the Cu(II)–primary tripeptide derivative system (too slow to allow conventional titrimetry). There is some dominance of the formation of oligonuclear (mostly dimeric or trimeric) complexes and, mainly with the secondary derivative, the formation of bis-hydroxamato intermediate complexes is also considerable.

5. There are only maximum three sites available for coordination for the studied half-sandwich type Ru(II) and Rh(III) cations. There is no doubt that with both cations and all four ligands the $(O,O)_{hydr}$ anchor-chelate can remain in the coordination sphere up to pH ca. 7 but is displaced by nitrogen donors, if there is no possibility for the formation of the hydroximate-(O,O) chelate, with the doubly deprotonated hydroxamic function. If, however, it can be formed, it remains in the coordination sphere, which is the case with the primary dipeptide derivative AlaAlaNHOH, and the N-donors can only coordinate to another metal ion. Consequently, dinuclear complexes predominate from slightly acidic conditions until the end of the investigated pH-range with both cations. In the most stable complex, the donor set $(NH_2, N_{amide}, N_{hydr})$ saturates the coordination sites of one metal, while the $(O,O)_{hydr}$ chelate and either a water, or above pH ca. 9–10, a hydroxide ion binds to another metal ion. On the contrary, mononuclear complexes dominate with the secondary counterpart, AlaAlaN(Me)OH, being the most stable an $(NH_2, N_{amide}, O_{hydr})$-coordinated complex with the $[(\eta^5\text{-Cp*})Rh(H_2O)_3]^{2+}$ cation. Due to the significantly higher affinity of $[(\eta^6\text{-}p\text{-cym})Ru(H_2O)_3]^{2+}$ toward hydrolysis, it forms a mixed hydroxido complex involving an (NH_2, N_{amide}) chelate and a monodentate OH^-.

6. The complex formation processes were too slow between $[(\eta^6\text{-}p\text{-cym})Ru(H_2O)_3]^{2+}$ and the two tripeptide derivatives, AlaGlyGlyNHOH and AlaGlyGlyN(Me)OH, above pH ca. 6, where the interaction with the N-donors started. Consequently, solution equilibrium measurements were possible only on the $[(\eta^5\text{-Cp*})Rh(H_2O)_3]^{2+}$-containing systems. With the secondary derivative containing three potential nitrogen donors, the initial $(O,O)_{hydr}$ chelate in the highly acidic pH range is partially replaced by the coordination of the NH_2 group (most probably together with the neighboring CO) above pH ca. 4. This results in the formation of dinuclear species with mixed $(O,O)_{hydr}$ and (NH_2, CO) coordination below pH ca. 7–7.5 as minor complexes, but mononuclear species with $(NH_2, N_{amide}, N_{amide})$ binding mode (having the hydroxamate function is uncoordinated) dominate even in this intermediate pH-range.

7. The primary AlaGlyGlyNHOH contains four potential N-donors, which is more than enough to saturate the coordination sphere of a $[(\eta^5\text{-Cp*})Rh(H_2O)_3]^{2+}$ cation. The results show a measurable competition between the C-terminal N_{amide} and N_{hydr} between pH ca. 7–10, but above this pH, the complex with the $(NH_2, N_{amide}, N_{amide})$ donor set, containing the hydroxamate function in uncoordinated form, has increasing dominance.

4. Materials and Methods

4.1. Materials and Stock Solutions

The ligands AlaAlaNHOH, AlaAlaN(Me)OH, AlaGlyGlyNHOH, and AlaGlyGlyN(Me)OH were synthesized as previously described [19–21]. The purity and the exact concentration of the ligand stock solutions were determined by pH-potentiometry using the Gran's method [33].

The metal ion stock solutions were prepared from $CuCl_2 \cdot 2H_2O$, $NiCl_2 \cdot 5H_2O$, $FeCl_3 \cdot 6H_2O$, and Na_2MoO_4 (Reanal, Hungary) using doubly deionised and ultra-filtered water obtained from a Milli-Q RG (Millipore, Burlington, MA, USA) water purification system. In the case of Fe(III), the stock solution also contained hydrochloric acid (~0.1 M). ZnO (Reanal, Hungary) was dissolved in diluted HCl to prepare Zn(II) stock solution. The metal ion concentrations were checked gravimetrically via precipitation of the quinolin-8-olate salts, Fe(III) was determined by complexometric titration. The acid content of the Fe(III) stock solution was also estimated using the Gran's method [33].

$RuCl_3 \cdot xH_2O$, α-terpinene were purchased from Aldrich (St. Louis, MO, USA), and $[(\eta^5\text{-Cp*})Rh(\mu^2\text{-Cl})Cl]_2$ was a commercial product from Strem Chemicals (Newburyport, MA, USA). These chemicals were used without further purification. $[(\eta^6\text{-}p\text{-cym})Ru(\mu^2\text{-Cl})Cl]_2$ was synthesized and purified according to a literature method [34]. The aqueous solutions of $[(\eta^6\text{-}p\text{-cym})Ru(H_2O)_3](NO_3)_2$ and $[(\eta^5\text{-Cp*})Rh(H_2O)_3](NO_3)_2$ were obtained by removal the chloride ions from the corresponding dimers using stoichiometric amount of $AgNO_3$. Metal ion and proton concentrations of these metal ion stock solutions were also checked with the aid of potentiometric titrations.

Carbonate-free KOH solutions of known concentrations (ca. 0.2 M during the pH-metric measurements and ca. 5 M to adjust the pH during the ^{17}O-NMR) were used as titrant. HCl and HNO_3 stock solutions were prepared from their concentrated solutions (both acids and the base were Merck products, Germany), and their concentrations were determined by pH-metric titrations.

4.2. Solution Studies

For all of the solution studies, doubly deionised and ultra-filtered water was obtained from a Milli-Q RG (Millipore) water purification system.

pH potentiometric measurements were carried out at 25.0 ± 0.1 °C, at an ionic strength of 0.20 M KNO_3 if the metal ion was either $[(\eta^6\text{-}p\text{-cym})Ru(H_2O)_3]^{2+}$ or $[(\eta^5\text{-Cp*})Rh(H_2O)_3]^{2+}$, while in all the other cases, it was at 0.20 M KCl. For the systems containing Ru(II) or Rh(III) and a dipeptide hydroxamic acid as ligand a Mettler Toledo (Switzerland) T50 titrator, if, however, the ligand was a tripeptide hydroxamic acid, a Mettler Toledo DL50 titrator was used for the pH-metric titrations. Both instruments were equipped with a Metrohm (Switzerland) double junction (6.0255.100) combined electrode. In all the other cases a Radiometer pHM 84 instrument equipped with Metrohm combined electrode (type 6.0234.100) and Metrohm 715 Dosimat burette was used for the pH-metry. The electrode systems were calibrated according to Irving et al. [35]. Therefore, the pH-meter readings could be converted into hydrogen ion concentrations. The water ionization constant was $pK_w = 13.75 \pm 0.01$ under the experimental conditions used. The initial volumes of the samples were 5.00, 10.00, or 15.00 mL, and the ligand concentrations were varied in the range of 1–5 mM and the metal ion to ligand ratios between 2:1–1:5. Typically, three to five ratios were measured in each system. The samples were stirred and completely deoxygenated by bubbling purified argon. Titrations were performed in the pH-range of 2.0–11.0 or until precipitation occurred in equilibrium controlled mode. pH equilibrium was assumed to be reached if a change in the measured potential was less than 0.01 mV within 11 s and 0.1 mV within 90 s for the Mettler Toledo DL50 and Mettler Toledo T50 titrators, respectively. The maximum waiting time for the metal ion–containing systems was 10 min in general, except the systems containing Ru(II) or Rh(III) half-sandwich cations, where it was 30 min due to the quite slow equilibrium processes. If the equilibrium was not reached within these times, the measured value was not used during the calculation.

In general, the overall stability constants calculated for the complexes relate to the equilibrium

$$pM + qH + rL \rightleftharpoons [M_pH_qL_r] \tag{5}$$

$$\beta_{pqr} = [M_pH_qL_r]/[M]^p[H]^q[L]^r \tag{6}$$

where "M" stands for Fe^{3+}, Ni^{2+}, Cu^{2+}, Zn^{2+}, $[(\eta^6\text{-}p\text{-cym})Ru(H_2O)_3]^{2+}$, or $[(\eta^5\text{-Cp*})Rh(H_2O)_3]^{2+}$ and "L" represents the completely deprotonated forms of the ligands. Because the charges are not always the same, they are omitted in Equation (5).

In the case of Mo(VI), however, the calculated stability constants refer to Equation (1) given in Section 2.3.

In all calculations, the stability constants were determined via fitting the titration curves by using the PSEQUAD and SUPERQUAD programs [36,37]. In the case of the systems, where measurable competition between the hydrolysis of the metal ions and the complexation processes can occur, the former was taken into account during the calculations by using the following literature data (where the Davies equation was used to take into account the different ionic strengths; negative stoichiometric number of H relates to the metal induced ionization of the coordinated water).

$[Fe(OH)]^{2+}$ $\log\beta_{1,-1,0} = -3.21$; $[Fe(OH)_2]^+$ $\log\beta_{1,-2,0} = -6.73$; $[Fe_2(OH)_2]^{4+}$ $\log\beta_{2,-2,0} = 4.09$; $[Fe_3(OH)_4]^{5+}$ $\log\beta_{3,-4,0} = -7.58$ [38].

$[HMoO_4]^-$ $\log\beta_{1,1,0} = 4.03$; $[H_2MoO_4]$ $\log\beta_{1,2,0} = 6.70$; $[H_8(MoO_4)_7]^{6-}$ $\log\beta_{7,8,0} = 53.18$; $[H_9(MoO_4)_7]^{5-}$ $\log\beta_{7,9,0} = 58.10$; $[H_{10}(MoO_4)_7]^{4-}$ $\log\beta_{7,10,0} = 62.11$; $[H_{11}(MoO_4)_7]^{3-}$ $\log\beta_{7,11,0} = 64.54$ [30].

$[\{(\eta^6\text{-}p\text{-cym})Ru\}_2(\mu^2\text{-OH})_3]^+$ ($\log\beta_{2,-3,0} = -9.16$) [32]

$[\{(\eta^5\text{-Cp*})Rh\}_2(\mu^2\text{-OH})_2]^{2+}$ ($\log\beta_{2,-2,0} = -8.53$); $[\{(\eta^5\text{-Cp*})Rh\}_2(\mu^2\text{-OH})_3]^+$ ($\log\beta_{2,-3,0} = -14.26$) [39].

For the Ru–AlaAlaNHOH system (where Ru stands for $[(\eta^6\text{-}p\text{-cym})Ru(H_2O)_3]^{2+}$), the corresponding hydrochloride salt of the ligand was used, therefore the studied samples also contain one equivalent of chloride ion as a second ligand.

^{1}H-NMR titrations were carried out on a Bruker (Billerica, MA, USA) Avance 400 instrument at 25.0 °C at an ionic strength of 0.20 M KNO$_3$ for the systems containing Ru(II) or Rh(III) half-sandwich cations and on a Bruker AM360 FT NMR instrument at 0.20 M KCl for the systems containing Zn(II) or Mo(VI). The chemical shifts are reported in ppm (δ_H) from TSP as internal standard. Titrations were performed using individual samples equilibrated for 1 hour prior to the measurements in D$_2$O (99.8%) at $c_L = 10.0$ mM in the case of dipeptide hydroxamic acid containing systems and $c_L = 5.0$ mM for the tripeptide hydroxamic acid containing ones. The metal ion to ligand ratios were 1:1 and 2:1, the pH of the samples was varied in the range of 2.0–11.5. The pH of the samples was set up with NaOD or DNO_3 solutions in D_2O. The pH* values (pH meter readings in D_2O solution of a pH-meter calibrated in H_2O according to Irving et al. [35]) were converted into pH values using the following equation: pH = 0.936×pH* + 0.412. [40].

On all the other systems, the ^{1}H-NMR measurements were made on Bruker AM 360 by using D_2O as solvent. For Mo(VI), DSS was used as standard, metal to ligand ratio was 1:3 in all samples, the analytical concentration of the ligand was 0.015 M.

For the Mo(VI)-containing systems, ^{17}O-NMR measurements were performed at 1:3 metal ion to ligand ratio at c_L = 0.15 M. The solvent was 90% H_2O 10% D_2O enriched for ^{17}O. Enrichment of the molybdate oxygen atoms to 3% was done by the addition of $H_2^{17}O$ (37.8 %, ISOTEC Inc., Matheson CO, USA) to the samples. The enrichment included the M=O oxygens, while the oxygens of the ligands were not involved in the ^{17}O isotope enrichment, being inert for oxygen exchange. Spectra were registered on a Bruker DRX 500 NMR equipment at 67.8 MHz. Spectral widths of 1200 ppm (81.4 kHz) were used, and data for the FID were accumulated in 8k blocks. A 40° pulse angle and 100 ms relaxation delays were used. The spectra were integrated after baseline correction by using WINNMR 960901 software. Chemical shifts refer to the signal of tap water, δ = 0 ppm.

Frozen solution EPR (Electron Paramagnetic Resonance) spectra in aqueous samples of the copper complexes were recorded on a Bruker EMX X-band spectrometer, operating at ~9.4 GHz, equipped with a HP 53150A microwave frequency counter using ^{63}CuSO$_4$ stock solution. Metallic copper was purchased from JV Isoflex (Moscow, Russia) containing 99.3% ^{63}Cu and 0.7% ^{65}Cu and converted into the sulfate. The samples for low-temperature measurements contained a few drops of ethylene glycol to ensure good glass formation. The metal ion to ligand ratios varied in the range 1:1–1:5 and $c_{Cu(II)}$ was 0.005 M; the pH of the samples was varied in the range of 3.4–10.2. Increasing the resolution and avoid the aggregation process 10 % ethylene glycol was added to the aqueous copper(II) complex samples.

An HP 8453 or Perkin Elmer Lambda 25 spectrophotometer was used to record the UV-Vis spectra over the range 250–800 nm for copper(II)-, iron(III)-, and nickel(II)-containing systems. The path length was 1 cm. Measurements for the iron(III)-containing samples were carried out on individual samples in which the 0.20 M KCl was partially or completely replaced by HCl. pH values, varying in the range ca. 0.7–1.6, were calculated from the HCl content. The metal ion concentrations were in the range 0.0004–0.0008 M, and the metal ion to ligand ratios were in the range 1:1–1:5. Spectrophotometric titrations were also performed with samples containing Fe(III), Cu(II) or Ni(II) in 0.0004–0.004 M concentrations at metal to ligand ratios ranging from 1:1 to 1:5. The spectrophotometric results were utilized to calculate the stability constants for the Fe(III) complexes formed below pH 2.0.

ESI-MS measurements were carried out on a Bruker micrOTOF-Q instrument in positive ion mode. The samples were prepared in water, at c_M = 0.3 mM. The metal ion to ligand ratios were 1:1 and 2:1 in all cases, the pH of the samples was set up according to the concentration distribution curves by using HNO_3 or KOH solutions. The temperature of the drying gas (N_2) was 180 °C, and the pressure of the nebulizing gas was 0.3 bar. The flow rate was 3 μL/min. The spectra were accumulated and recovered by a digitalizer at a sampling rate of 2 GHz. DataAnalysis (version 3.4) was used for the calculations.

Supplementary Materials: The following are available online at http://www.mdpi.com/1420-3049/24/21/3941/s1: **Figure S1**. EPR spectra recorded at different pH values for the (a) ^{63}Cu(II)–AlaGlyGlyNHOH and (b) ^{63}Cu(II)–AlaGlyGlyN(Me)OH systems at 1:1 and 1:2 metal ion to ligand ratios, respectively ($c_{Cu(II)}$ = 5.00 mM); **Figure S2**. pH dependence on the low-field region of ^{1}H-NMR spectra of [(η^6-p-cym)Ru(H_2O)$_3$]$^{2+}$–AlaAlaNHOH system at 1:1 metal ion to ligand ratio (c_L = 10.0 mM); **Figure S3**. Measured and calculated ESI-MS spectra of [$M_2H_{-2}L$]+ formed in [(η^6-p-cym)Ru(H_2O)$_3$]$^{2+}$–AlaAlaNHOH system at pH = 8.01; **Figure S4**. pH dependence on the ^{1}H-NMR spectra of (a) [(η^5-Cp*)Rh(H_2O)$_3$]$^{2+}$–AlaGlyGlyN(Me)OH = 2:1 system and (b) CH_3 signals of Cp* ligand at different pH values (region of the methyl protons is shown with reduced intensity for an easier interpretation); **Table S1**. Observed and calculated m/z values of the species formed in the investigated half-sandwich cation–dipeptide hydroxamic acid systems.

Author Contributions: A.O., L.B., E.M.N., and D.S. performed experimental work and were involved in calculations and evaluation of the data. A.O. wrote the first version of the Materials and Methods part of the paper,

E.F. and P.B. directed the project, supervised the work. E.F. wrote the draft version of the paper (Introduction, Results, and Discussion), which was corrected and completed by the team of the co-authors.

Funding: This research was funded by the EU, co-financed by the European Regional Development Fund under project GINOP-2.3.2-15-2016-00008, and funded by the Hungarian Scientific Research Fund (OTKA K112317).

Acknowledgments: The authors thank Ildikó Nagy for performing the experimental work on the Mo(VI)-containing systems.

Conflicts of Interest: The authors declare no conflict of interest.

References

1. Codd, R. Traversing the coordination chemistry and chemical biology of hydroxamic acids. *Coord. Chem. Rev.* **2008**, *252*, 1387–1408. [CrossRef]
2. Gupta, S.P.; Sharma, A. The Chemistry of Hydroxamic Acids. In *Hydroxamic acids: A unique Family of Chemicals with Multiple Biological Activities*; Gupta S.P, Ed.; Springer: Berlin, Germany, 2013; pp. 1–17.
3. Albrecht-Gary, A.M.; Crumbliss, A.L. Coordination chemistry of siderophores: thermodynamics and kinetics of iron chelation and release. In *Metal Ions in Biological Systems*; Sigel, A., Sigel, H., Eds.; Marcel Dekker: New York, NY, USA, 1998; Volume 35, pp. 239–327.
4. Muri, E.M.F.; Nieto, M.J.; Sindelar, R.D.; Williamson, J.S. Hydroxamic acids as pharmacological agents. *Curr. Med. Chem.* **2002**, *9*, 1631–1653. [CrossRef] [PubMed]
5. Marmion, C.J.; Parker, J.P.; Nolan, K.B. Hydroxamic acids: An Important Class of Metalloenzyme Inhibitors. In *Comprehensive Inorganic Chemistry II: From Elements to Applications*, 2nd ed.; Reedijk, J., Poeppelmeier, K.R., Eds.; Elsevier Ltd.: Amsterdam, The Netherlands, 2013; Volume 3, pp. 683–708. [CrossRef]
6. Marmion, C.J.; Murphy, T.; Docherty, J.R.; Nolan, K.B. Hydroxamic acids are nitric oxide donors. Facile formation of ruthenium(II)-nitrosyls and NO-mediated activation of guanylate cyclase by hydroxamic acids. *Chem. Commun.* **2000**, 1153–1154. [CrossRef]
7. Kohli, R. Intra-and intermolecular hydrogen bonding in formohydroxamic acid. In *Hydrogen bonding abilities of hydroxamic acid and its isosteres*; Anchor Academic Publishing: Hamburg, Germany, 2016; pp. 58–112.
8. Carrott, M.J.; Fox, O.D.; LeGurun, G.; Jones, C.J.; Mason, C.; Taylor, R.J.; Andrieux, F.P.L.; Boxall, C. Oxidation–reduction reactions of simple hydroxamic acids and plutonium(IV) ions in nitric acid. *Radiochim. Acta* **2008**, *96*, 333–343. [CrossRef]
9. Farkas, E.; Enyedy, É.A. Interaction between iron(II) and hydroxamic acids: oxidation of iron(II) to iron(III) by desferrioxamine B under anaerobic conditions. *J. Inorg. Biochem.* **2001**, *83*, 107–114. [CrossRef]
10. Kurzak, B.; Kozlowski, H.; Farkas, E. Hydroxamic and aminohydroxamic acids and their complexes with metal ions. *Coord. Chem. Rev.* **1992**, *114*, 169–2000. [CrossRef]
11. Farkas, E.; Csóka, H.; Bell, G.; Brown, D.A.; Cuffe, L.P.; Fitzpatrick, N.J.; Glass, W.K.; Errington, W.; Kemp, T.J. Oxygen *versus* nitrogen co-ordination in complexes of Mo^{VI} and hydroxamate derivatives of α-amino acids: equilibrium, structural and theoretical studies. *J. Chem. Soc. Dalton Trans.* **1999**, *16*, 2789–2794. [CrossRef]
12. Parajdi-Losonczi, P.L.; Bényei, A.C.; Kováts, É.; Timári, I.; Muchova Radosova, T.; Novohradsky, V.; Kasparkova, J.; Buglyó, P. [(η^6-*p*-cymene)Ru(H$_2$O)$_3$]$^{2+}$ binding capability of aminohydroxamates — A solution and solid state study. *J. Inorg. Biochem.* **2016**, *160*, 236–245. [CrossRef]
13. Parajdi-Losonczi, P.L.; Buglyó, P.; Skakalova, H.; Kasparkova, J.; Lihi, N.; Farkas, E. Half-sandwich type rhodium(III)-aminohydroxamate complexes: the role of the position of the amino group in metal binding. *New J. Chem.* **2018**, *42*, 7659–7670. [CrossRef]
14. Kurzak, B.; Farkas, E.; Glowiak, T.; Kozlowski, H. X-Ray and potentiometric studies on a pentanuclear copper(II) complex with β-alaninehydroxamic acid. *J. Chem. Soc., Dalton Trans.* **1991**, *2*, 163–167. [CrossRef]
15. Tegoni, M.; Remelli, M. Metallacrowns of copper(II) and aminohydroxamates: Thermodynamics of self assembly and host–guest equilibria. *Coord. Chem. Rev.* **2012**, *56*, 289–315. [CrossRef]
16. Ostrowska, M.; Fritsky, I.O.; Gumienna-Kontecka, E.; Pavlishchu, A.V. Metallacrown-based compounds: Applications in catalysis, luminescence, molecular magnetism, and adsorption. *Coord. Chem. Rev.* **2016**, *327*, 304–332. [CrossRef]
17. Farkas, E.; Kiss, I. Complexes of peptidehydroxamates. Complex formation between transition metals and L-prolyl-L-leucylglycinehydroxamic acid [*N*-hydroxy-7-methyl-4-oxo-5-(pyrrolidine-2'-carboxamido)-3-

azaoctanamide] and L-prolyl-L-leucinehydroxamic acid [N-hydroxy-4-methyl-2-(pyrrolidine-2'-carboxamido)pentanamide]. *J. Chem. Soc. Dalton Trans.* **1990**, *3*, 749–753. [CrossRef]

18. Farkas, E.; Csapó, E.; Buglyó, P.; Damante, C.A.; Di Natale, G. Metal binding ability of histidine-containing peptidehydroxamic acids: Imidazole versus hydroxamate coordination. *Inorg. Chim. Acta* **2009**, *362*, 753–762. [CrossRef]

19. Buglyó, P.; Nagy, E.M.; Farkas, E.; Sóvágó, I.; Sanna, D.; Micera, G. New insights into the metal ion-peptidehydroxamate interactions: Metal complexes of primary hydroxamic acid derivatives of common dipeptides in aqueous solution. *Polyhedron* **2007**, *26*, 1625–1633. [CrossRef]

20. Buglyó, P.; Nagy, E.M.; Sóvágó, I.; Ozsváth, A.; Sanna, D.; Farkas, E. Metal ion binding capability of secondary (N-methyl) versus primary (N-H) dipeptide hydroxamic acids. *Polyhedron* **2016**, *110*, 172–181. [CrossRef]

21. Ozsváth, A.; Farkas, E.; Diószegi, R.; Buglyó, P. Versatility and trends in the interaction between Pd(II) and peptide hydroxamic acids. *New. J. Chem.* **2019**, *43*, 8239–8249. [CrossRef]

22. Moore, W.M.; Spilburg, C.A. Purification of human collagenases with a hydroxamic acid affinity column. *Biochemistry* **1986**, *25*, 5189–5195. [CrossRef]

23. Melchart, M.; Sadler, P.J. Ruthenium Arene Anticancer Complexes. In *Bioorganometallics: Biomolecules, Labeling, Medicine*; Jaouen, G., Ed.; John Wiley & Sons: Hoboken, NJ, USA, 2005; pp. 39–64. [CrossRef]

24. Mészáros, J.P.; Poljarevic, J.M.; Gál, G.T.; May, N.V.; Spengler, G.; Enyedy, É.A. Comparative solution and structural studies of half-sandwich rhodium and ruthenium complexes bearing curcumin and acetylacetone. *J. Inorg. Biochem.* **2019**, *195*, 91–100. [CrossRef]

25. Tejada-Jimenez, M.; Chamizo-Ampudia, A.; Calatrava, V.; Galvan, A.; Fernandez, E.; Llamas, A. From the Eukaryotic Molybdenum Cofactor Biosynthesis to the Moonlighting Enzyme mARC. *Molecules* **2018**, *23*, 3287. [CrossRef]

26. Leimkühler, S.; Wuebbens, M.M.; Rajagopalan, K.V. The history of the discovery of the molybdenum cofactor and novel aspects of its biosynthesis in bacteria. *Coord. Chem. Rev.* **2011**, *255*, 1129–1144. [CrossRef] [PubMed]

27. Enyedy, É.A.; Csóka, H.; Lázár, I.; Micera, G.; Garibba, E.; Farkas, E. Effects of side-chain aminonitrogen donor atoms on metal complexation of aminohydroxamic acids: New diaminohydroxamates chelating Ni(II) more strongly than Fe(III). *J. Chem. Soc. Dalton Trans.* **2002**, *13*, 2632–2640. [CrossRef]

28. Yokoi, H. ESP and optical absorption studies of various bis(N-salicylidenealkylaminato)copper(II) complexes with terahedrally-distoted coordination geometry. *Bull. Chem. Soc. Japan* **1974**, *47*, 3037–3040. [CrossRef]

29. Yokoi, H.; Addison, A.W. Spectroscopic and redox properties of pseudotetrahedral copper(II) complexes. Their relation to copper proteins. *Inorg. Chem.* **1977**, *16*, 1341–1349. [CrossRef]

30. Farkas, E.; Csóka, H.; Tóth, I. New insights into the solution equilibrium of molybdenum(VI)-hydroxamate systems: ^{1}H and ^{17}O-NMR spectroscopic study of Mo(VI)-desferrioxamine B and Mo(VI)-monohdroxamic acid systems. *Dalton Trans.* **2003**, *8*, 1645–1652. [CrossRef]

31. Buglyo, P.; Parajdi-Losonczi, P.L.; Benyei, A.C.; Lihi, N.; Biro, L.; Farkas, E. Versatility of Coordination Modes in Complexes of Monohydroxamic Acids with Half-Sandwich Type Ruthenium, Rhodium, Osmium and Iridium Cations. *Chem. Select* **2017**, *26*, 8127–8136. [CrossRef]

32. Bíró, L.; Farkas, E.; Buglyó, P. Hydrolytic behaviour and chloride ion binding capability of [Ru(η^6-p-cym)(H$_2$O)$_3$]$^{2+}$: A solution equilibrium study. *Dalton Trans.* **2012**, *41*, 285–299. [CrossRef]

33. Gran, G. Determination of the Equivalent Point in Potentiometric Titrations. *Acta Chem. Scand.* **1950**, *4*, 559–577. [CrossRef]

34. Bennett, M.A.; Smith, A.K. Arene ruthenium(II) complexes formed by dehydrogenation of cyclohexadienes with ruthenium(III) trichloride. *J. Chem. Soc. Dalton Trans.* **1974**, 233–241. [CrossRef]

35. Irving, H.M.; Miles, M.G.; Pettit, L.D. A study of some problems in determining the stoicheiometric proton dissociation constants of complexes by potentiometric titrations using a glass electrode. *Anal. Chim. Acta* **1967**, *38*, 475–488. [CrossRef]

36. Zékány, I.; Nagypál, I. PSEQUAD: A Comprehensive Program for the Evaluation of Potentiometric and/or Spectrophotometric Equilibrium Data Using Analytical Derivatives. In *Computational Methods for the Determination of Formation Constants*; Leggett, D.J., Ed.; Plenum: New York, NY, USA, 1985; pp. 291–352.

37. Gans, P.; Sabatini, A.; Vacca, A. SUPERQUAD: An improved general program for computation of formation constants from potentiometric data. *J. Chem. Soc. Dalton Trans.* **1985**, *6*, 1195–1200. [CrossRef]

38. Baes, C.F.; Mesmer, R.E. Iron. In *The Hydrolysis of Cations*; John Wiley & Sons: Hoboken, NJ, USA, 1976; pp. 226–237.

39. Dömötör, O.; Aicher, S.; Schmidlehner, M.; Novak, M.S.; Roller, A.; Jakupec, M.A.; Kandioller, W.; Hartinger, C.G.; Keppler, B.K.; Enyedy, É.A. Antitumor pentamethylcyclopentadienyl rhodium complexes of maltol and allomaltol: synthesis, solution speciation and bioactivity. *J. Inorg. Biochem.* **2014**, *134*, 57–65. [CrossRef] [PubMed]
40. Krezel, A.; Bal, W. A formula for correlating pK_a values determined in D_2O and H_2O. *J. Inorg. Biochem.* **2004**, *98*, 161–166. [CrossRef] [PubMed]

Sample Availability: Samples of the compounds are not available from the authors.

 © 2019 by the authors. Licensee MDPI, Basel, Switzerland. This article is an open access article distributed under the terms and conditions of the Creative Commons Attribution (CC BY) license (http://creativecommons.org/licenses/by/4.0/).

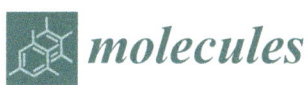

Article

Modeling Solid State Stability for Speciation: A Ten-Year Long Study

Roberta Risoluti [1], Giuseppina Gullifa [1], Elena Carcassi [1], Francesca Buiarelli [1], Li W. Wo [2] and Stefano Materazzi [1,*]

[1] Department of Chemistry, "Sapienza" University of Rome, p.le A.Moro 5, 00185 Roma, Italy
[2] Department of Chemistry, Illinois State University, 100 N University St, Normal, IL 61761, USA
* Correspondence: stefano.materazzi@uniroma1.it; Tel.: +39-0649913616; Fax: +39-06490631

Received: 23 June 2019; Accepted: 13 August 2019; Published: 20 August 2019

Abstract: Speciation studies are based on fundamental models that relate the properties of biomimetic coordination compounds to the stability of the complexes. In addition to the classic approach based on solution studies, solid state properties have been recently proposed as supporting tools to understand the bioavailability of the involved metal. A ten-year long systematic study of several different complexes of imidazole substituted ligands with transition metal ions led our group to the definition of a model based on experimental evidences. This model revealed to be a useful tool to predict the stability of such coordination complexes and is based on the induced behavior under thermal stress. Several different solid state complexes were characterized by Thermally Induced Evolved Gas Analysis by Mass Spectrometry (TI-EGA-MS). This hyphenated technique provides fundamental information to determine the solid state properties and to create a model that relates stability to coordination. In this research, the model resulting from our ten-year long systematic study of complexes of transition metal ions with imidazole substituted ligands is described. In view of a systematic addition of information, new complexes of Cu(II), Zn(II), or Cd(II) with 2-propyl-4,5-imidazoledicarboxylic acid were precipitated, characterized, and studied by means of Thermally Induced Evolved Gas Analysis performed by mass spectrometry (TI-EGA-MS). The hyphenated approach was applied to enrich the information related to thermally induced steps, to confirm the supposed decomposition mechanism, and to determine the thermal stability of the studied complexes. Results, again, allowed supporting the theory that only two main characteristic and common thermally induced decomposition behaviors join the imidazole substituted complexes studied by our group. These two behaviors could be considered as typical trends and the model allowed to predict coordination behavior and to provide speciation information.

Keywords: speciation; biomimetic complexes; evolved gas analysis; TI-EGA-MS

1. Introduction

Speciation studies can be related by setting up fundamental models based on properties of biomimetic coordination compounds that provide the stability of the complexes in order to understand the bioavailability of the involved metal.

Speciation models are mainly based on the classic approach by studies in different solution conditions. It is also well known that the thermal stability of a complex in the solid state is inversely proportional to the stability of the same complex in aqueous solution.

Metal complexes containing imidazoledicarboxylate ligands have been extensively studied because of their interesting properties. They are recognized to be realistic models as biomimetic simulators because of their characteristics, such as versatile structures useful for flexible tailoring. Additional interest has been demonstrated because of promising applications in gas storage, catalysis, optoelectronics, sensors, magnetism, luminescence, environment, and porous materials [1–33]. In consulting the literature, it is usual to find characterizations of new coordination compounds or complexes that report the synthesis, the elemental analysis, IR spectroscopic, and sometimes NMR or X-ray resulting information. More frequently, additional information is obtained from the solid state precipitates by means of thermal behavior. It is now globally recognized that the thermal stress induced on the complexes is able to provide kinetic and chemical decomposition information of the examined samples. This approach in itself is not sufficient to explain complex releasing steps. The most recent approach on-line couples FTIR or MS spectroscopies to increase the information and correctly characterizes the releasing (or decomposition) steps. The obtained data from the Thermally Induced Evolved Gas Analysis (TI-EGA) are becoming valuable supporting information that proposes a more complete characterization of the study of thermally induced decomposition mechanisms [34–41]. Our group reported these advantages in several reviews [42,43], enhancing the very different fields of application. This hyphenated approach is recognized as a very useful tool to propose decomposition mechanisms for precipitated complexes [44–48]. To step ahead, our group recently suggested new trends in thermal analysis [49–55] also comparing a new approach by portable microNIR, both oriented on the application of chemometrics [56,57].

A ten-year long systematic study of several different complexes of imidazole substituted ligands with transition metal ions led our group to the definition of a model based on experimental evidences. This model is revealed to be a useful tool to predict the stability of such coordination complexes and is based on the induced behavior under thermal stress. Several different solid state complexes were characterized by Thermally Induced Evolved Gas Analysis by Mass Spectrometry (TI-EGA-MS). This hyphenated technique provides fundamental information to determine the solid state properties and to create a model that relates stability to coordination.

The results of our ten-year long systematic study on several different complexes of substituted imidazole ligands with transition metal ions gave us the experimental evidence of two characteristic reproducible decomposition pathways. A predictive model was consequently proposed by our group. The TI-EGA-MS results allowed us to propose, for all these complexes, preliminary low-temperature thermally induced steps related to the loss of water molecules and counter ions, already present, followed by two different reproducible discriminating trends:

- The rupture of side chains, to give a five- or six-member ring as intermediate, compatibly with the percent weight loss and the TI-EGA-MS information. This behavior was recorded with ligands, such as N,N'-bis-(2-hydroxybenzylidene)-1,1-diaminobutane, 2-aminomethyl-benzimidazole, imidazole-4,5-dicarboxylic acid, and similar structures;
- The total loss of substitutions, with an imidazole 1:2 or 1:4 complex remaining as intermediate, before the last decomposition step involving the metal oxide. This behavior was recorded with ligands, such as (1-methylimidazol-2-yl)ketone, dopamine, and derived structures. All these studies are described in the references [57–68] and are the experimental evidences on which the proposed model is based. This thermally induced behavior, and the consequently derived model, is proposed as a tool to provide stability information on the complexes to be related to speciation studies.

The robustness of this predictive model needs additional examples to be continuously inserted. This study of new solid state complexes of Cu(II), Zn(II), and Cd(II) with 2-propyl-4,5-imidazoledicarboxylic acid was carried out with two main goals: i) To predict the stability from the solid state characteristics and ii) to add experimental evidences to the model.

Complexes were precipitated and characterized following previously reported procedure to be correctly compared. On the basis of the resulting characteristics, a predicted behavior and consequent stability was predicted by the model. The model prediction was successfully confirmed by the results of the Thermally Induced Mass Spectrometry Evolved Gas Analysis (TI-EGA-MS). Results, again, showed that between the two main common thermally induced decomposition behaviors, the one predicted by the model joined the substituted imidazole complexes studied by our group and could be considered as typical trends for these structures.

2. Results and Discussion

The results from the elemental analysis of the precipitated complexes are reported in Table 1. Calculated and experimentally measured element percents are in good agreement.

Table 1. Elemental analysis results for the precipitated complexes. Cu, Zn, or Cd (Metal%) were determined by ICP-OES.

Complex	C/%		H/%		N/%		Metal/%	
	Found	Calculated	Found	Calculated	Found	Calculated	Found	Calculated
$Cu(H_2PIDC)_2(H_2O)_2$	39.1	39.3	4.7	4.5	11.8	11.4	12.2	12.1
$Zn(H_2PIDC)_2(H_2O)_2$	39.3	39.3	4.7	4.5	11.5	11.4	11.9	12.1
$Cd(H_2PIDC)_2(H_2O)_2$	27.2	27.4	4.5	4.0	7.9	8.0	21.1	21.3

As for similar complexes, reported by Yang and coworkers [69], FTIR spectra confirmed the main common absorption band (KBr, cm^{-1}): 2975 (m), 1720 (s), 1540 (s), 1390 (s), 1280 (s), 1100 (m), 860 (m), 775 (m), 695 (w), 660 (m), 510 (m).

The Solid State Model, on the basis of these characteristics, predicted these complexes belonging to the first group described in the introduction.

Thermally induced releasing steps of the precipitated $Cu(H_2PIDC)_2(H_2O)_2$, $Zn(H_2PIDC)_2(H_2O)_2$, and $Cd(H_2PIDC)_2(H_2O)_2$ were comparatively studied by thermally induced evolved gas analysis by mass spectrometry (TI-EGA-MS) to confirm the decomposition mechanism proposed by the model. In Figure 1, the thermoanalytical profiles of the three complexes, registered while heating the precipitates, are overlapped to compare the releasing steps under the oxidant (air) purging flow.

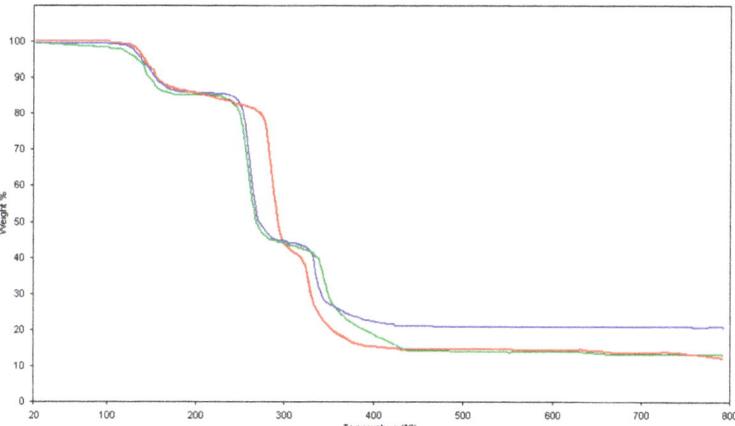

Figure 1. Thermally induced releasing profiles of the $Cu(H_2PIDC)_2(H_2O)_2$ (blue curve), $Cd(H_2PIDC)_2(H_2O)_2$ (red curve), and $Zn(H_2PIDC)_2(H_2O)_2$ (green curve): Air flow at 100 mL min^{-1}; heating rate 5 °C min^{-1}.

As previously reported for similar complexes, the thermally induced behavior was confirmed to be based on three main steps (see Table 1) with a first release of the water molecules and of only one side chain of the ligand. This hypothesis can be based on the molecular structure of this complex that shows one side chain in the external position, consequently easier to be removed.

The consequent Evolved Gas Analysis by Mass Spectrometry confirmed the release of the two water molecules by detecting fragments at $m/z = 17$ and 18, and of the side chain by $m/z = 28$, in the temperature range of 100–200 °C, as shown in Figure 2. The behavior was not influenced when the oxidant flow (air) was changed to inert flow (N_2).

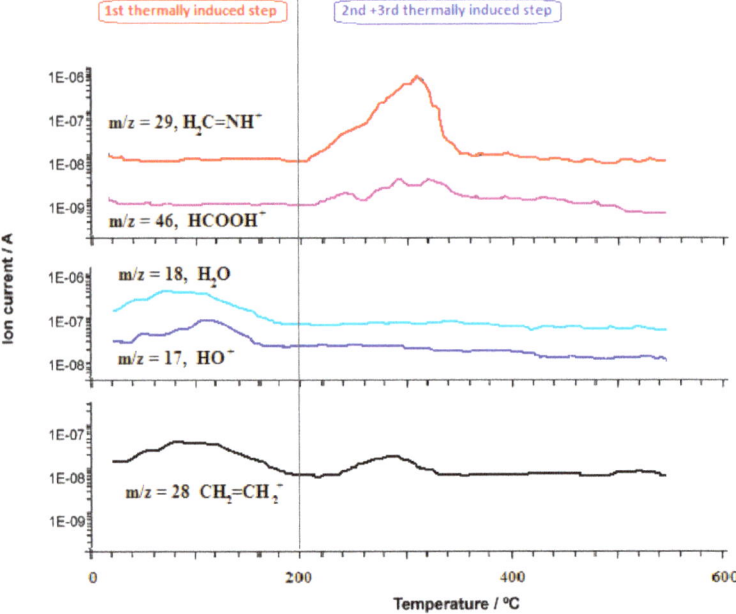

Figure 2. Representative curves of Thermally Induced Evolved Gas Analysis by Mass Spectrometry: *m/z* traces commonly recorded as a function of the temperature for all the analyzed complexes.

In the second releasing process (200–300 °C), the presence of fragments at *m/z* = 28, 29, and 46 when nitrogen is the reacting flow (Figure 2) and the calculated percent weight loss, proved the rupture of the ligand ring, as depicted in Figure 3, and the temporary consequent rearrangement. The final third thermally induced step (300–500 °C) led to the complete decomposition of the residual compound to obtain the metal oxide.

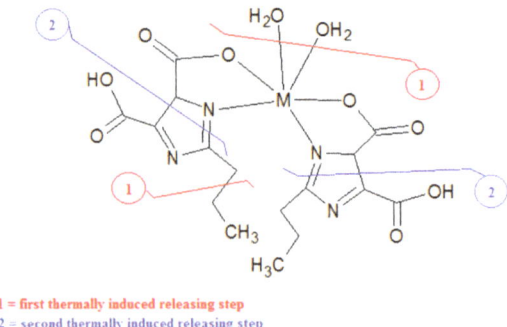

Figure 3. Scheme of the general decomposition mechanism.

By matching the MS fragmentation and the correspondence between percent weight loss calculated and percent weight loss experimentally recorded (Table 2), the proposed decomposition mechanism is clearly supported.

148

Table 2. Temperature range of the main thermal steps and the corresponding percent weight loss.

Complex	First TG Step 100–190 °C Weight Loss %		Second TG Step 230–300 °C Weight Loss %		Third TG Step 300–450 °C Weight Loss %	
	Found	Calculated	Found	Calculated	Found	Calculated
$Cu(H_2PIDC)_2(H_2O)_2$	13.3	13.1	45.0	45.8	25.7	26.0
$Zn(H_2PIDC)_2(H_2O)_2$	13.0	13.1	46.9	45.8	24.0	26.0
$Cd(H_2PIDC)_2(H_2O)_2$	11.6	11.2	43.0	43.3	24.3	24.2

The thermal behavior of the complexes was also verified by an inert purging flow (nitrogen) to check the differences when the pyrolysis took place instead of oxidation. Only the final step showed a different shape due to the uncompleted reaction to give the metal oxides.

No effects due to the inert atmosphere were detected up to 300 °C.

Consequently, the results clearly showed that the studied complexes of transition metal ions with 2-propyl-4,5-imidazoledicarboxylic acid belong to the first group described in the introduction.

The model correctly predicted the corresponding group.

3. Experimental and Methods

3.1. Materials

The ligand 2-propyl-4,5-imidazoledicarboxylic acid (H_3PIDC) and the copper, zinc, and cadmium salts were purchased from Sigma-Aldrich-Merck Co. (St. Louis, MO, USA). All the reagents were of A.R. grade and used without further purification. The conditions already reported for the previously published similar complexes were strictly followed.

3.2. Instrumental

Elemental and spectroscopic analyses, thermoanalytical characterization, and consequent Thermally Induced Evolved Gas Analysis by Mass Spectrometry (TI-EGA-MS) were performed as previously reported [68,70,71].

4. Conclusions

This study of newly synthesized transition metal complexes is aimed to contribute to a larger systematic investigation to support the two-way characteristic decomposition path that is strictly related to the structural stability of the precipitated complexes.

The ten-year long based model correctly predicted the characteristics of the precipitated complexes, anticipating what was experimentally confirmed.

Author Contributions: Conceptualization, R.R. and S.M.; methodology, R.R. and F.B.; software, R.R. and G.G.; validation, R.R. and E.C.; formal analysis, G.G., L.W.W. and E.C.; investigation, G.G., L.W.W. and F.B.; data curation, R.R. and S.M.; writing—original draft preparation, R.R. and S.M.; writing—review and editing, R.R. and S.M.; visualization, S.M.; supervision, R.R. and S.M.; project administration, S.M.

Funding: This research received no external funding.

Conflicts of Interest: The authors declare no conflict of interest.

References

1. Rajendiran, T.M.; Kirk, M.L.; Setyawati, I.A.; Caudle, M.T.; Kampf, J.W.; Pecoraro, V.W. Isolation of the first ferromagnetically coupled Mn(III/IV) complex. *Chem. Commun.* **2003**, 824–825. [CrossRef]
2. Bayon, J.C.; Net, G.; Rasmussen, P.G.; Kolowich, J.B. Dinuclear rhodium and iridium complexes of dicarboxyimidazolates; crystal structure of [NBu$_4$][(cod)Rh(dcbi)Rh(cod)]·2Pr^{i}OH. *J. Chem. Soc. Dalton Trans.* **1987**, 3003–3007. [CrossRef]

3. Zou, R.-Q.; Sakurai, H.; Xu, Q. Preparation, Adsorption Properties, and Catalytic Activity of 3D Porous Metal–Organic Frameworks Composed of Cubic Building Blocks and Alkali-Metal Ions. *Angew. Chem. Int. Ed.* **2006**, *45*, 2542. [CrossRef] [PubMed]
4. Marchetti, L.; Sabbieti, M.G.; Materazzi, S.; Hurley, M.M.; Menghi, G. Effects of phthalate esters on actin cytoskeleton of Py1a rat osteoblasts. *Histol. Histopathol.* **2002**, *17*, 1061–1066. [CrossRef] [PubMed]
5. Liu, Y.; Cheng, D.; Li, Y.-X.; Zhang, J.-D.; Yang, H.-X. A new one-dimensional Cd^{II} coordination polymer incorporating 2,2'-(1,2-phenylene)bis(1*H*-imidazole-4,5-dicarboxylate). *Acta Crystallogr. Sect. C Struct. Chem.* **2018**, *74*, 1128–1132. [CrossRef] [PubMed]
6. Liu, Y.; Kravtsov, V.C.; Eddaoudi, M. Template-Directed Assembly of Zeolite-like Metal–Organic Frameworks (ZMOFs): A usf-ZMOF with an Unprecedented Zeolite Topology. *Angew. Chem. Int. Ed.* **2008**, *47*, 8446. [CrossRef]
7. Wang, W.; Wang, R.; Liu, L.; Wu, B. Coordination Frameworks Containing Magnetic Single Chain of Imidazoledicarboxylate-Bridged Cobalt(II)/Nickel(II): Syntheses, Structures, and Magnetic Properties. *Cryst. Growth Des.* **2018**, *18*, 3449–3457. [CrossRef]
8. Wang, R.; Liu, L.; Lv, L.; Wang, X.; Chen, R.; Wu, B. Synthesis, Structural Diversity, and Properties of Cd Metal–Organic Frameworks Based on 2-(5-Bromo-pyridin-3-yl)-1H-imidazole-4,5-dicarboxylate and N-Heterocyclic Ancillary Ligands. *Cryst. Growth Des.* **2017**, *17*, 3616–3624. [CrossRef]
9. Wang, S.; Zhang, L.; Li, G.; Huo, Q.; Liu, Y. Assembly of two 3-D metal–organic frameworks from Cd(II) and 4,5-imidazoledicarboxylic acid or 2-ethyl-4,5-imidazoledicarboxylic acid. *Cryst. Eng. Comm.* **2008**, *10*, 1662. [CrossRef]
10. Bai, X.-Y.; Ji, W.-J.; Li, S.-N.; Jiang, Y.-C.; Hu, M.-C.; Zhai, Q.-G. Nonlinear Optical Rod Indium-Imidazoledicarboxylate Framework as Room-Temperature Gas Sensor for Butanol Isomers. *Cryst. Growth Des.* **2017**, *17*, 423–427. [CrossRef]
11. Catauro, M.; Tranquillo, E.; Risoluti, R.; Vecchio Ciprioti, S. Sol-Gel Synthesis, Spectroscopic and Thermal Behavior Study of SiO_2/PEG Composites Containing Different Amount of Chlorogenic Acid. *Polymers* **2018**, *10*, 682. [CrossRef] [PubMed]
12. Gangu, K.K.; Maddila, S.; Mukkamala, S.B.; Jonnalagadda, S.B. Synthesis, characterisation and catalytic activity of 4, 5-imidazoledicarboxylate ligated Co(II) and Cd(II) metal-organic coordination complexes. *J. Mol. Struct.* **2017**, *1143*, 153–162. [CrossRef]
13. Catauro, M.; Naviglio, D.; Risoluti, R.; Vecchio Ciprioti, S. Sol-gel synthesis and thermal behavior of bioactive ferrous citrate-silica hybrid materials. *J. Therm. Anal. Calorim.* **2018**, *133*, 1085–1092. [CrossRef]
14. Fei, H.; Lin, Y.; Xu, T. Cobalt imidazoledicarboxylate coordination complex microspheres: Stable intercalation materials for lithium and sodium-ion batteries. *Ionics* **2017**, *23*, 1949–1954. [CrossRef]
15. Song, Y.; Lin, C.-S.; Wei, Q.; Wu, Z.-F.; Huang, X.-Y. Three-Dimensional Non-Centrosymmetric Ba(II)/Li(I)–Imidazolecarboxylate Coordination Polymers: Second Harmonic Generation and Blue Fluorescence. *Cryst. Growth Des.* **2016**, *16*, 6654–6662. [CrossRef]
16. Jing, X.-M.; Xiao, L.-W.; Wei, L.; Dai, F.-C.; Ren, L.-L. Solvent directed assembly of two zinc(II)-2-(4-pyridyl)-4,5-imidazoledicarboxylate frameworks. *Inorg. Chem. Commun.* **2016**, *71*, 78–81. [CrossRef]
17. Perrino, C.; Marconi, E.; Tofful, L.; Farao, C.; Materazzi, S.; Canepari, S. Thermal stability of inorganic and organic compounds in atmospheric particulate matter. *Atmos. Environ.* **2012**, *54*, 36. [CrossRef]
18. Jia, Y.; Li, Y.; Zhou, R.; Song, J. The Advance of Imidazoledicarboxylate Derivatives-Based Coordination Polymers. *Prog. Chem.* **2016**, *28*, 482–496. [CrossRef]
19. Pang, Q.; Tu, B.; Ning, E.; Li, Q.; Zhao, D. Distinct Packings of Supramolecular Building Blocks in Metal–Organic Frameworks Based on Imidazoledicarboxylic Acid. *Inorg. Chem.* **2015**, *54*, 9678–9680. [CrossRef] [PubMed]
20. Liu, Y.; Kravtsov, V.; Walsh, R.D.; Poddar, P.; Srikanthc, H.; Eddaoudi, M. Directed assembly of metal–organic cubes from deliberately predesigned molecular building blocks. *Chem. Commun.* **2004**, 2806–2807. [CrossRef] [PubMed]
21. Dai, C.; Zhou, X.; Jing, X.; Li, G.; Huo, Q.; Liu, Y. Assembly of two Cu-based coordination polymers from 2-(pyridine-3-yl)-1H-4,5-imidazoledicarboxylate ligand. *Inorg. Chem. Commun.* **2015**, *52*, 69–72. [CrossRef]
22. Sabbieti, M.G.; Agas, D.; Santoni, G.; Materazzi, S.; Menghi, G.; Marchetti, L. Involvement of p53 in phthalate effects on mouse and rat osteoblasts. *J. Cell. Biochem.* **2009**, *107*, 316–327. [CrossRef] [PubMed]

23. Li, S.-M.; Cao, W.; Zheng, X.-J.; Jin, L.-P. Self-assembly and characterization of Ca–Zn heterometallic MOFs with 4,5-imidazoledicarboxylate. *Polyhedron* **2014**, *83*, 122–129. [CrossRef]
24. Liu, L.; Zhang, Z.; Zhao, Z.; Niu, S.; Song, A.; Peng, Y. Syntheses, Crystal Structures, and Luminescent Properties of Two Cadmium(II) Complexes with CdS Network and (3,4)-Connected Topology. *Anorg. Allg. Chem.* **2014**, *640*, 2520–2524. [CrossRef]
25. Sergi, M.; Gentili, A.; Perret, D.; Marchese, S.; Materazzi, S.; Curini, R. MSPD Extraction of Sulphonamides from Meat followed by LC Tandem MS Determination. *Chromatographia* **2007**, *65*, 757–761. [CrossRef]
26. Luo, Z.-R.; Yin, X.-H.; Zhao, J.-H.; Gao, P. Coordination Polymers with the Ligand (2-propyl-4,5-imidazoledicarboxylic acid): Synthesis, Structural Characteristics, and Properties Studies. *Synth. React. Inorg. Met. Org. Nano Met. Chem.* **2013**, *43*, 662–670. [CrossRef]
27. Yue, S.; Li, N.; Bian, J.; Hou, T.; Ma, J. Synthesis, crystal structure and luminescent properties of transition metals complexes based on imidazole derivatives. *Synth. Met.* **2012**, *162*, 247. [CrossRef]
28. Gentili, A.; Caretti, F.; D'Ascenzo, G.; Mainero Rocca, L.; Marchese, S.; Materazzi, S.; Perret, D. Simultaneous Determination of Trichothecenes A, B, and D in Maize Food Products by LC-MS-MS. *Chromatographia* **2007**, *66*, 669–676. [CrossRef]
29. Liu, Y.; Kravtsov, V.; Larsena, R.; Eddaoudi, M. Molecular building blocks approach to the assembly of zeolite-like metal–organic frameworks (ZMOFs) with extra-large cavities. *Chem. Commun.* **2006**, 1488–1490. [CrossRef]
30. Migliorati, V.; Ballirano, P.; Gontrani, L.; Materazzi, S.; Ceccacci, F.; Caminiti, R. A Combined Theoretical and Experimental Study of Solid Octyl and Decylammonium Chlorides and of Their Aqueous Solutions. *J. Phys. Chem. B* **2013**, *117*, 7806. [CrossRef]
31. Nouar, F.; Eckert, J.; Eubank, J.F.; Forster, P.; Eddaoudi, M. Zeolite-like Metal–Organic Frameworks (ZMOFs) as Hydrogen Storage Platform: Lithium and Magnesium Ion-Exchange and H_2-(rho-ZMOF) Interaction Studies. *J. Am. Chem. Soc.* **2009**, *131*, 2864. [CrossRef] [PubMed]
32. Rumyantseva, M.; Nasriddinov, A.; Vladimirova, S.; Tokarev, S.; Fedorova, O.; Krylov, I.; Drozdov, K.; Baranchikov, A.; Gaskov, A. Photosensitive Organic-Inorganic Hybrid Materials for Room Temperature Gas Sensor Applications. *Nanomaterials* **2018**, *8*, 671. [CrossRef] [PubMed]
33. Silva, M.O.D.; Carneiro, M.L.B.; Siqueira, J.L.N.; Báo, S.N.; Souza, A.R. Development of a Promising Antitumor Compound Based on Rhodium(II) Succinate Associated with Iron Oxide Nanoparticles Coated with Lauric Acid/Albumin Hybrid: Synthesis, Colloidal Stability and Cytotoxic Effect in Breast Carcinoma Cells. *J. Nanosci. Nanotechnol.* **2018**, *18*, 3832–3843. [CrossRef] [PubMed]
34. Shahbazi, S.; Stratz, S.A.; Auxier, J.D.; Hanson, D.E.; Marsh, M.L.; Hall, H.L. Characterization and thermogravimetric analysis of lanthanide hexafluoroacetylacetone chelates. *J. Radioanal. Nucl. Chem.* **2017**, *311*, 617–626. [CrossRef] [PubMed]
35. Liu, N.; Guo, X.; Navrotsky, A.; Shi, L.; Wu, D. Thermodynamic complexity of sulfated zirconia catalysts. *J. Catal.* **2016**, *342*, 158–163. [CrossRef]
36. Veselá, P.; Slovák, V.; Zelenka, T.; Koštejn, M.; Mucha, M. The influence of pyrolytic temperature on sorption ability of carbon xerogel based on 3-aminophenol-formaldehyde polymer for Cu(II) ions and phenol. *J. Anal. Appl. Pyrolysis* **2016**, *121*, 29–40. [CrossRef]
37. Baksi, A.; Cocke, D.L.; Gomes, A.; Gossage, J.; Riggs, M.; Beall, G.; McWhinney, H. Characterization of Copper-Manganese-Aluminum-Magnesium Mixed Oxyhydroxide and Oxide Catalysts for Redox Reactions. *Charact. Miner. Met. Mater.* **2016**, *2016*, 151–158. [CrossRef]
38. Aiello, D.; Materazzi, S.; Risoluti, R.; Thangavel, H.; Di Donna, L.; Mazzotti, F.; Casadonte, F.; Siciliano, C.; Sindona, G.; Napoli, A. A major allergen in rainbow trout (Oncorhynchus mykiss): Complete sequences of parvalbumin by MALDI tandem mass spectrometry. *Mol. BioSyst.* **2015**, *11*, 2373–2382. [CrossRef]
39. Oliani, W.L.; Komatsu, L.G.H.; Lugao, A.B.; Rangari, V.K.; Parra, D.F. Natural Aging Effects in HMS-Polypropylene Synthesized by Gamma Radiation in Acetylene Atmosphere. In *TMS Annual Meeting & Exhibition*; Springer: Cham, Switzerland, 2016; pp. 151–158.
40. Duemichen, E.; Braun, U.; Senz, R.; Fabian, G.; Sturm, H. Assessment of a new method for the analysis of decomposition gases of polymers by a combining thermogravimetric solid-phase extraction and thermal desorption gas chromatography mass spectrometry. *J. Chromatogr. A* **2014**, *1354*, 117–128. [CrossRef]

41. Dovgaliuk, I.; Ban, V.; Sadikin, Y.; Černý, R.; Aranda, L.; Casati, N.; Devillers, M.; Filinchuk, Y. The First Halide-Free Bimetallic Aluminum Borohydride: Synthesis, Structure, Stability, and Decomposition Pathway. *J. Phys. Chem. C* **2014**, *118*, 145–153. [CrossRef]
42. Szymańska, I.B.; Piszczek, P.; Szłyk, E. Gas phase studies of new copper(I) carboxylates compounds with vinylsilanes and their application in Chemical Vapor Deposition (CVD). *Polyhedron* **2009**, *28*, 721–728. [CrossRef]
43. Risoluti, R.; Fabiano, M.A.; Gullifa, G.; Vecchio Ciprioti, S.; Materazzi, S. FTIR-evolved gas analysis in recent thermoanalytical investigations. *Appl. Spectr. Rev.* **2017**, *52*, 39. [CrossRef]
44. Materazzi, S.; Risoluti, R. Evolved Gas Analysis by Mass Spectrometry. *Appl. Spectr. Rev.* **2014**, *49*, 635. [CrossRef]
45. Humphrie, T.D.; Sheppard, D.A.; Li, G.; Rowles, M.R. Complex hydrides as thermal energy storage materials: Characterisation and thermal decomposition of $Na_2Mg_2NiH_6$. *J. Mater. Chem. A* **2018**, *6*, 9099–9108. [CrossRef]
46. Lin, Y.; Zheng, M.; Ye, C.; Power, I.M. Thermogravimetric analysis–mass spectrometry (TGA–MS) of hydromagnesite from Dujiali Lake in Tibet, China. *J. Therm. Anal. Calorim.* **2018**, *133*, 1429–1437. [CrossRef]
47. Fernández-Alonso, S.; Corrales, T.; Pablos, J.L.; Catalina, F. A Switchable fluorescence solid sensor for Hg^{2+} detection in aqueous media based on a photocrosslinked membrane functionalized with (benzimidazolyl)methyl-piperazine derivative of 1,8-naphthalimide. *Sens. Actuators B Chem.* **2018**, *270*, 256–262. [CrossRef]
48. Kumar, A.; Chae, P.S. Fluorescence tunable thiophene-bis(benzimidazole)-based probes for cascade trace detection of Hg^{2+} and lysine: A molecular switch mimic. *J. Nanosci. Nanotechnol.* **2018**, *18*, 3832–3843. [CrossRef]
49. Zhang, H.; Zheng, J.; Chao, Y.; Zhang, K.; Zhu, Z. Surface engineering of FeCo-based electrocatalysts supported on carbon paper by incorporating non-noble metals for water oxidation. *New J. Chem.* **2018**, *42*, 7254–7261. [CrossRef]
50. Materazzi, S.; Risoluti, R.; Gullifa, G.; Fabiano, M.A.; Frati, P.; Santurro, A.; Scopetti, M.; Fineschi, V. New frontiers in thermal analysis. A TG/Chemometrics approach for postmortem interval estimation in vitreous humor. *J. Therm. Anal. Calorim.* **2017**, *130*, 549–557. [CrossRef]
51. Risoluti, R.; Materazzi, S.; Sorrentino, F.; Maffei, L.; Caprari, P. Thermogravimetric analysis coupled with chemometrics as a powerful predictive tool for ß-thalassemia screening. *Talanta* **2016**, *159*, 425. [CrossRef] [PubMed]
52. Risoluti, R.; Gregori, A.; Schiavone, S.; Materazzi, S. "Click and Screen" Technology for the Detection of Explosives on Human Hands by a Portable MicroNIR–Chemometrics Platform. *Anal. Chem.* **2018**, *90*, 4288. [CrossRef] [PubMed]
53. Materazzi, S.; Peluso, G.; Ripani, L.; Risoluti, R. High-throughput prediction of AKB48 in emerging illicit products by NIR spectroscopy and chemometrics. *Microchem. J.* **2017**, *134*, 277. [CrossRef]
54. Materazzi, S.; Risoluti, R.; Pinci, S.; Romolo, F.S. New insights in forensic chemistry: NIR/Chemometrics analysis of toners for questioned documents examination. *Talanta* **2017**, *174*, 673. [CrossRef] [PubMed]
55. Materazzi, S.; Gregori, A.; Ripani, L.; Apriceno, A.; Risoluti, R. Cocaine profiling: Implementation of a predictive model by ATR-FTIR coupled with chemometrics in forensic chemistry. *Talanta* **2017**, *166*, 328. [CrossRef] [PubMed]
56. Risoluti, R.; Materazzi, S.; Gregori, A.; Ripani, L. Early detection of emerging street drugs by near infrared spectroscopy and chemometrics. *Talanta* **2016**, *153*, 407. [CrossRef] [PubMed]
57. Materazzi, S.; Risoluti, R.; Napoli, A. EGA-MS study to characterize the thermally induced decomposition of Co(II), Ni(II), Cu(II) and Zn(II) complexes with 1,1-diaminobutane-Schiff base. *Thermochim. Acta* **2015**, *606*, 90. [CrossRef]
58. Materazzi, S.; Risoluti, R.; Finamore, J.; Napoli, A. Divalent Transition Metal Complexes of 2-(Pyridin-2-yl)imidazole: Evolved Gas Analysis Predicting Model to Provide Characteristic Coordination. *Microchem. J.* **2014**, *115*, 27. [CrossRef]
59. Materazzi, S.; Napoli, A.; Finamore, J.; Risoluti, R.; D'Arienzo, S. Characterization of thermally induced mechanisms by mass spectrometry-evolved gas analysis (EGA-MS): A study of divalent cobalt and zinc biomimetic complexes with N-heterocyclic dicarboxylic ligands. *Int. J. Mass Spectrom.* **2014**, *365/366*, 372. [CrossRef]

60. Materazzi, S.; Foti, C.; Crea, F.; Risoluti, R.; Finamore, J. Biomimetic complexes of divalent cobalt and zinc with N-heterocyclic dicarboxylic ligands. *Thermochim. Acta* **2014**, *580*, 7. [CrossRef]
61. Papadopoulos, C.; Cristóvão, B.; Ferenc, W.; Hatzidimitriou, A.; Vecchio Ciprioti, S.; Risoluti, R.; Lalia-Kantouri, M. Thermoanalytical, magnetic and structural investigation of neutral Co(II) complexes with 2,2′-dipyridylamine and salicylaldehydes. *J. Therm. Anal. Calorim.* **2016**, *123*, 717. [CrossRef]
62. Risoluti, R.; Piazzese, D.; Napoli, A.; Materazzi, S. Study of [2-(2′-pyridyl)imidazole] complexes to confirm two main characteristic thermoanalytical behaviors of transition metal complexes based on imidazole derivatives. *J. Anal. Appl. Pyrolysis* **2016**, *117*, 82. [CrossRef]
63. Risoluti, R.; Gullifa, G.; Fabiano, M.A.; Iona, R.; Zuccatosta, F.; Wo, L.W.; Materazzi, S. Divalent Transition Metal Complexes of 2-(Pyridin-2-yl)imidazole: Evolved Gas Analysis Predicting Model to Provide Characteristic Coordination. *Russ. J. Gen. Chem.* **2017**, *87*, 2915. [CrossRef]
64. Risoluti, R.; Gullifa, G.; Fabiano, M.A.; Wo, L.W.; Materazzi, S. Biomimetic complexes of Cd(II), Mn(II), and Zn(II) with 1,1-diaminobutane–Schiff base. EGA/MS study of the thermally induced decomposition. *Russ. J. Gen. Chem.* **2017**, *87*, 564. [CrossRef]
65. Risoluti, R.; Gullifa, G.; Fabiano, M.A.; Wo, L.W.; Materazzi, S. Biomimetic complexes of Cd(II), Mn(II), and Zn(II) with 2-aminomethylbenzimidazole. EGA/MS characterization of the thermally induced decomposition. *Russ. J. Gen. Chem.* **2017**, *87*, 300. [CrossRef]
66. Risoluti, R.; Gullifa, G.; Fabiano, M.A.; Materazzi, S. Biomimetic complexes of Co(II), Mn(II), and Ni(II) with 2-propyl-4,5-imidazoledicarboxylic acid. EGA–MS characterization of the thermally induced decomposition. *Russ. J. Gen. Chem.* **2015**, *85*, 2374. [CrossRef]
67. Materazzi, S.; Curini, R.; D'Ascenzo, G. Thermoanalytical study of benzimidazole complexes with transition metal ions: Copper (II) complexes. *Thermochim. Acta* **1996**, *286*, 1–15. [CrossRef]
68. Materazzi, S.; Vecchio, S.; Wo, L.W.; De Angelis Curtis, S. TG–MS and TG–FTIR studies of imidazole-substituted coordination compounds: Co(II) and Ni(II)-complexes of bis(1-methylimidazol-2-yl)ketone. *Thermochim. Acta* **2012**, *543*, 183. [CrossRef]
69. De Angelis Curtis, S.; Kurdziel, K.; Materazzi, S.; Vecchio, S. Crystal structure and thermoanalytical study of a manganese(II) complex with 1-allylimidazole. *J. Therm. Anal. Calorim.* **2008**, *92*, 109. [CrossRef]
70. Yang, Z.; Chen, N.; Wang, C.; Yan, L.; Li, G. Syntheses, Crystal Structures, and Properties of Four Complexes Constructed from 2-Propyl-1*H*-Imidazole-4,5- Dicarboxylic Acid. *Synth. React. Inorg. Met. Org. Nano Met. Chem.* **2012**, *42*, 336. [CrossRef]
71. Bretti, C.; Crea, F.; De Stefano, C.; Foti, C.; Materazzi, S.; Vianelli, G. Thermodynamic Properties of Dopamine in Aqueous Solution. Acid–Base Properties, Distribution, and Activity Coefficients in NaCl Aqueous Solutions at Different Ionic Strengths and Temperatures. *J. Chem. Eng. Data* **2013**, *58*, 2835–2847. [CrossRef]

Sample Availability: Samples of the compounds are not available from the authors.

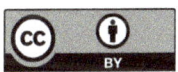

© 2019 by the authors. Licensee MDPI, Basel, Switzerland. This article is an open access article distributed under the terms and conditions of the Creative Commons Attribution (CC BY) license (http://creativecommons.org/licenses/by/4.0/).

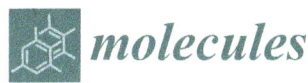

Article

Associated Effects of Cadmium and Copper Alter the Heavy Metals Uptake by *Melissa Officinalis*

Dorota Adamczyk-Szabela [1,*], Katarzyna Lisowska [1], Zdzisława Romanowska-Duda [2] and Wojciech M. Wolf [1]

1. Institute of General and Ecological Chemistry, Lodz University of Technology, 90-924 Lodz, Zeromskiego 116, Poland
2. Department of Plant Ecophysiology, Faculty of Biology and Environmental Protection, University of Lodz, 90-237 Lodz, Banacha 12/16, Poland
* Correspondence: dorota.adamczyk@p.lodz.pl; Tel.: +48-42-631-31-32

Academic Editors: Francesco Crea and Alberto Pettignano
Received: 12 June 2019; Accepted: 2 July 2019; Published: 4 July 2019

Abstract: Lemon balm (*Melissa officinalis*) is a popular herb widely used in medicine. It is often cultivated in soils with substantial heavy metal content. Here we investigate the associated effects of cadmium and copper on the plant growth parameters augmented by the manganese, zinc, and lead uptake indicators. The concentration of all elements in soil and plants was determined by the HR-CS FAAS with the ContrAA 300 Analytik Jena spectrometer. Bioavailable and total forms calculated for all examined metals were augmented by the soil analyses. The index of chlorophyll content in leaves, the activity of net photosynthesis, stomatal conductance, transpiration rate, and intercellular concentration of CO_2 were also investigated. Either Cd or Cu acting alone at high concentrations in soil are toxic to plants as indicated by chlorophyll indices and gas exchange parameters. Surprisingly, this effect was not observed when both metals were administered together. The sole cadmium or copper supplementations hampered the plant's growth, lowered the leaf area, and altered the plant's stem elongation. Analysis of variance showed that cadmium and copper treatments of lemon balm significantly influenced manganese, lead, and zinc concentration in roots and above ground parts.

Keywords: *Melissa officinalis*; herbs; heavy metals interactions; photosynthesis indicators; HR-CS FAAS

1. Introduction

Plants utilize diverse strategies for the uptake of heavy metals from soil. This issue has been thoroughly investigated over years yielding a continuously growing number of publications [1,2]. One of the most important questions is related to the way in which particular metals enter and further migrate in the plant body. Several mechanisms and strategies have been reported [3]. However, we should bear in mind that real soil is a complex matrix in which components promptly interact with one another [4]. This issue is of particular relevance when heavy metals uptake and further migration are concerned. In this study we describe the combined impact of copper and cadmium on manganese, lead, and zinc uptake by the lemon balm (*Melissa officinalis* L.).

Despite remarkable progress in modern medicinal chemistry herbal therapies, almost 80% of the world's population relies on herbal medicine [5]. Therefore, herbs are important commodities on the global market. In particular, the production of dry herbal raw material in Poland approaches 20,000 tons annually, giving this country a leading position in Europe [6]. *Melissa officinalis*, also known as lemon balm, honey balm, common balm or balm mint, is a perennial herbaceous plant in the mint family *Lamiaceae*. This plant is native to south-central Europe, the Mediterranean Basin, Iran, and Central Asia, but now has been naturalized in both Americas and elsewhere [7]. It is widely used in medicine all over the world. Its leaves contain flavonoids, beneficial volatile compounds, triterpenes, and polyphenols. *M. officinalis* possesses sedative, antibacterial, antiviral, and antifungal activities [8]. It is not demanding and is an easy-to-grow herb, which can be cultivated in diverse soils and climatic conditions. The perspective applications of either extracts or essential oils may be related to the antioxidant activities as confirmed by several recent publications [9]. In view of those reports, lemon balm may be a useful source of rosmarinic acid and other phenolic compounds. According to Dastmalchi et al. [10], the former is responsible for the anti- acetylcholinesterase activity of *M. officinalis* extracts and may be applied in controlling Alzheimer's disease [11]. Those extracts were also administered in multidimensional cancer therapies [12].

The diverse conditions of lemon balm cultivation inflict changes in the constitution of this particular plant and affect its medical value [13]. Furthermore, the latter may be also affected by the processing method and storage conditions of the harvested herbs [14]. Especially, heavy metals in soil and their either uptake or accumulation by plants should be carefully controlled. The EU regulations as applied to herbs are restricted to toxic elements, i.e., cadmium, lead, and chromium only [15,16]. Unfortunately, metals widely regarded as beneficial may also be stressful to plants at ambient concentrations.

Cadmium and copper are classified as priority pollutants. Copper is essential for the plant's growth. However, its elevated concentrations in soil may lead to toxicity symptoms and hamper proper plant development [17]. Cadmium is a toxic element. Indeed, our recent study showed that its supplementation to soil reduced the growth of the lemon balm (*Melissa officinalis L.*) plant and decreased all relevant photosynthesis indicators [18]. Copper and cadmium associated interactions have been scarcely studied so far. To the best of our knowledge, their impact on the uptake of heavy metals widely distributed in the soil environment has not been investigated yet. Copper and cadmium are reported to enter the plant cell through either a competing or synergistic way, respectively [19]. Verification of this hypothesis for plants cultivated in real soil environments is of practical relevance when migrations of metals originating from wastes, sewage, or fertilizers are concerned.

In this publication we show the influence of copper and cadmium on manganese, lead, and zinc uptake by lemon balm (*Melissa officinalis L.*). Both former metals are prone to associated interactions. Nevertheless, their combined impact on heavy metals uptake by plants has not been investigated so far.

2. Results and Discussion

The investigated soil was slightly acidic (pH = 6.1) with the organic matter content at the 26% level. This is typical for the organic arable lands widely encountered in central Poland. The Mn, Cu, Zn, Cd, Pb bioavailable (89.2 ± 4; 2.78 ± 0.04; 19.6 ± 0.8; 0.14 ± 0.01; 8.70 ± 0.30 $\mu g\ g^{-1}$, respectively) and total (143 ± 3; 5.54 ± 0.4; 46.4 ± 1.9; 0.21 ± 0.02; 12.7 ± 0.3 $\mu g\ g^{-1}$, respectively) forms were below limits as specified in international regulations [20,21]. Metals content in the lemon balm cultivated in soil treated with Cd, Cu, or mixtures of both metals are presented in Figure 1.

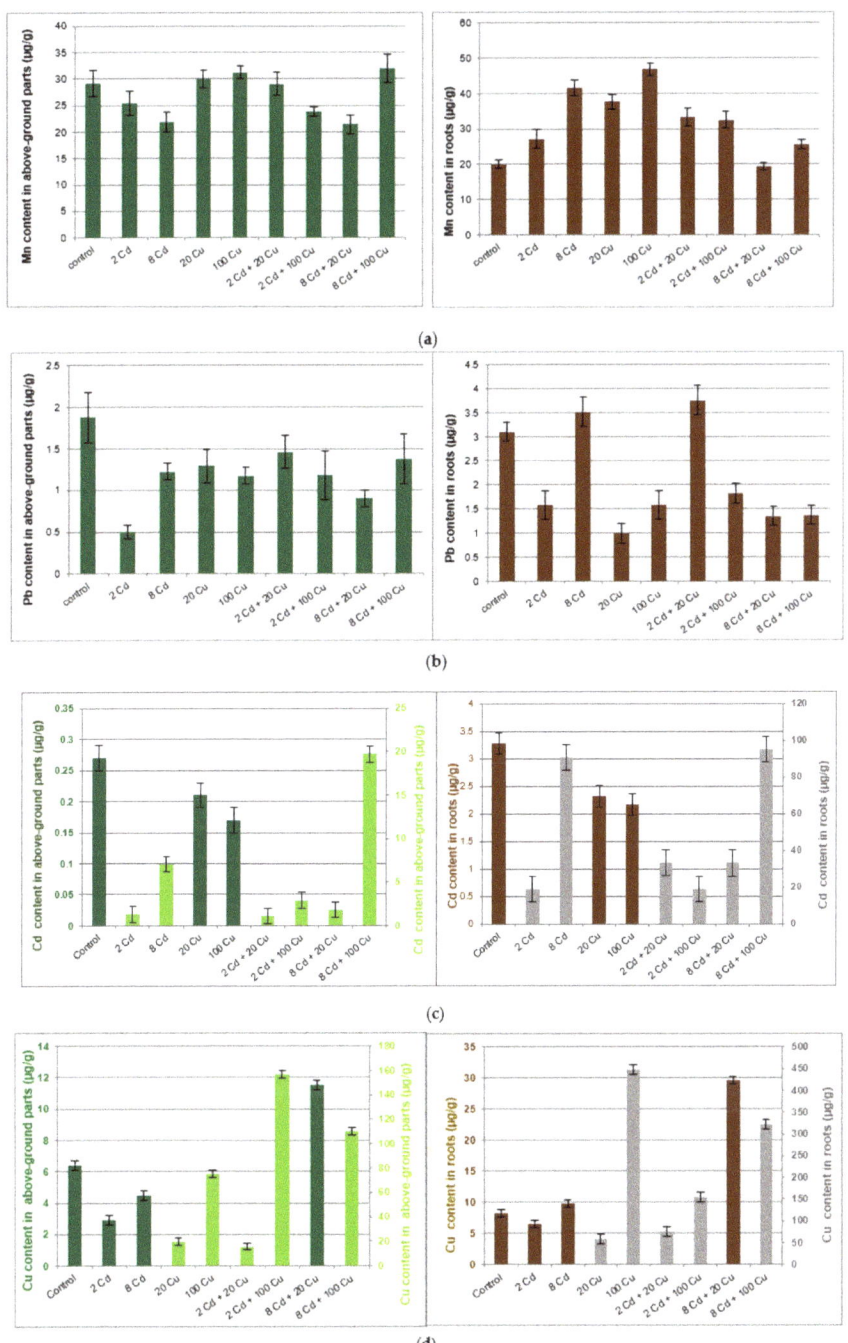

Figure 1. *Cont.*

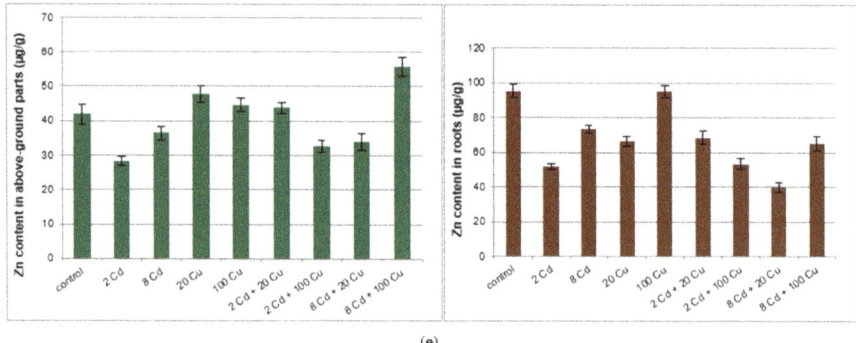

(e)

Figure 1. Manganese (**a**); lead (**b**); copper (**c**); cadmium (**d**); zinc (**e**) content (μg/g) in above ground parts and roots of the *Melissa officinalis* plant displayed against the Cd and Cu doses as used for the soil supplementation. 2 Cd = 2 μg/g cadmium; 8 Cd = 8 μg/g cadmium; 20 Cu = 20 μg/g copper; 100 Cu = 100 μg/g copper. In (**c**) and (**d**) dark bars show lower metal concentrations and are related to the left scale axis while pale bars (higher concentrations) are represented by the right axis.

Melissa officinalis cultivated in the untreated reference soil accumulated all investigated metals mostly in roots. The important exception was manganese, which to a large extent migrated to the above ground parts of the plant. The copper treatment at either 20 μg g^{-1} or 100 μg g^{-1} had a significant impact on the Mn, Pb, Cd, and Zn content in roots only. The cadmium supplementation (2 and 8 μg g^{-1}) reduced Mn, Pb, Cu, and Zn uptake by the above ground part of the *Melissa officinalis* plant as compared to that in the control sample. Surprisingly, Cd uptake by either roots or above ground parts of lemon balm was inversely proportional to the Cu concentration in soil. However, the Cu concentration in plant tissues was not directly related to the Cd content in soil.

The chlorophyll content in leaves, the activity of net photosynthesis, stomatal conductance transpiration rate, and intercellular CO_2 concentration (Figure 2) indicate that lemon balm exhibited diverse photosynthesis activities. Either Cd or Cu acting alone at high concentrations in soil (8 and 20 μg g^{-1}, respectively) are toxic to plants as indicated by chlorophyll indices and gas exchange parameters. Surprisingly, this effect was not observed when both metals were administered together. The sole cadmium or copper supplementations hampered the plant's growth, lowered the leaf area, and altered the plant's stem elongation. The important exception was the lowest 2 μg g^{-1} Cd dose, which increased the leaf area and the stem length (Figure 3) while at the same time prompted the leaves' green colour to fade. The inhibition of chlorophyll synthesis upon the Cd administration in soil has been recognized and it is sometimes related to hampering the Mg uptake by particular plants [22]. Remarkably, the higher Cd doses did not affect either the plant's growth or the leaf area as compared to the control species. It is generally accepted that Cd alters physiological processes in leaves [23]. The majority of reports emphasize the negative effects leading to the biomass decline. However, contradictory statements do also exist. In particular, Piršelová et al. [24] showed that in the faba bean plant (*Vicia faba* cv. Aštar) Cd administration to soil resulted in the decrease of either fresh or dry root weight, but at the same time it prompted the increase of shoots fresh biomass. A similar rise of fresh shoots weight was also observed by Shah et al. [25] in shisham (*Dalbergia sissoo* Roxb.). The Cd toxicity in plants has been a subject of numerous investigations [26,27]. Unfortunately it is species dependent and the final conclusions are often contradictory and by all means are far from clarity [28,29].

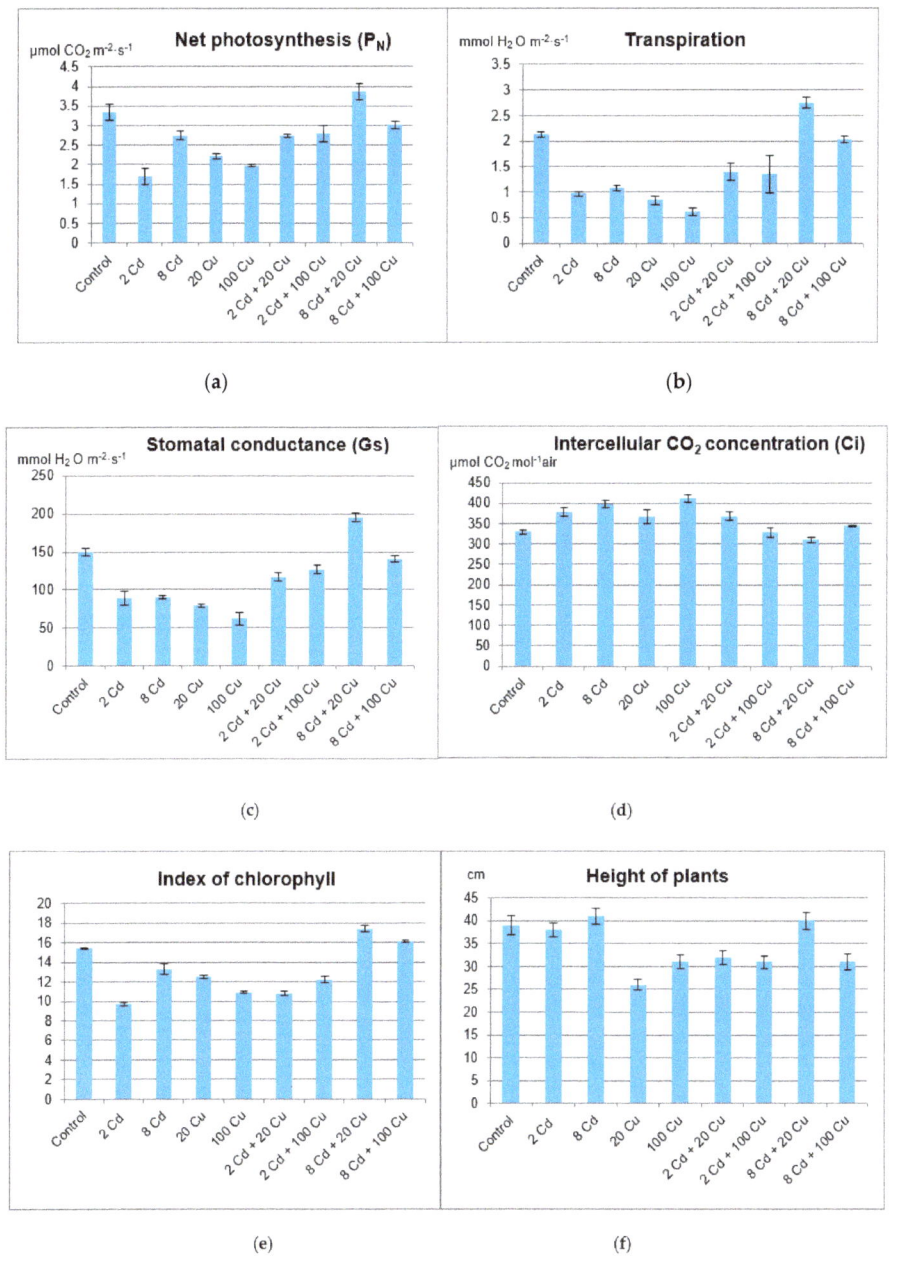

Figure 2. Net photosynthesis (**a**); transpiration (**b**); stomatal conductance (**c**); intercellular CO_2 concentration (**d**); index of chlorophyll content (**e**); height of the plant (**f**) for lemon balm grown on soil either with or without Cd and Cu treatment. 2 Cd = 2 µg/g cadmium; 8 Cd = 8 µg/g cadmium; 20 Cu = 20 µg/g copper; 100 Cu = 100 µg/g copper.

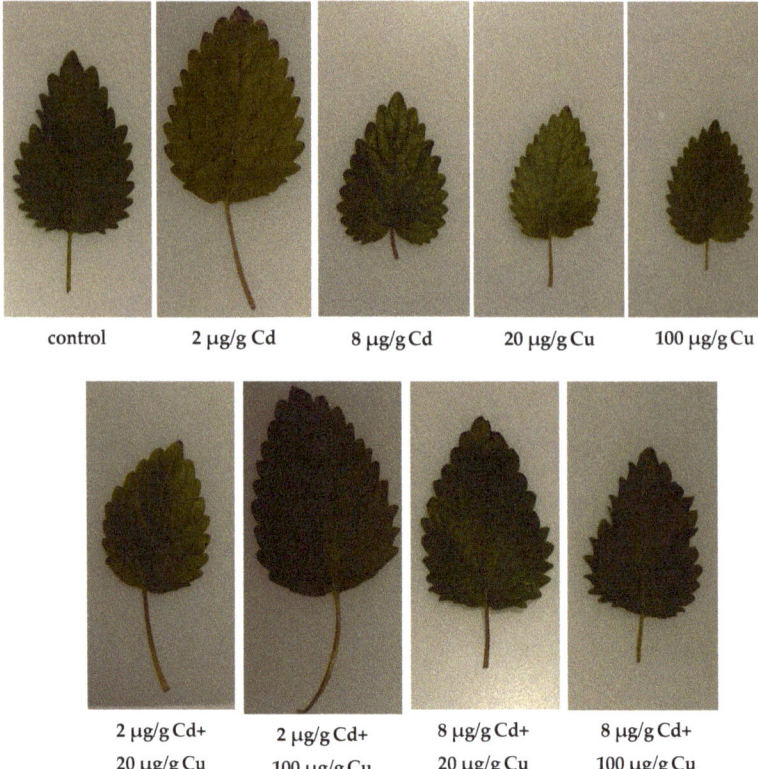

Figure 3. Representative leaves of *Melissa officinalis* cultivated in soils either with or without Cd and Cu treatment.

The two-way ANOVA (Table 1) shows that significant, combined Cd and Cu interactions are triggered by the Mn, Pb, and Zn as present in soil. Correlations between Cd and Cu in soil and plant environment are quite well recognized and documented in the scientific literature [30,31]. However, the associated interactions involving more heavy metals as present in the soil environment has not been studied as yet.

Table 1. Two-way ANOVA parameters* for Mn, Pb, and Zn contents in above ground parts and in roots of *Melissa officinalis* across eight soil supplementations as described in the Materials and Methods section.

Source of variation	SS	df	Roots MS	F	p	Test F
Samples	7961.42	8	995.18	207.72	6.35×10^{-62}	2.0252
Metals	96,997.42	2	48,498.71	10,123.28	1.40×10^{-123}	3.0803
Interactions	9687.58	16	605.47	126.38	3.59×10^{-62}	1.7380
Source of variation	SS	df	Above ground parts MS	F	p	Test F
Samples	2514.20	8	314.28	106.00	1.49×10^{-47}	2.0252
Metals	36,578.72	2	18,289.36	6168.95	4.70×10^{-112}	3.0803
Interactions	2080.99	16	130.06	43.87	9.17×10^{-40}	1.7380

*SS—sum of squares; df—degrees of freedom; MS—mean square; p—probability value; F—calculated Snedecor's F parameter; Test F—Snedecor's F critical value.

Cd and Cu may influence either metals uptake from the soil or their further migration within the plant body. The former may be analyzed by the transfer coefficient (TC) and bioaccumulation factor (BAF). They are defined as ratios of particular element concentrations in root and shoot, respectively, related to their content in the soil environment [32–34]. Metal distribution inside the plant body was assessed by the translocation factor (TF), which is the ratio of element concentration in the above ground part of the plant to that in roots [35–37].

The TC calculated for lemon balm plants cultivated in the reference, untreated soil was in the series Cd > Zn > Cu > Pb > Mn. The TF for the untreated soil followed the order Mn > Cu > Pb > Zn > Cd. Increase of Cd content in soil from 2 to 8 $\mu g\ g^{-1}$ changed the position of Cu, Zn, and Pb in both series, giving the orders Cd > Cu > Zn > Mn > Pb and Mn > Zn > Cu > Pb > Cd, respectively. The BAF calculated for plants cultivated in the untreated soil was in the order Cd > Cu > Zn > Mn > Pb, which was significantly altered upon the Cd and Cu administration.

The uptake and transport of ballast metals Cd and Pb take place on a competitive basis with micro- and macroelements for trans-membrane carriers characterized by a broad specificity. Upon ion deficit in the cell, those transporters are synthesized and further activated in biological membranes. As non-specific carriers, they also transport ballast elements in excess. Cadmium entering root cells probably uses broad-spectrum transporters for copper and zinc. Therefore, the uptake of this metal in the presence of increased doses of cadmium decreases.

3. Materials and Methods

3.1. Soil Analysis

Soil samples were collected in May 2017 from the topsoil according to the standard procedure [38] on agricultural land located at 51°22' N, 19°49' E (Włodzimierzów village, Piotrków Trybunalski district, Poland). All samples were dried and sifted (<2 mm). Soil pH was measured in 1 mol L^{-1} KCl solution by the potentiometric method [39]. The gravimetric method for the determination of soil organic matter by the mass loss at 550 °C was applied [40,41]. The bioavailable forms of metals were determined in 0.5 mol·L^{-1} HCl solutions [42]. The total metal contents were measured in samples mineralized with the Multiwave 3000 instrument (Anton Paar GmbH, Graz, Austria). A mixture of concentrated HNO_3 (6 mL) and HCl (2 mL) was applied. Metal concentrations were determined by the HR-CS FAAS with the ContrAA 300 (Analytik Jena spectrometer, Jena, Germany).

3.2. Preparation of Plant Material

Lemon balm was cultivated under laboratory conditions by the pot method [43]. A single pot contained 200 g of soil. The first series consisted of five pots and was cultivated as a reference without metals addition. The subsequent eight series (five samples each) were augmented with $Cd(NO_3)_2$ or $Cu(NO_3)_2$ solutions to the final metal concentrations in soil: (I) 2 $\mu g\ g^{-1}$ Cd; (II) 8 $\mu g\ g^{-1}$ Cd; (III) 20 $\mu g\ g^{-1}$ Cu; (IV) 100 $\mu g\ g^{-1}$ Cu; (V) 2 $\mu g\ g^{-1}$ Cd and 20 $\mu g\ g^{-1}$ Cu; (VI) 2 $\mu g\ g^{-1}$ Cd and 100 $\mu g\ g^{-1}$ Cu; (VII) 8 $\mu g\ g^{-1}$ Cd and 20 $\mu g\ g^{-1}$ Cu; (VIII) 8 $\mu g\ g^{-1}$ Cd and 100 $\mu g\ g^{-1}$ Cu. Seeds of *Melissa officinalis* (P.H. Legutko company, Jutrosin, Poland) were sown in an amount of 0.1 g (approximately 80 seeds) per pot. All pots were kept in a growth chamber at controlled temperatures 23 °C ± 2 °C (day) and 16 °C ± 2 °C (night). The relative humidity was limited to 70–75% while the photosynthetic active radiation (PAR) during the 16 h photoperiod was restricted to 400 $\mu mol\ m^{-2}\ s^{-1}$. All plants were regularly watered by demineralized water. After three months, the above ground parts of the plants were cut, and the roots were separated from the soil and washed with demineralized water. The entire harvest was dried at 45 °C, homogenized, and grounded.

3.3. Determination of Metals in Basil

The dried lemon balm samples (0.5 g) were mineralized in concentrated HNO_3 (6 mL) and HCl (1 mL) acid solutions with a microwave (Anton Paar Multiwave 3000). Metal contents were determined by the HR-CS FAAS with the ContrAA 300 Analytik Jena spectrometer. The certified reference material INCT-MPH-2 (a mixture of selected Polish herbs) was used for the validation of the analytical methodology (Table 2) [44].

Table 2. Metals concentration in the certified reference material ($p = 0.95$; $n = 6$).

Metal	Certified Value µg g^{-1}	Found µg g^{-1}	Recovery %
Manganese	191 ± 12	188 ± 8	98
Lead	2.16 ± 0.23	2.13 ± 0.13	98
Copper	7.77 ± 0.53	7.50 ± 0.38	96
Cadmium	0.199 ± 0.015	0.206 ± 0.007	103
Zinc	33.5 ± 2.1	34.2 ± 0.7	102

3.4. Melissa Plant Growth and Its Physiological Activity

Plant height was measured from the soil surface up to the highest part of the leaf. Index of chlorophyll content was evaluated using the Konica Minolta SPAD-502, Tokyo, Japan, a methodology in which the chlorophyll concentration is determined by measuring the leaf absorbance in the red and near-infrared regions. Gas exchange (activity of net photosynthesis, stomatal conductance, intercellular concentration of carbon dioxide, and transpiration) was determined with the gas analyzer apparatus TPS-2 (Portable Photosynthesis System, Amesbury, MA, USA) [45–48]. All measurements were made in triplicate on separate plants.

3.5. Data Analysis

All analyses were repeated five times. Bartlett's and Hartley's tests were used to confirm the equality of investigated population variance (STATISTICA, version 10 PL, package). The normality of the data was tested using the Shapiro-Wilk test [49,50]. Two-way ANOVA was used to evaluate the combined effect of the cadmium or copper supplementation in soil on the accumulation of manganese, lead, and zinc by the lemon balm plant. All calculations were performed at the 0.95 probability level.

4. Conclusions

Our results showed that additive cadmium–copper interactions modified manganese, lead, and zinc uptake by *Melissa officinalis*. This issue is of particular importance when herbs are grown in soils with diverse and not fully controlled heavy metals concentrations. Either Cd or Cu acting alone at high concentrations in soil (8 and 20 µg g^{-1}, respectively) is toxic to plants as indicated by chlorophyll indices and gas exchange parameters. Surprisingly, this effect was not observed when both metals were administered together. The maximum permissible concentrations (MPC) commonly used in agriculture and environmental protection assessment strategies usually accounts for single-metal toxicities and do not acknowledge additive effects. This issue has not been fully recognized by the environmental protection bodies at either national or European levels.

Author Contributions: Conceptualization, D.A.-S. and W.M.W.; Methodology, D.A.-S. and Z.R.-D.; Validation, D.A.-S.; Formal analysis, D.A.-S. and K.L.; Investigation, D.A.-S.; K.L and Z.R.-D.; Writing—original draft preparation, D.A.-S.; Writing—review and editing, D.A.-S. and W.M.W.; Visualization, D.A.-S. and K.L.; Supervision, D.A.-S. and W.M.W.

Funding: This research was funded by Regional Fund for Environmental Protection and Water Management in Łódź, Poland, grant numbers: 804/BNID/2016 and 58/BN/D2018. Additional funding from the Institute of General and Ecological Chemistry of Łódź University of Technology is also acknowledged.

Conflicts of Interest: The authors declare no conflict of interest. The founding sponsors had no role in the design of the study, in the collection, analyses, or interpretation of data, in the writing of the manuscript, or in the decision to publish the results.

References

1. Bernal, M.; Ramiro, M.V.; Cases, R.; Picorel, R.; Yruela, I. Excess copper effect on growth, chloroplast ultrastructure, oxygen-evolution activity and chlorophyll fluorescence in Glycine max cell suspensions. *Physiol. Plant.* **2006**, *127*, 312–325. [CrossRef]
2. Dubey, S.; Shri, M.; Gupta, A.; Rani, V.; Chakrabarty, D. Toxicity and detoxification of heavy metals during plant growth and metabolism. *Environ. Chem. Lett.* **2018**, *3*, 1–24. [CrossRef]
3. Sattelmacher, B. The apoplast and its significance for plant mineral nutrition. *New Phytol.* **2001**, *149*, 167–192. [CrossRef]
4. Babula, P.; Adam, V.; Opatrilova, R.; Zehnalek, J.; Havel, L.; Kizek, R. Uncommon heavy metals, metalloids and their plant toxicity: A review. *Environ. Chem. Lett.* **2008**, *6*, 189–213. [CrossRef]
5. Cass, H. Herbs for the nervous system: Ginko, kava, valerian, passionflower. *Semin. Integr. Med.* **2004**, *2*, 82–88. [CrossRef]
6. Jambor, J. Growing herbs and herbal processing in Poland—Current state and development perspectives. *Herba Pol.* **2007**, *53*, 22–24.
7. Miraj, S.; Rafieian, K.; Kiani, S. *Melissa officinalis* L.: A review study with an antioxidant prospective. *J. Evid. Based Complement. Alter Med.* **2017**, *22*, 385–394. [CrossRef] [PubMed]
8. Dastmalchia, K.; Dormana, H.J.D.; Oinonena, P.P.; Darwisd, Y.; Laakso, I.; Hiltunen, R. Chemical composition and in vitro antioxidative activity of a lemon balm (*Melissa officinalis* L.) extract. *LWT* **2008**, *41*, 391–400. [CrossRef]
9. Mihajlov, L.; Ilieva, V.; Markova, N.; Zlatkovski, V. Organic cultivation of lemon ballm (*Melissa officinalis*) in Macedonia. *J. Agric. Sci. Technol. B* **2013**, *3*, 769–775.
10. Dastmalchi, K.; Ollilainen, V.; Lackman, P.; Boije af Gennas, G.; Dorman, D.H.J.; Jarvinen, P.P.; Yli-Kauhaluoma, J.; Hiltunen, R. Acetylcholinesterase inhibitory guided fractionation of *Melissa officinalis* L. *Bioorg. Med. Chem.* **2009**, *17*, 867–871. [CrossRef] [PubMed]
11. Mahboubi, M. *Melissa officinalis* and rosmarinic acid in management of memory functions and Alzheimer disease. *Asian Pac. J. Trop. Biomed.* **2019**, *9*, 47–52. [CrossRef]
12. Shakeri, A.; Sahebkar, A.; Javadi, B. *Melissa officinalis* L.—A review of its traditional uses, phytochemistry and pharmacology. *J. Ethnopharm.* **2016**, *188*, 204–228. [CrossRef] [PubMed]
13. Tabatabaei, S.J. Effects of cultivation systems on the growth, and essential oil content and composition of valerian. *J. Herbs Spices Med. Plants* **2008**, *14*, 54–67. [CrossRef]
14. Peirce, A. *The American Pharmaceutical Association Practical Guide to Natural Medicines*; William Morrow and Company: New York, NY, USA, 1999.
15. *WHO Guidelines for Assessing Quality of Herbal Medicines with Reference to Contaminants and Residues*; WHO Library Cataloguing-in-Publication Data; WHO: Geneva, Switzerland, 2007.
16. Alloway, B.J. The General Monograph Herbal Drugs (1433). *Pharmeuropa* **2008**, *20*, 302–303.
17. Miotto, A.; Ceretta, C.A.; Brunetto, G.; Nicoloso, F.T.; Girotto, E.; Farias, J.G.; Tiecher, T.L.; De Conti, L.; Trentin, G. Copper uptake, accumulation and physiological changes in adult grapevines in response to excess copper in soil. *Plant. Soil* **2014**, *374*, 593–610. [CrossRef]
18. Adamczyk-Szabela, D.; Lisowska, K.; Romanowska-Duda, Z.; Wolf, W.M. Combined cadmium-zinc interactions alter manganese, lead, copper uptake by *Melissa officinalis*. In *Scientific Reports*, under review.
19. Küpper, H.; Andresen, E. Mechanisms of metal toxicity in plants. *Metallomics* **2016**, *8*, 269–285.
20. Directive, C. Council Directive 86/278/EEC of 12 June 1986 on the protection of the environment, and in particular of the soil, when sewage sludge is used in agriculture. *Offic. J. Eur. Comm.* **1986**, *118*, 0006–0012.
21. IUSS Working Group. *WRB World Reference Base for Soil Resources (2006)*; World Soil Resources Reports No. 103; FAO: Rome, Italy, 2006.
22. Parmar, P.; Kumari, N.; Sharma, V. Structural and functional alterations in photosynthetic apparatus of plants under cadmium stress. *Bot. Stud.* **2013**, *54*, 45. [CrossRef]
23. Xie, Y.; Hu, L.; Du, Z.; Sun, X.; Amombo, E.; Fan, J.; Fu, J. Effects of cadmium exposure on growth and metabolic profile of Bermudagrass (*Cynodon dactylon* L. Pers.). *PLoS ONE* **2014**, *29*, e115279. [CrossRef]
24. Piršelová, B.; Kuna, R.; Lukáč, P.; Havrlentová, M. Effect of cadmium on growth, photosynthetic pigments, iron and cadmium accumulation of faba bean (*Vicia Faba* cv. Aštar). *Agriculture (Polnohospodárstvo)* **2016**, *62*, 72–79. [CrossRef]

25. Shah, F.R.; Ahmad, N.; Masood, K.R.; Zahid, D.M. The influence of cadmium and chromium on the biomass production of shisham (*Dalbergia Sissoo* Roxb.) seedlings. *Pak. J. Bot.* **2008**, *40*, 1341–1348.
26. Ibrahim, M.H.; Kong, Y.C.; Zain, N.A.M. Effect of cadmium and copper exposure on growth, secondary metabolites and antioxidant activity in the medicinal plant Sambung Nyawa (*Gynura procumbens* (Lour.) Merr.). *Molecules* **2017**, *22*, 1623. [CrossRef]
27. Feng, J.; Lin, Y.; Yang, Y.; Shena, Q.; Huanga, J.; Wang, S.; Zhu, X.; Li, Z. Tolerance and bioaccumulation of Cd and Cu in Sesuvium portulacastrum. *Ecotoxicol. Environ. Saf.* **2018**, *147*, 306–312. [CrossRef] [PubMed]
28. Balestri, M.; Ceccarini, A.; Forino, L.M.C.; Zelko, I.; Martinka, M.; Lux, A.; Castiglione, M.R. Cadmium uptake, localization and stress-induced morphogenic response in the fern *Pteris vittata*. *Planta* **2014**, *239*, 1055–1064. [CrossRef] [PubMed]
29. De Maria, S.; Puschenreiter, M.; Rivelli, A.R. Cadmium accumulation and physiological response of sunflower plants to Cd during the vegetative growing cycle. *Plant. Soil Environ.* **2013**, *59*, 254–261. [CrossRef]
30. Burzyński, M.; Migocka, M.; Kłobus, G. Cu and Cd transport in cucumber (*Cucumis sativus* L.) root plasma membranes. *Plant. Sci.* **2005**, *168*, 1609–1614. [CrossRef]
31. Žaltauskaite, J.; Šliumpaite, I. Evaluation of toxic effects and bioaccumulation of cadmium and copper in Spring Barley (*Hordeum vulgare* L.) *Environ. Res. Eng. Manag.* **2013**, *2*, 51–58. [CrossRef]
32. Chen, H.; Yuan, X.; Li, T.; Hu, S.; Ji, J.; Wang, C. Characteristics of heavy metal transfer and their influencing factor in different soil-crop systems of the industrialization region, China. *Ecotoxicol. Environ. Saf.* **2016**, *126*, 193–201. [CrossRef]
33. Galal, T.M.; Shehata, H.S. Bioaccumulation and translocation of heavy metals by *Plantago major* L. grown in contaminated soils under the effect of traffic pollution. *Ecol. Indic.* **2015**, *48*, 244–251. [CrossRef]
34. Liu, K.; Lv, J.; He, W.; Zhang, H.; Cao, Y.; Dai, Y. Major factors influencing cadmium uptake from the soil into wheat plants. *Ecotoxicol. Environ. Saf.* **2015**, *113*, 207–213. [CrossRef]
35. Skiba, E.; Kobyłecka, J.; Wolf, W.M. Influence of 2,4-D and MCPA herbicides on uptake and translocation of heavy metals in wheat (*Triticum aestivum* L.). *Environ. Poll.* **2017**, *220*, 882–890. [CrossRef] [PubMed]
36. Testiati, E.; Parinet, J.; Massiani, C.; Laffont-Schwob, I.; Rabier, J.; Pfeifer, H.-R.; Lenoble, V.; Masotti, V.; Prudent, P. Trace metal and metalloid contamination levels in soils and two native plant species of a former industrial site: Evaluation of the phytostabilization potential. *J. Hazard. Mater.* **2013**, *248–249*, 131–141. [CrossRef] [PubMed]
37. Xiao, R.; Bai, J.; Lu, Q.; Zhao, Q.; Gao, Z.; Wen, X.; Liu, X. Fractionation, transfer and ecological risks of heavy metals in riparian and ditch wetlands across a 100-year chronosequence of reclamation in estuary of China. *Sci. Total Environ.* **2015**, *517*, 66–75. [CrossRef]
38. PN-ISO 10381-4:2007. Soil Quality—Sampling—Part 4: Rules for Procedure During the Research Areas of Natural, Semi-Natural and Cultivated. 2007. Available online: http://sklep.pkn.pl/pn-iso-10381-4-2007p.html (accessed on 15 May 2019).
39. PN-ISO 10390:1997. Agricultural Chemical Analysis of the Soil. Determination of pH. 1997. Available online: http://sklep.pkn.pl/pn-iso-10390-1997p.html (accessed on 20 April 2019).
40. ASTM D2974-00. *Standard Test Methods for Moisture, Ash, and Organic Matter of Peat and Other Organic Soils. Method D 2974–00*; American Society for Testing and Materials: West Conshohocken, PA, USA, 2000.
41. Schumacher, B.A. *Methods for the Determination of Total Organic Carbon (TOC) in Soils and Sediments*; United States Environmental Protection Agency Environmental Sciences Division National Exposure Research Laboratory: Las Vegas, NV, USA, 2002.
42. PN-ISO 11259:2001. Soil Quality—A Simplified Description of the Soil. 2001. Available online: http://sklep.pkn.pl/pn-iso-11259-2001p.html (accessed on 5 May 2019).
43. Adamczyk-Szabela, D.; Markiewicz, J.; Wolf, W.M. Heavy metal uptake by herbs. IV. Influence of soil pH on the content of heavy metals in *Valeriana officinalis* L. *Water Air Soil Pollut.* **2015**, *226*, 106–114. [CrossRef] [PubMed]
44. Dybczyński, R.; Danko, B.; Kulisa, K.; Maleszewska, E.; Polkowska- Motrenko, H.; Samczyński, Z.; Szopa, Z. Preparation and preliminary certification of two new Polish CRMs for inorganic trace analysis. *J. Radioanal. Nucl. Chem.* **2004**, *259*, 409–413. [CrossRef]
45. Grzesik, M.; Romanowska-Duda, Z.B. Ability of Cyanobacteria and microalgae in improvement of metabolic activity and development of willow plants. *Pol. J. Environ. Stud.* **2015**, *24*, 1003–1006. [CrossRef]

46. Piotrowski, K.; Romanowska-Duda, Z.B.; Grzesik, M. How Biojodis and cyanobacteria alleviate the negative influence of predicted environmental constraints on growth and physiological activity of corn plants. *Pol. J. Environ. Stud.* **2016**, *25*, 741–751. [CrossRef]
47. Kalaji, M.H.; Carpentier, R.; Allakhverdiev, S.I.; Bosa, K. Fluorescence parameters as an early indicator of light stress in barley. *J. Photochem. Photobiol. B* **2012**, *112*, 1–6. [CrossRef]
48. Kalaji, M.H.; Schansker, G.; Ladle, R.J.; Goltsev, V.; Bosa, K.; Allakhverdiev, S.I.; Brestic, M.; Bussotti, F.; Calatayud, A.; Dąbrowski, P.; et al. Frequently asked questions about chlorophyll fluorescence, the sequel. *Photosynth. Res.* **2016**, *122*, 121–127. [CrossRef]
49. Goodson, D.Z. *Mathematical Methods for Physical and Analytical Chemistry*; Wiley & Sons: Hoboken, NJ, USA, 2011.
50. Razali, N.M.; Wah, Y.B. Power comparisons of Shapiro–Wilk, Kolmogorov–Smirnov, Lilliefors and Anderson–Darling tests. *J. Stat. Model. Anal.* **2011**, *2*, 21–33.

Sample Availability: Samples of the compounds are not available from the authors.

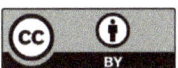

© 2019 by the authors. Licensee MDPI, Basel, Switzerland. This article is an open access article distributed under the terms and conditions of the Creative Commons Attribution (CC BY) license (http://creativecommons.org/licenses/by/4.0/).

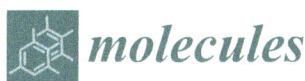

Article

Increased Aluminum Content in Certain Brain Structures is Correlated with Higher Silicon Concentration in Alcoholic Use Disorder

Cezary Grochowski [1,2,*], Eliza Blicharska [3], Jacek Bogucki [4], Jędrzej Proch [5], Aleksandra Mierzwińska [6], Jacek Baj [1], Jakub Litak [2], Arkadiusz Podkowiński [2], Jolanta Flieger [3], Grzegorz Teresiński [6], Ryszard Maciejewski [1], Przemysław Niedzielski [5] and Piotr Rzymski [7]

1. Department of Anatomy, Medical University of Lublin, Jaczewskiego 4, 20-090 Lublin, Poland; jacek.baj@me.com (J.B.); maciejewski.r@gmail.com (R.M.)
2. Department of Neurosurgery and Pediatric Neurosurgery, Medical University of Lublin, Jaczewskiego 8, 20-954 Lublin, Poland; jakub.litak@gmail.com (J.L.); apodkowinski@wp.pl (A.P.)
3. Department of Analytical Chemistry, Medical University of Lublin, Chodźki 4a, 20-093 Lublin, Poland; bayrena@o2.pl (E.B.); jolanta.flieger@umlub.pl (J.F.)
4. Department of Clinical Genetics, Medical University of Lublin, Radziwiłłowska 11, 20-080 Lublin, Poland; jacekbogucki@wp.pl
5. Faculty of Chemistry, Department of Analytical Chemistry, Adam Mickiewicz University in Poznań, 89B Umultowska Street, 61-614 Poznan, Poland; jed.proch@gmail.com (J.P.); pnied@amu.edu.pl (P.N.)
6. Department of Forensic Medicine, Medical University of Lublin, 8b Jaczewskiego St, 20-090 Lublin, Poland; mierzwinska.aa@gmail.com (A.M.); grzegorz.teresinski@umlub.pl (G.T.)
7. Department of Environmental Medicine, Poznan University of Medical Sciences, 61-701 Poznan, Poland; rzymskipiotr@ump.edu.pl
* Correspondence: cezary.grochowski@o2.pl; Tel.: +48-81448-6020

Academic Editors: Francesco Crea and Alberto Pettignano
Received: 8 April 2019; Accepted: 1 May 2019; Published: 3 May 2019

Abstract: Introduction: Alcohol overuse may be related to increased aluminum (Al) exposure, the brain accumulation of which contributes to dementia. However, some reports indicate that silicon (Si) may have a protective role over Al-induced toxicity. Still, no study has ever explored the brain content of Al and Si in alcoholic use disorder (AUD). Materials and methods: To fill this gap, the present study employed inductively coupled plasma optical emission spectrometry to investigate levels of Al and Si in 10 brain regions and in the liver of AUD patients ($n = 31$) and control ($n = 32$) post-mortem. Results: Al content was detected only in AUD patients at mean ± SD total brain content of 1.59 ± 1.19 mg/kg, with the highest levels in the thalamus (4.05 ± 12.7 mg/kg, FTH), inferior longitudinal fasciculus (3.48 ± 9.67 mg/kg, ILF), insula (2.41 ± 4.10 mg/kg) and superior longitudinal fasciculus (1.08 ± 2.30 mg/kg). Si content displayed no difference between AUD and control, except for FTH. Positive inter-region correlations between the content of both elements were identified in the cingulate cortex, hippocampus, and ILF. Conclusions: The findings of this study suggest that AUD patients may potentially be prone to Al-induced neurodegeneration in their brain—although this hypothesis requires further exploration.

Keywords: aluminum; silicon; ICP-OES; trace elements; brain trace element concentration; brain toxicity

---

1. Introduction

Aluminum (Al), the most abundant metal and third most common element in the Earth's crust, is increasingly used for various purposes in a number of sectors within the pharmaceutical (e.g., as antacids, phosphate binders, buffered aspirins, adjuvant) cosmetics (e.g., in antiperspirants) and food (e.g., as a packing material, food additive) industries. The majority of Al is continuously extracted from existing ores, with recycling processes accounting only to 40% of its overall supply [1]. This results in a rise in environmental and circulating levels of Al, and as estimated, its exposures have increased at least 30-fold over the last 50 years—with a mean of 11 kg of Al being currently refined for every human, annually [2].

There is no specific biological role identified for Al, and its ion (Al^{3+}) is known to reveal toxic action. Accumulating evidence from in vitro and in vivo experimental studies, as well as epidemiological observations, demonstrate that increased exposures to Al can lead to a number of adverse health effects [3]. Al has been postulated to induce oxidative stress in various cell types [4,5], interfere with estrogen receptors [6], support osteomalacia via phosphate deficiency, impair calcium uptake and engender dysfunctional osteoblast proliferation [7], as well as to alter iron homeostasis by disrupting intestinal Fe absorption and normal tissue ferritin levels [8]. Of highest concern is that studies on Al uptake have revealed a neurotoxic action that is potentially implicated in different neurodegenerative disorders, including encephalopathy, Alzheimer's disease and multiple sclerosis [9–11]. As shown in experimental animals, Al can lead to accumulation of Aβ and tau protein, and induction of neuronal apoptosis in the brain [12,13], and impair learning and memory functions [14,15]. Acute exposures to Al in human were associated with cognitive impairment, such as agitation, confusion, or myoclonic jerk [16,17], while occupationally exposed subjects revealed disruption in memory and concentration [18,19]. Thus, research has assessed its content in human bones [20,21], in organs, such as the brain [22] and uterus [23,24], as well as in fluids including urine [25], serum [26], breast milk [27], and semen [28].

A number of activities are known to significantly increase Al exposure. These include specific industrial and agriculture occupations, first-hand and second-hand smoking, and the use of recreational drugs. such as heroin or cocaine. Furthermore, selected food products have been shown to have high Al content, e.g., jellyfish, fried twisted cruller, or microalgal supplements if Al compounds were used to harvest the biomass [29–31]. Al is known to be poorly absorbed in the gastrointestinal tract at levels of 0.1–1.0% of the oral dose, and in healthy subjects, most of the absorbed pool is readily excreted from the body in the urine. However, some factors, such as consumption of citric acid in the form of fruit juices, markedly increase Al absorption. Hence, under sustained exposure of the gastrointestinal tract, or/and under certain conditions, particularly renal failure, increased Al accumulation in the body can occur. This effect is particularly noticeable in the central nervous system [32].

Some additional factors, such as excessive consumption of ethanol, have been suggested to increase Al bioavailability due to increased permeability of the intestinal mucosa [33]. However, experimental studies have shown that silicon (Si) may be protective against aluminum accumulation in the brain [34,35]. It has been previously hypothesized that alcoholic amnesia and dementia may also arise from increased Al exposures in individuals through the excessive consumption of ethanol beverages [33] and that Al accumulation may be regulated by Si availability. Thus, the aim of the present study is to compare Al and Si content in different regions of the brain of individuals with alcohol use disorder (AUD) and in control subjects and to assess whether levels of these two elements in the brain and liver reveal any association. To the best of our knowledge, this is the first, albeit preliminary study to demonstrate that AUD patients may face increased Al accumulation in their brains.

2. Results

2.1. Demographic Characteristic

The studied AUD and control group consisted of 31 and 32 subjects, respectively. Their demographic data are summarized in Table 1.

Table 1. Demographic characteristic of studied subjects enrolled in this study.

Parameter	Control (n = 32)	AUD (n = 31)	p-Value
Age [years] (mean ± SD)	49.4 ± 19.5	47.9 ± 13.1	0.74
Sex [n/%]			
Female	12 (37.5%)	8 (25.8%)	0.32
Male	20 (62.5%)	23 (74. 2)	
Weight [kg] (mean ± SD)	79.4 ± 21.3	77.9 ± 15.7	0.82
BMI [kg/m^2] (mean ± SD)	26.7 ± 5.6	26.8 ± 6.2	0.65

2.2. Al Content

The total (mean ± SD) content of Al in the brain of the AUD subjects was 1.59 ± 1.19 mg/kg. Al was identified in every studied area, albeit at levels decreasing in the following order: FTH > ILF > INS > SLF > ACC > CA > HPC > PCG > NAc > PFC. All control samples displayed Al content below detection limits. The Al levels in the liver displayed no significant difference between AUD and control subjects (Table 2).

Table 2. Content of Al in alcohol use disorder (AUD) (n = 31) and control (n = 32) subjects in different brain structures and in the liver (mg/kg).

		% < LOD	N > LOD	Mean	± SD	Median	Min	Max	CV	p-Value
PFC	AUD	54.8	14	0.49	0.44	0.27	0.01	1.4	0.20	-
	Control	96.9	1	-	-	-	-	-	-	
PCG	AUD	45.1	17	0.95	1.5	0.46	0.04	6.6	2.4	-
	Control	96.9	1	-	-	-	-	-	-	
ACC	AUD	41.9	18	1.0	1.3	0.54	0.03	5.0	1.8	-
	Control	100	0	-	-	-	-	-	-	
HPC	AUD	67.7	10	0.98	0.59	0.98	0.08	1.9	0.34	-
	Control	96.9	1	-	-	-	-	-	-	
CA	AUD	54.8	14	0.99	1.5	0.39	0.04	5.7	2.2	-
	Control	96.9	1	-	-	-	-	-	-	
FTH	AUD	51.6	15	4.0	12.7	0.31	0.04	49.7	161.	-
	Control	96.9	1	-	-	-	-	-	-	
SLF	AUD	58.1	13	1.1	2.3	0.21	0.01	8.3	5.3	-
	Control	96.9	1	-	-	-	-	-	-	
ILF	AUD	51.6	15	3.5	9.7	0.41	0.02	37.4	93.5	-
	Control	93.7	2	-	-	-	-	-	-	
NAc	AUD	71.0	9	0.65	0.79	0.30	0.05	2.4	0.63	-
	Control	90.6	3	-	-	-	-	-	-	
INS	AUD	74.	8	2.4	4.1	0.40	0.05	12.1	16.8	-
	Control	100	0	-	-	-	-	-	-	
Liver	AUD	51.6	15	1.5	3.0	0.42	0.02	12.0	9.0	0.173
	Control	81.2	16	0.31	0.22	0.30	0.06	0.92	0.09	

A number of significant, mostly positive correlations in Al content in various brain regions of the AUD subjects were identified. INS content was, however, negatively correlated with PFC and ILF. Additionally, the liver levels of Al revealed a positive correlation with that found in PFC, PCG, FTH, SLF, and ILF (Table 3).

Table 3. Spearman correlation coefficient for Al content in various brain structures and the liver of AUD subjects. Asterisks indicate $p < 0.05$ analysis of Al concentration. Correlation coefficients marked with * are significant at $p < 0.05$.

	Al-PFC	Al-PCG	Al-ACC	Al-HPC	Al-CA	Al-FTH	Al-SLF	Al-ILF	Al-liver	Al-NAc	Al-INS
Al-PCG	0.43 *										
Al-ACC	0.283	0.574 *									
Al-HPC	−0.049	0.269	0.071								
Al-CA	0.627 *	0.291	0.340	0.021							
Al-FTH	0.393 *	0.339	0.167	0.084	0.561 *						
Al-SLF	0.265	0.585 *	0.178	0.233	0.068	0.505 *					
Al-ILF	0.529 *	0.419 *	0.402 *	−0.323	0.526 *	0.238	0.073				
Al-liver	0.406 *	0.632 *	0.277	0.239	0.349	0.421 *	0.556 *	0.511 *			
Al-NAc	−0.194	0.185	−0.106	0.377 *	0.087	−0.013	0.257	−0.146	0.083		
Al-INS	−0.414 *	0.155	−0.032	0.403 *	−0.158	−0.118	0.124	−0.417*	−0.024	0.655 *	

2.3. Si Content

Si was identified above detection limits at varying frequency in all brain regions of both AUD and control subjects at total mean ± SD content of 32.1 ± 11.3 and 5.6 ± 2.6 mg/kg, respectively ($p < 0.001$, Mann-Whitney U test). In both groups, Si levels displayed high variance of observed levels. In AUD subjects, Si mean content decreased in the following order: FTH > INS > ACC > CA > PCG > SLF > NAc > HPC > ILF > PFC, while in control, a strikingly different order was observed: PFC > SLF > ACC > PCG > HPC > NAc > FTH > INS > CA > ILF. However, the only significant difference in Si content between the AUD and the control group was found for FTH. Liver content of Si did not differ between groups (Table 4).

Table 4. Content of Si in AUD ($n = 31$) and control ($n = 32$) subjects in different brain structures and in the liver (mg/kg).

		% < LOD	N > LOD	Mean	± SD	Median	Min	Max	CV	p-Value
PFC	AUD	35.5	20	13.5	37.9	2.5	0.02	171.	1439.	0.474
	Control	43.7	18	11.6	1.5	30.2	0.03	125.	911.	
PCG	AUD	12.9	27	31.1	73.1	4.4	0.02	367.	5351.	0.164
	Control	53.1	15	5.9	3.1	9.9	0.11	39.8	97.5	
ACC	AUD	9.7	28	40.8	129.	3.9	0.12	683.	16738.	0.326
	Control	65.6	11	6.5	1.8	8.1	0.12	20.2	65.1	
HPC	AUD	41.9	18	25.9	47.2	3.8	0.37	183.	2231.	0.076
	Control	50.0	16	5.2	1.8	7.3	0.13	26.8	54.1	
CA	AUD	25.8	23	34.9	94.1	2.4	0.12	436.	8856.	0.094
	Control	56.2	14	3.2	1.5	6.2	0.11	24.2	38.7	
FTH	AUD	25.8	23	51.1	151.	3.4	0.03	532.	22698.	0.020
	Control	50.0	16	3.7	1.0	6.5	0.02	23.6	42.1	
SLF	AUD	29..0	22	27..0	53..7	4..2	0..13	225..	2880..	0..887
	Control	68..7	10	8.0..	2..8	10..5	0..19	32..9	111..	
ILF	AUD	29..0	22	22.0	43..9	5..8	0..04	192..	1931..	0..149
	Control	56.250	14	2.5	2.2	2.4	0.06	9.7	5.7	
NAc	AUD	41.9	18	26.1	80.8	1.8	0.02	341.	6526.	0.759
	Control	53.1	15	5.0.	2.3	6.7	0.24	19.0	45.1	
INS	AUD	41.9	18	50.0	127.	4.5	0.12	506.	16264.	0.149
	Control	40.6	19	3.6	1.62	4.9	0.09	17.1	24.2	
Liver	AUD	12.9	27	31.3	115.	2.6	0.14	598.	13322.	0.096
	Control	18.7	26	6.0	1.9	17.3	0.07	89.2	299.9	

A number of significant correlations in Si content in various brain areas were identified in the AUD group. Additionally, Si levels in the PFC, PCG, ACC, CA, and FTH were positively correlated with that found in the liver (Table 5).

Table 5. Spearman correlation coefficient for Si content in various brain structures of AUD subjects and in their liver. Asterisks indicate $p < 0.05$.

	Si-PFC	Si-PCG	Si-ACC	Si-HPC	Si-CA	Si-FTH	Si-SLF	Si-ILF	Si-liver	Si-NAc	Si-INS
Si-ACC	0.150										
Si-HPC	0.285	0.788 *									
Si-CA	−0.338	−0.036	−0.043								
Si-FTH	0.316	0.632 *	0.717 *	−0.040							
Si-SLF	0.167	0.429 *	0.457 *	−0.008	0.640 *						
Si-ILF	−0.088	0.464 *	0.315	0.104	0.274	0.506 *					
Si-liver	0.467 *	0.624 *	0.742 *	−0.078	0.694 *	0.422 *	0.289				
Si-NAc	0.208	0.244	0.266	−0.043	0.393 *	0.405 *	0.530 *	0.385 *			
Si-INS	−0.579 *	−0.104	−0.145	0.180	0.022	0.032	0.026	−0.302	−0.066		
Si-ACC	−0.490 *	0.095	0.024	0.288	−0.034	0.222	0.378 *	−0.164	0.184	0.581 *	
Total Si	0.067	0.767 *	0.706 *	0.158	0.691 *	0.615 *	0.656 *	0.525 *	0.507 *	0.038	0.333

In the control group, Si content in all brain areas was significantly and positively intercorrelated. A similar observation was made for Al content in the liver, and that found in every studied brain area (Table 3). The conducted analysis revealed the existence of a series of (22) positive, statistically significant r-Spearman correlation coefficients, attesting to the existence of a positive correlation. The highest value of the correlation coefficient was observed in the correlation between the amount of silicon in the Si-PCG and the Si-ACC. In the liver, four statistically significant positive correlation coefficients were noted—with the Si-CA, Si-FTH, Si-SLF, and Si-ILF (Table 6).

Table 6. Spearman correlation coefficient for Al content in various brain structures and the liver of AUD subjects. Asterisks indicate $p < 0.05$.

	Si-PFC	Si-PCG	Si-ACC	Si-HPC	Si-CA	Si-FTH	Si-SLF	Si-ILF	Si-liver	Si-NAc	Si-INS
Si-PCG	0.719 *										
Si-ACC	0.405 *	0.538 *									
Si-HPC	0.632 *	0.647 *	0.510 *								
Si-CA	0.733 *	0.824 *	0.611 *	0.758 *							
Si-FTH	0.553 *	0.510 *	0.350 *	0.421 *	0.556 *						
Si-SLF	0.385 *	0.370 *	0.283	0.261	0.422 *	0.608 *					
Si-ILF	0.470 *	0.623 *	0.431 *	0.521 *	0.705 *	0.447 *	0.584 *				
Si-liver	0.590 *	0.515 *	0.249	0.288	0.457 *	0.364 *	0.452 *	0.494 *			
Si-NAc	0.669 *	0.693 *	0.515 *	0.489 *	0.661 *	0.642 *	0.573 *	0.599 *	0.512 *		
Si-INS	0.502 *	0.673 *	0.542 *	0.569 *	0.648 *	0.426 *	0.332	0.613 *	0.396 *	0.507 *	
Total Si	0.762 *	0.781 *	0.488 *	0.681 *	0.767 *	0.763 *	0.618 *	0.678 *	0.502 *	0.783 *	0.717 *

There were also two statistically significant, negative correlation coefficients seen, indicating the existence of a negative correlation between the amount of silicon in the Si-PFC and Si-NAc and Si-INS. Likewise, a number of correlations in Si content in various areas were identified in the control group.

2.4. Association Between Al and Si Content

Several significant positive correlations between Al and Si content in the different brain regions of AUD subjects were identified (Table 7). Inter-region correlations were found for ACC, HPC, and ILF. The liver content of both elements was also found to be significantly associated.

Table 7. Spearman correlation coefficient calculated for Al and Si content in different brain regions of AUD subjects.

Si	AUD Group Al									
	PFC	PCG	ACC	HPC	CA	FTH	SLF	ILF	NAc	INS	Liver
PFC	0.379	−0.055	0.437	−0.200	−0.013	−0.163	0.033	0.720	0.485	−0.800	0.045
PCG	0.608	0.267	0.541	0.672	0.235	−0.207	−0.219	0.349	0.200	−0.214	0.050
ACC	0.582	0.094	0.581	0.783	0.379	−0.019	−0.097	0.460	0.238	−0.107	0.274
HPC	0.381	−0.063	0.783	0.666	−0.006	0.233	−0.133	−0.187	−0.095	0.285	0.230
CA	0.604	0.191	0.438	0.500	0.481	−0.157	−0.090	0.661	0.714	0.250	0.225
FTH	0.836	0.142	0.287	0.607	−0.063	0.461	0.200	−0.081	−0.371	0.600	0.482
SLF	0.054	0.217	0.100	−0.116	−0.172	0.327	0.296	0.524	−0.500	0.750	0.112
ILF	0.223	0.279	0.502	0.321	0.167	−0.159	−0.466	0.560	0.392	−0.085	0.055
NAc	0.000	0.154	−0.218	−0.095	−0.023	−0.200	0.533	−0.023	−0.100	0.035	0.761
INS	0.485	0.442	0.600	0.428	0.428	0.333	0.714	0.285	−0.404	0.595	0.216
Liver	0.293	0.342	−0.007	0.309	−0.188	0.138	0.216	0.132	−0.190	0.142	0.678

3. Discussion

This is the first study to demonstrate that Al content is significantly increased in the brains of AUD subjects. Considering that Al has been implicated in neurodegenerative processes, this appears to be a clinically relevant observation. As noted previously, chronic Al exposure can cause the accumulation of AβP, impair spatial learning memory and induce conformational changes to proteins related to neurodegeneration. These include tau, PHF-tau, synuclein, amylin, ABri, microglobulin, and APP [36–41]. A recent study reported brain Al levels of subjects suffering from Alzheimer's disease and multiple sclerosis, the content of which is in excess of 10 and 50 mg/kg, respectively [11]. The present study found that compared to control, mean brain content of Al in AUD subjects was by order of magnitude higher and exceeded 7 mg/kg.

Studies on animal models have demonstrated the neurotoxicity of chronic exposure to low doses of aluminum. This causes brain aging acceleration through the induction of inflammatory processes, such as an increase in inflammatory cytokines and amyloid precursor proteins, as well as enhanced glial activation. There are several theories explaining the toxicity of aluminum in relation to the brain tissue. It is suggested that its insoluble complexes stimulate the activation of glial cells and magnify the activity of macrophages. These effects were confirmed by studies in rats in which deposits of the element within the striatum and associated renal gliosis were observed [42]. Within the striatum, excessive proliferation of astrocytes and microglia was found in patients with chronic renal failure who had used aluminum gels [43]. Abou-Donia's research also suggests the direct toxicity of the element to the brain tissue. Such conclusions were drawn while treating dialysis encephalopathy with deferoxamine [44]. In a study conducted by Petrik et al. on a mouse model where aluminum-containing adjuvants were injected, inflammation and loss of cells within the motor cortex and spinal cord were detected, and memory deficits were described [45]. Symptoms of encephalopathy have also been observed among aluminum industry workers [46]. Moreover, progressive cognitive dysfunction, as well as ataxia, dysarthria, and seizures, have been noted among people taking drugs through the intravenous route caused by the preparation of a methadone solution in an aluminum dish [47].

During the consumption of water containing elevated concentrations of this element, significant deficits in cognitive functions were detected among the population [48]. This was confirmed also in the animal model, where behavioral disorders [49], as well as changes in cognitive and morphological functions in the central nervous system, were demonstrated [50].

Memory impairment due to aluminum poisoning was first described in 1921. This was subsequently confirmed by Rondeau et al., who in a 15-year cohort study, demonstrated that daily intake of high doses of aluminum correlates with an increased risk of cognitive decline and dementia. Herein, Al intake brought about the death of neurons and glial cells, and, consequently, deficits in spatial memory, emotional deficits, and impaired memory and learning processes [51].

There are many papers reporting an increased risk of developing Alzheimer's disease by drinking water with a high concentration of aluminum. McLachlan et al., in their study, showed that people living in areas where the concentration of this element in water was above 100 µg/l have a higher risk of suffering from Alzheimer's disease [50], which was also confirmed by a study by Rondeau et al. [51]. A meta-analysis by Flaten [52], as well as a study carried out after 15 years on a large population, confirmed the association of the development of Alzheimer's disease with high aluminum content in drinking water [51].

Increased Al content in AUD subjects leads to the hypothesis that this metal could plausibly add to neurodegeneration processes involved in alcoholic amnesia and dementia in subjects over-consuming ethanol. This could partially be due to increased absorption of Al in the gastrointestinal tract due to altered permeability of intestinal mucosa [33] and/or its increased retention because of renal failure, both of which have been observed in AUD subjects [53]. One should further note that various alcoholic beverages can contain detectable content of Al. Herein, the highest values are found in red and white wine [54] by way of its binding to tartaric acid and other organic acids that can increase the bioavailability of the element [55]. As suggested by some authors, Al content in wine should not exceed 0.5 mg/L. Increased Al content was also found in beers stored in aluminum cans [56]. It is thus plausible that increased Al accumulation in the brain of AUD subjects results from ethanol-induced binge intake, as well as from general elevated oral exposures to this metal.

In addition, the present study also investigated brain Si content.

Silicic acid has not been found to interfere with organic molecules in biological systems. However, it is able to react with Al_3^+ (at pH ≥ 5). As found, there was no statistically significant difference in Si content in brain regions between AUD and control subjects, with the exception of FTH. Previous research has shown that AUD subjects display positive inter-region correlations between Al and Si levels in ILF, HPC, and ACC. It remains unknown whether Si may immobilize Al in these areas or alter its toxicity—these hypotheses require further exploration in experimental models. Silicic acid has not been found to interfere with organic molecules in biological systems. However, it is able to react with Al^{3+} (at pH ≥ 5).

The daily intake of Al is about 20mg, and silicon absorption has been evaluated at 20–50 mg. Water and other drinks can provide 19% of daily intake [36].

Using an Atlantic salmon model, Exley et al. were the first to suggest the protective effect of silicon in Al. As demonstrated, fish exposed to water with high Al concentration and low Si concentration were observed to be intoxicated. Moreover, whole-body Al content was assessed as being higher in those fishes [57]. And some additional studies report that the greater amount of absorbed Al was of a temporary situation, some Al was permanently stored in tissue. This resulted in a delay before excretion [58]. The preliminary work by Belia and Roberts claims that an increased intake of silicic acid can mobilize Al and decrease the tissue storage concentration [59]. Moreover, studies conducted by Desouky et al. in which the accumulation of Al in snail cells was investigated, revealed co-accumulation of Si, even without exogenous Si supplementation [60].

Although silicic acid was noted to reduce Al uptake in the intestine [61], there are several different routes of Al uptake—dermal, olfactory and respiratory. White et al. report that Si-Al interactions occur within the tissues in vivo [62]. They also concluded that, in spite of normalization of Al levels after nine days, there were no behavioral improvements at day 15, which suggest long-term Al effects on nervous tissue. Currently, there are no known mechanisms of Si transportation into the tissue, however, because of the small dimensions of $Si(OH)_4$ and its neutral charge it is possible for silicic acid to enter into the cells through passive diffusion. Moreover, chronic alcohol consumption causes changes in cytoskeletal and tight junction assembly, thus the dysfunction of blood-brain barrier and increased porosity.

In our study, increased Si levels accompanied increased Al levels in three out of 10 analyzed brain structures. Herein, the Si concentration levels were several times higher than Al levels. Of note, studies report high Si concentration in beer [63], which may have protective properties in this group.

However, while these findings imply that AUD patients may be more prone to Al-induced toxic effects in the brain, it should be underlined that the Al content was not explored here in the context of neurodegenerative changes in brain regions or cognitive function impairment. This would require experimental in vivo research and/or intravital neuroimaging of Al in the brain, neither of which has been done. Moreover, the nature of Al and Si association in selected brain regions in AUD remains unknown, and whether the latter may affect the activity of the former is purely speculative.

4. Material and Methods

4.1. Subjects

The research material consisted of brain and liver tissue samples taken from individuals reported to the autopsies in the Department of Forensic Medicine at the Medical University of Lublin in Poland. Samples were collected from 31 subjects (23 male, 8 female) with AUD, with inclusion criteria of chronic alcohol abuse in their medical history, no history of mental disorders and alcohol level > 2‰ in blood confirmed at the time of the section. Samples were also collected from 31 control subjects (21 male and 10 female). The inclusion criteria for this group were the absence of documented alcoholic and neurodegenerative disorder history, macroscopically unaltered brain tissue, and blood alcohol level of <2‰ as confirmed at the time of the section. The competent prosecutor's office consented to the collection of tissues, and the study was approved by the Local Bioethical Committee of the Medical University of Lublin (approval No. KE-0254/2018). In addition, the work described in this article has been carried out in accordance with The Code of Ethics of the World Medical Association (Declaration of Helsinki) for experiments involving humans; Uniform Requirements for manuscripts submitted to Biomedical journals.

4.2. Sample Tissue Collection and Procedure

Samples were collected by qualified pathologists in accordance with the analytical protocol. In order to prevent contamination of the tissue sample, all materials in contact with the samples were previously decontaminated with 5% (v/v) suprapure nitric acid solution and thoroughly washed with ultrapure water (Milli-Q, Millipore, Raleigh, NC, USA, resistivity 18.2 MΩ·cm).

After removing the brain from the cranium, the excess of the blood was thoroughly washed with ultrapure water. Meninges were removed with plastic tweezers, and the brain tissue was washed again with ultrapure water to minimize samples contamination with blood or cerebrospinal fluid.

For analysis, 0.5 g of tissue samples were harvested in ten anatomical locations using disinfected plastic knives. Ten areas of the brain were selected: frontal cortex (Broadmann area no. 11, PFC), postcentral gyrus (Broadmann area no. 1, PCG), dorsal anterior cingular cortex (Broadmann area no. 32, ACC), the foot of the hippocampus (HPC), the head of the caudate nucleus (CA), the frontal part of the thalamus (FTH), superior longitudinal fasciculus (SLF), inferior longitudinal fasciculus (ILF) and the nucleus accumbens (NAc), frontal part of the insula (INS).

Additionally, liver samples were collected by dissecting 0.5 g from the 6th segment. All tissue samples were thoroughly rinsed with deionized water and drained on sterile blotting paper. All of the collected samples were weighed. The tissue sample was then put into sterile polypropylene containers (Bionovo), and, afterwards, the initial decay of the organic matrix through the use of 2 mL of 65% suprapure HNO_3 was performed. The mass loss of the samples was limited, and samples were digested directly after sampling without preliminary drying.

In the last stage of the experiment, each sample was quantitatively transferred to close Teflon containers and digested at 180 °C utilizing the microwave digestion system Mars 6 (CEM, Matthews, NC, USA). After digestion, samples were diluted with water to meet a total volume of 10.0 mL using scaled test-tubes.

4.3. Analytical Procedures

The inductively coupled plasma optical emission spectrometer Agilent 5110 ICP-OES (Agilent, Santa Clara, CA, USA) was employed for Al and Si determination. The synchronous vertical dual view (SVDV) of the plasma was accomplished by using dichroic spectral combiner (DSC) technology. This allows axial and radial view analysis simultaneously. In doing so, radio frequency (RF) power was 1.2 kW, nebulizer gas flow—0.7 L min−1, auxiliary gas flow—1.0 L min−1, plasma gas flow—12.0 L min−1, charge coupled device (CCD) temperature was −40 °C, viewing height for radial plasma observation was 8 mm, while accusation time was 5 s. The analysis was repeated three times. The following wavelengths were applied: Al—396.152 nm, Si—288.158 nm. ICP commercial analytical standards (Romil, Cambridge, UK) were used for calibration. Detection limits were determined through 3-sigma criteria and were on the level of 0.01 (mg/kg) wet weight (*w/w*) for all elements determined. The uncertainty for the complete analytical process (including sample preparation) was at the level of 20%. Traceability was assessed by comparison with reference materials. A recovery of 80–120% was considered acceptable for all the elements determined.

4.4. Statistical Analysis

All statistical analyses were performed with the use of Statistica v.13.3 (StatSoft Polska Sp. zo.o., Kraków, Poland). The assumption of Gaussian distribution was not met ($p < 0.05$, Shapiro-Wilk test), thus non-parametric methods were then applied. Herein, differences between two and three independent groups were assessed via the Mann-Whitney U test, Pearson's chi^2 and Kruskal-Wallis ANOVA, respectively. The correlation between two variables was evaluated with Spearman Rs coefficient. A *p*-value of $s < 0.05$ was considered to be statistically significant.

5. Conclusions

The present study demonstrated for the first time that AUD patients are characterized by increased Al content in various brain regions, with the highest content identified in FTH, ILF, and INS. Considering that Al has neurodegenerative potential, and cognitive impairments in alcoholics are linked to ethanol-induced neurodegeneration and alcohol dependence, these findings appear to be clinically relevant. Furthermore, we saw that AUD patients did not display significantly increased levels of brain Si, an element previously postulated to have a protective role over toxicity expressed by Al. Thus, an association between both elements in ACC, HPC, and ILF was observed—the nature of these correlations remains, however, yet to be explored. Our findings are in favor of a hypothesis that has been previously put forward that alcohol overuse may contribute to increased Al exposure and that this element may potentially add to the neurodegenerative outcomes observed in AUD patients, such as dementia. Further research is required to investigate the mechanisms of neurotoxicity of Al under ethanol exposure and to explore whether Al accumulation can be decreased in AUD subjects.

Author Contributions: Conceptualization, C.G., R.M. and E.B.; methodology, E.B., J.P., P.R., P.N.; software, J.B., J.P.; validation, A.M., J.B.A., J.L. and A.P.; formal analysis, A.P.; investigation, A.M., J.B.A., J.P.; resources, E.B., J.P.; data curation, J.B.; writing—original draft preparation, C.G., P.R; writing—review and editing, P.R., A.P., J.L. and J.F.; visualization, A.M., J.L.; supervision, R.M., J.F. , P.N., P.R. and G.T.; project administration, R.M..; funding acquisition, E.B.

Funding: This research received no external funding.

Conflicts of Interest: The authors declare no conflict of interest.

References

1. Schlesinger, M.E. *Aluminum Recycling*; CRC Press: Boca Raton, FL, USA, 2013.
2. Exley, C. Human exposure to aluminium. *Environ. Sci. Process. Impacts* **2013**, *15*, 1807–1816. [CrossRef]
3. Exley, C. The toxicity of aluminium in humans. *Morphologie* **2016**, *100*, 51–55. [CrossRef] [PubMed]
4. Yuan, C.Y.; Lee, Y.J.; Hsu, G.S. Aluminum overload increases oxidative stress in four functional brain areas of neonatal rats. *J. Biomed. Sci.* **2012**, *19*, 51. [CrossRef]
5. Cheraghi, E.; Golkar, A.; Roshanaei, K.; Alani, B. Aluminium-induced oxidative stress, apoptosis and alterations in testicular tissue and sperm quality in Wistar rats: Ameliorative effects of curcumin. *Int. J. Fertil. Steril.* **2017**, *11*, 166–175.
6. Darbre, P.D.; Mannello, F.; Exley, C. Aluminium and breast cancer: Sources of exposure, tissue measurements and mechanisms of toxicological actions on breast biology. *J. Inorg. Biochem.* **2013**, *128*, 257–261. [CrossRef] [PubMed]
7. Gura, K.M. Aluminum contamination in products used in parenteral nutrition: Has anything changed? *Nutrition* **2010**, *26*, 585–594. [CrossRef]
8. Rosenlöf, K.; Fyhrquist, F.; Tenhunen, R. Erythropoietin, aluminium, and anaemia in patients on haemodialysis. *Lancet* **1990**, *335*, 247–249. [CrossRef]
9. Rondeau, V.; Commenges, D.; Jacqmin-Gadda, H.; Dartigues, J.-F. Relation between aluminum concentrations in drinking water and Alzheimer's disease: An 8-year follow-up study. *Am. J. Epidemiol.* **2000**, *152*, 59–66. [CrossRef]
10. Nakamura, H.; Rose, P.; Blumer, J.; Reed, M. Acute encephalopathy due to aluminum toxicity successfully treated by combined intravenous deferoxamine and hemodialysis. *J. Clin. Pharmacol.* **2000**, *40*, 296–300. [CrossRef] [PubMed]
11. Mold, M.; Chmielecka, A.; Rodriguez, M.R.R.; Thom, F.; Linhart, C.; King, A.; Exley, C. Aluminium in Brain Tissue in Multiple Sclerosis. *Int. J. Environ. Res. Public Health* **2018**, *15*, 1777. [CrossRef]
12. Walton, J.R. An aluminium-based rat model for Alzheimer disease exhibits oxidative damage, inhibition of PP2A activity, hyperphosphorylated tau and granulovascuolar degeneration. *J. Inorg. Biochem.* **2007**, *101*, 1275–1284. [CrossRef]
13. Ribes, D.; Colomina, M.T.; Vicens, P.; Domingo, J.L. Effects of oral aluminium exposure on behavior and neurogenesis in a transgenic mouse model of Alzheimer's disease. *Exp. Neurol.* **2008**, *214*, 293–300. [CrossRef]
14. Miu, A.C.; Andreescu, C.E.; Vasiu, R.; Oleanu, A.I. A behavioural and histological study of the effects of long-term exposure of adult rats to aluminium. *Int. J. Neurosci.* **2003**, *113*, 1197–1211. [CrossRef]
15. Jing, Y.; Wang, Z.; Song, Y. Quantitative study of aluminium-induced changes in synaptic ultrastructure in rats. *Synapse* **2004**, *52*, 292–298. [CrossRef]
16. Bakir, A.A.; Hryhorczuk, D.O.; Berman, E.; Dunea, G. Acute fatal hyperaluminemic encephalopathy in undialyzed and recently dialyzed uremic patients. *Trans Am. Soc. Artif. Intern. Organs* **1986**, *32*, 171–176.
17. Nayak, P. Aluminium: Impacts and disease. *Environ. Res.* **2002**, *89*, 101–115. [CrossRef]
18. Riihimäki, V.; Hänninen, H.; Akila, R.; Kovala, T.; Kuosma, E.; Paakkulainen, H.; Valkonen, S.; Engström, B. Body burden of aluminium in relation to central nervous system function among metal inert-gas welders. *Scand. J. Work Environ. Health* **2000**, *26*, 118–130. [CrossRef] [PubMed]
19. Giorgianni, C.; Faranda, M.; Brecciaroli, R.; Beninato, G.; Saffioti, G.; Muraca, G.; Congia, P.; Catanoso, R.; Agostani, G.; Abbate, C. Cognitive disorders among welders exposed to aluminium. *G. Ital. Med. Lav. Ergon.* **2003**, *25*, 102–103. [PubMed]
20. Hongve, D.; Johansen, D.; Andruchow, E.; Bjertness, E.; Becher, G.; Alexander, J. Determination of aluminium in samples from bone and liver of elderly Norwegians. *J. Trace Elem. Med. Biol.* **1996**, *10*, 6–11. [CrossRef]
21. Zioła-Frankowska, A.; Dąbrowski, M.; Kubaszewski, Ł.; Rogala, P.; Frankowski, M. Factors affecting the aluminium content of human femoral head and neck. *J. Inorg. Biochem.* **2015**, *152*, 167–173. [CrossRef] [PubMed]
22. Mold, M.; Umar, D.; King, A.; Exley, C. Aluminium in brain tissue in autism. *J. Trace Elem. Med. Biol.* **2018**, *46*, 76–82. [CrossRef]
23. Rzymski, P.; Niedzielski, P.; Rzymski, P.; Tomczyk, K.; Kozak, L.; Poniedziałek, B. Metal accumulation in the human uterus varies by pathology and smoking status. *Fertil. Steril.* **2016**, *105*, 1511–1518. [CrossRef]

24. Rzymski, P.; Niedzielski, P.; Poniedziałek, B.; Tomczyk, K.; Rzymski, P. Identification of toxic metals in human embryonic tissues. *Arch. Med. Sci.* **2018**, *14*, 415–421. [CrossRef]
25. Ogawa, M.; Kayama, F. A study of the association between urinary aluminum concentration and pre-clinical findings among aluminum-handling and non-handling workers. *J. Occup. Med. Toxicol.* **2015**, *10*, 13. [CrossRef] [PubMed]
26. Röllin, H.B.; Nogueira, C.; Olutola, B.; Channa, K.; Odland, J.Ø. Prenatal Exposure to Aluminum and Status of Selected Essential Trace Elements in Rural South African Women at Delivery. *Int. J. Environ. Res. Public Health* **2018**, *15*, 1494. [CrossRef] [PubMed]
27. Poniedziałek, B.; Rzymski, P.; Piet, M.; Gasecka, M.; Stroin' ska, A.; Niedzielski, P.; Mleczek, M.; Rzymski, P.; Wilczak, M. Relation between polyphenols, malondialdehyde, antioxidant capacity, lactate dehydrogenase and toxic elements in human colostrum milk. *Chemosphere* **2018**, *191*, 548–554. [CrossRef] [PubMed]
28. Klein, J.P.; Mold, M.; Mery, L.; Cottier, M.; Exley, C. Aluminum content of human semen: Implications for semen quality. *Reprod. Toxicol.* **2014**, *50*, 43–48. [CrossRef]
29. Rzymski, P.; Niedzielski, P.; Kaczmarek, N.; Jurczak, T.; Klimaszyk, P. The multidisciplinary approach to safety and toxicity assessment of microalgae-based food supplements following clinical cases of poisoning. *Harmful Algae* **2015**, *46*, 34–42. [CrossRef]
30. Rzymski, P.; Budzulak, J.; Niedzielski, P.; Klimaszyk, P.; Proch, J.; Kozak, L.; Poniedziałek, B. Essential and toxic elements in commercial microalgal food supplements. *J. Appl. Phycol.* **2018**. [CrossRef]
31. Zhang, H.; Tang, J.; Huang, L.; Shen, X.; Zhang, R.; Chen, J. Aluminium in food and daily dietary intake assessment from 15 food groups in Zhejiang Province, China. *Food Addit. Contam. Part B Surveill.* **2016**, *9*, 73–78. [CrossRef]
32. Yokel, R.A.; McNamara, P.J. Aluminium toxicokinetics: An updated minireview. *Pharmacol Toxicol.* **2001**, *88*, 159–167. [CrossRef]
33. Davis, W.M. Is aluminium an etiologic contributor to alcoholic amnesia and dementia? *Med. Hypotheses* **1993**, *41*, 341–343. [CrossRef]
34. Carlisle, E.M.; Curran, M.J. Effect of dietary silicon and aluminum on silicon and aluminum levels in rat brain. *Alzheimer Dis. Assoc. Disord.* **1987**, *1*, 83–89. [CrossRef] [PubMed]
35. Davenward, S.; Bentham, P.; Wright, J.; Crome, P.; Job, D.; Polwart, A.; Exley, C. Silicon-rich mineral water as a non-invasive test of the 'aluminum hypothesis' in Alzheimer's disease. *J. Alzheimers Dis.* **2013**, *33*, 423–430. [CrossRef] [PubMed]
36. Chaussidon, M.; Netter, P.; Kessler, M.; Membre, H.; Fener, P.; Delons, S.; Albarède, F. Dialysis-associated arthropathy: Secondary ion mass spectrometry evidence of aluminum silicate in β-microglobulin amyloid synovial tissue and articular cartilage. *Nephron* **1993**, *65*, 559–563. [CrossRef] [PubMed]
37. Muma, N.A.; Singer, S.M. Aluminum-induced neuropathology: Transient changes in microtubule-associated proteins. *Neurotoxicol. Teratol.* **1996**, *18*, 679–690. [CrossRef]
38. Murayama, H.; Shin, R.W.; Higuchi, J.; Shibuya, S.; Muramoto, T.; Kitamoto, T. Interaction of aluminum with PHFtau in Alzheimer's disease neurofibrillary degeneration evidenced by desferrioxamine-assisted chelating autoclave method. *Am. J. Pathol.* **1999**, *155*, 877–885. [CrossRef]
39. Uversky, V.N.; Fink, A.L. Metal-triggered structural transformations, aggregation, and fibrillation of human α-synuclein: A possible molecular link between parkinson's disease and heavy metal exposure. *J. Biol. Chem.* **2001**, *276*, 44284–44296. [CrossRef]
40. Khan, A.; Ashcroft, A.E.; Korchazhkina, O.V.; Exley, C. Metal-mediated formation of fibrillar ABri amyloid. *J. Inorg. Biochem.* **2004**, *98*, 2006–2010. [CrossRef]
41. Rodella, L.F.; Ricci, F.; Borsani, E.; Stacchiotti, A.; Foglio, E.; Favero, G.; Rezzani, R.; Mariani, C.; Bianchi1, R. Aluminium exposure induces Alzheimer's disease-like histopathological alterations in mouse brain. *Histol. Histopathol.* **2008**, *23*, 433–439.
42. Polizzi, S.; Pira, E.; Ferrara, M.; Bugiani, M.; Papaleo, A.; Albera, R.; Palmi, S. Neurotoxic effects of aluminium among foundry workers and Alzheimer's disease. *Neurotoxicology* **2002**, *23*, 761–774. [CrossRef]
43. Shafer, U.; Seifert, M. Oral intake of aluminum from foodstuffs, food additives, food packaging, cookware and pharmaceutical preparations with respect to dietary regulations. *Trace Elem. Electrolytes* **2006**, *23*, 150–161. [CrossRef]
44. Abou-Donia, M.B. Metals. In *Neurotoxicology*; CRC Press: Boca Raton, FL, USA, 1992; pp. 363–393.

45. Petrik, M.S.; Wong, M.C.; Tabata, R.C.; Garry, R.F.; Shaw, C.A. Aluminum adjuvant linked to Gulf War illness induces motor neuron death in mice. *Neuromol. Med.* **2007**, *9*, 83–100. [CrossRef]
46. Phan, K.L. Functional neuroanatomy of emotion: A meta-analysis of emotion activation studies in PET and fMRI. *Neuroimage* **2002**, *16*, 331–348. [CrossRef] [PubMed]
47. Floresco, S.B. The nucleus accumbens: An interface between cognition, emotion, and action. *Annu. Rev. Psychol.* **2015**, *66*, 25–52. [CrossRef]
48. Alfrey, A.C.; Legendre, G.R.; Kaehny, W.D. The dialysis encephalopathy syndrome—possible aluminium intoxication. *N. Engl. J. Med.* **1976**, *294*, 184–188. [CrossRef] [PubMed]
49. Bouras, C.; Giannakopoulos, P.; Good, P.F.; Hsu, A.; Hof, P.R.; Perl, D.P. A laser microprobe mass analysis of trace elements in brain mineralizations and capillaries in Fahr's disease. *Acta Neuropathol.* **1996**, *92*, 351–357. [CrossRef]
50. McLachlan, D.R.C.; Bergeron, C.; Smith, J.E.; Boomer, D.; Rifat, S.L. Risk for neuropathologically confirmed Alzheimer's disease and residual aluminum in municipal drinking water employing weighted residential histories. *Neurology* **1996**, *46*, 401–405. [CrossRef]
51. Rondeau, V.; Jacqmin-Gadda, H.; Commenges, D.; Helmer, C.; Dartigues, J.F. Aluminum and silica in drinking water and the risk of Alzheimer's disease or cognitive decline: Findings from 15-year follow-up of the PAQUID cohort. *Am. J. Epidemiol.* **2009**, *169*, 489–496. [CrossRef]
52. Flaten, T.P. Aluminium as a risk factor in Alzheimer's disease, with emphasis on drinking water. *Brain Res. Bull.* **2001**, *55*, 187–196. [CrossRef]
53. Varga, Z.; Matyas, C.; Paloczi, J.; Pacher, P. Alcohol Misuse, and Kidney Injury: Epidemiological Evidenc and Potential Mechanisms. *Alcohol Res. Curr. Rev.* **2017**, *38*, 283–288.
54. Lopez, F.F.; Cabrera, C.; Luisa Lorenzo, M.; Carmen Lopez, M. Aluminium levels in wine, beer and other alcoholic beverages consumed in Spain. *Sci. Total Environ.* **1998**, *220*, 1–9. [CrossRef]
55. Pennington, J.A.T.; Jones, J.W. *Aluminium in Health: A Critical Review*; Fitelman, H.J., Ed.; CRC Press: Boca Raton, FL, USA, 1989.
56. Minoia, C.; Sabbioni, E.; Ronchi, A.; Gatti, A. Trace element reference values in tissues from inhabitans of the Euro- pean community influence of dietary factors. *Sci. Total Environ.* **1994**, *141*, 181–195. [CrossRef]
57. Exley, C.; Chappell, J.S.; Birchall, J.D. A mechanism for acute aluminium toxicity in fish. *J. Theor. Biol.* **1991**, *151*, 417–428. [CrossRef]
58. Schlatter, C.; Steinegger, A.F. Messung der Aluminiumexposition an Arbeitsplatzen in der Aluminiumprimarindustrie. *Erzmetall* **1991**, *44*, 326–331.
59. Chadwick, D.J.; Whelan, J. *Aluminium in Biology and Medicine*; Wiley: Hoboken, NJ, USA, 2008; pp. 58–59, ISBN 978-0-470-51431-3.
60. Desouky, M.; Jugdaohsingh, R.; McCrohan, C.R.; White, K.N.; Powell, J.J. Aluminium-dependent regulation of intracellular silicon in the aquatic invertebrate Lymnaea stagnalis. *Proc. Natl. Acad. Sci. USA* **2002**, *99*, 3394–3399. [CrossRef]
61. Edwardson, J.A.; Moore, P.B.; Ferrier, I.N.; Lilley, J.S.; Newton, G.W.A.; Barker, J.; Templar, J.; Day, J.P. Effect of silicon on gastrointestinal absorption of aluminium. *Lancet* **1993**, *342*, 211–212. [CrossRef]
62. White, K.N.; Ejim, A.I.; Walton, R.C.; Brown, A.P.; Jugdaohsingh, R.; Powell, J.J.; McCrohan, C.R. Avoidance of aluminum toxicity in freshwater snails involves intracellular silicon-aluminum biointeraction. *Environ. Sci. Technol.* **2008**, *42*, 2189–2194. [CrossRef]
63. Casey, T.R.; Bamforth, C.W. Silicon in beer and brewing. *J. Sci. Food Agric.* **2010**, *90*, 784–788. [CrossRef]

Sample Availability: Not Available.

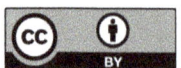

© 2019 by the authors. Licensee MDPI, Basel, Switzerland. This article is an open access article distributed under the terms and conditions of the Creative Commons Attribution (CC BY) license (http://creativecommons.org/licenses/by/4.0/).

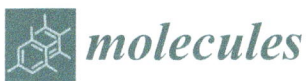

Article

Analysis of Hazardous Elements in Children Toys: Multi-Elemental Determination by Chromatography and Spectrometry Methods

Katarzyna Karaś and Marcin Frankowski *

Department of Water and Soil Analysis, Faculty of Chemistry, Adam Mickiewicz University in Poznań, Umultowska 89 b, 61-614 Poznań, Poland; katarzyna.karas@amu.edu.pl
* Correspondence: marcin.frankowski@amu.edu.pl

Received: 23 October 2018; Accepted: 15 November 2018; Published: 19 November 2018

Abstract: This paper presents the results of determination of hazardous metal (Cd, Cu, Cr, Hg, Mn, Ni, Pb, Zn) and metalloid (As, Sb) levels in toys available in the Polish market. Two independent sample preparation methods were used to determine the concentration and content of the metals and metalloids. The first one is defined by the guidelines of the EN-71 standard and undertook extraction in 0.07 mol/L HCl. This method was used to conduct speciation analysis of Cr(III) and Cr(VI), as well as for the determination of selected metals and metalloids. The second method conducted mineralization in a HNO_3 and H_2O_2 mixture using microwave energy to determine the content of metals and metalloids. Determination of chromium forms was made using the high-performance liquid chromatography inductively coupled plasma mass spectrometry (HPLC-ICP-MS) method, while those of metals and metalloids were made using the ICP-MS technique. Additionally, in order to determine total content of chromium in toys, an energy dispersive X-ray fluorescence spectrometer (EDX) was used. The results of the analyses showed that Cr(VI) was not detected in the toys. In general, the content of heavy metals and metalloids in the studied samples was below the migration limit set by the norm EN-71.

Keywords: chromium speciation; hazardous elements; toys safety; migration; ICP-MS

1. Introduction

The amount of heavy metals in the environment is still increasing mainly due to anthropogenic activities that include industrial processes, power engineering, communication development, and the use of fertilizers and pesticides [1]. News about contamination of heavy metals in toy materials continues to be alarming. Some of them like arsenic (As), chromium (Cr), mercury (Hg), lead (Pb), selenium (Se), and zinc (Zn) are commonly used as coloring agents and catalysts to provide desired softness, brightness, and flexibility [2–6]. The maximum levels of metal contamination should be strictly regulated and kept at the lowest level that are technically feasible or are of no toxicological concern because of the toxicity and effects of bioaccumulation. It causes a variety of diseases, disorders, impairments, and organ malfunctions. This is important especially for children because they are considered more susceptible to hazardous metal substances compared to adults; they have higher basal metabolic rates, higher comparative uptakes of food, and lower toxins elimination rates. Moreover, children's organs or tissues are developing, and thus, more sensitive to perturbed cellular processes [7–9]. Children typically spend a large amount of time playing with toys; toxic chemicals can be transferred from contaminated surfaces or soil to the hand and then ingested via hand-to-mouth activity. Threat of ingestion is common with children especially during the oral stage, which spans from birth until the age of 6 [10–13]. For children less than six years old, object mouthing is a common behavior and mouthing frequency and duration are especially high for infants (6–12 months) and toddlers (1–3 years). The knowledge of the total metal concentration in a solid sample is not sufficient to predict metal reactivity and effects on human health; indeed, metals can be present in various forms with different chemical properties and consequently different potential toxicity for humans [14]. One of the important elements is chromium, which has various oxidation states from II to VI [15]. Each of the forms presents different chemical properties and toxicity. The two most widespread forms of chromium in the environment are Cr(III) and Cr(VI). The intermediate states Cr(II), Cr(IV), and Cr(V) are unstable products in oxidation and reduction reactions of trivalent and hexavalent chromium, respectively. In various physiochemical processes, the different forms of chromium might undergo specific transformations, changing from one into another [16]. The inorganic trivalent form of chromium (Cr(III)) is relatively nontoxic and is an essential element in mammalian diets, especially in human beings [17,18]. It is a necessary microelement, which is involved in carbohydrate, lipid, and protein metabolism. By contrast, at the cellular level, hexavalent chromium (Cr(VI)) is a highly active carcinogen [19,20]. It can penetrate biological membranes and is recognized as a toxic substance. The ability to diffuse through the cell membranes is possible due to structural similarity of CrO_4^{2-} ion to anions as SO_4^{2-} or PO_4^{3-}, which are transported by their respective ion exchange channels [16,21]. Cr(VI) could reduce the amount of mitochondrial DNA (mtDNA) and inhibit mitochondrial electron transport chain complex I, resulting in perturbation of mitochondrial respiration and redox homeostasis. Human oral exposure to Cr(VI) produces hepatotoxicity and there is evidence that Cr(VI) accumulation occurs by oral exposure route mostly in the liver, which is the largest detoxification organ. Moreover, Cr(VI) may cause primary liver cancer and increase the risk of deterioration of cancer patients [7]. In Europe, toys must meet the criteria and requirements set by the European Commission Toys Safety Directive to carry the CE (Conformité Européenne) mark. All European Union member states have transposed this directive into law. The presence of Cr(VI) in toys sold in the European Union (EU) is strictly limited by the Toy Safety Directive (2009/48/EC) which ensures the safety of children by minimizing their exposure to potentially hazardous or toxic toy products, bearing in mind the young children's tendency to mouth objects [22–25]. Part 3 of the standard—EN71-3+A1:2014-12—entitled "Migration of certain elements" subsequently outlines the migration limits of 18 elements from various categories of toy products, to enable the testing of toys for its compliance with legal provisions [24–27]. Toy materials are divided into three categories:

I: Dry, brittle powder-like or pliable materials;
II: Liquid or sticky materials;
III: Coatings and scraped-off materials.

Chromium has separate migration limits for Cr(III) and Cr(VI), which are 9.4 and 0.005 mg/kg, respectively [23]. Different analytical systems have been used for speciation analysis. The first group consists of methods requiring pretreatment, which are UV–visible spectrophotometry, atomic absorption spectrometry (AAS), inductively coupled plasma optical emission spectrometry (ICP-OES), and inductively coupled plasma mass spectrometry (ICP-MS). The other methods consists of hyphenated techniques such as flow injection analyzer (FIA), coupling of liquid chromatography with inductively coupled plasma mass spectrometry (LC-ICP-MS) with different separation modes, and capillary electrophoresis (CE). The second group involves solid techniques such as X-ray photoelectron spectroscopy (XPS), X-ray absorption near-edge spectroscopy (XANES), X-ray diffraction (XRD), and low-energy-electron-induced X-ray spectroscopy (LLEIXS) [15]. As the chromium species content in such samples is rather low, the coupling of liquid chromatography with inductively coupled plasma mass spectrometry (HPLC–ICP-MS) is a most often used technique, which is based on the combination of a separation method with an element-selective detection system [28]. Anion exchange columns and columns, which have both anion and cation exchange capabilities, are especially used for chromium speciation analysis [29]. High Performance Liquid Chromatography Inductively Coupled Plasma Mass Spectrometry (HPLC-ICP-MS) is often used in analyses of different environmental matrices such as natural water, soils, sediments, etc. [30]. In this study, for the first time, this technique was used to analyze samples of toys. The choice of this method is also justified by the fact that the ICP-MS analytical technique is one of the most sensitive and robust techniques, which offers pronounced advantages for its elemental specificity, wide linear dynamic range, and significantly low detection limits [31]. This method is also one of the most powerful analytical techniques for the collection of elemental information, offering LODs in the low- to sub-ng/L range for most elements. A wide linear dynamic range, multielement capabilities, survivable spectra, and the possibility of high sample throughput further characterizes this technique [30].

The objectives of this study are: (1) application of energy dispersive X-ray fluorescence spectrometry to determine the total content of chromium in toys; (2) development of a method for speciation analysis of chromium (III and VI) in toys; (3) determination of chromium, metals (Cd, Cu, Hg, Mn, Ni, Pb, Zn), and metalloids (As, Sb) by ICP-MS in HCl extracts and after microwave-assisted mineralization in HNO_3/H_2O_2 mixture; and (4) assess the safety of toys particularly intended for younger children based on the requirements contained in EN71-3 norm Part 3: Migration of certain elements.

2. Results and Discussion

2.1. Application of Energy Dispersive X-ray Fluorescence Spectrometry to Determine Total Content of Chromium in Toys

Despite the use of nondestructive methods that did not require any sample preparation and measuring the toy material in different places and pieces several times, the results from the analysis showed that chromium was not detected in any toy material in mg/kg levels. But the fact that the chromium content was not found at such a level does not mean that it does not exist at all. The need to confirm this assumption was the starting point for the speciation analysis of chromium.

2.2. Method Development for Speciation Analysis of Chromium

A series of standard solutions containing 5, 10, 20, 50, and 100 ng/L Cr(VI), and 10 times higher concentrations of Cr(III) were prepared. The Cr species were completely resolved on anion exchange Hamilton PRPX-100 250 mm × 4.1 mm (10 μm) column with retention times of 6.1 min for Cr(III) and 9.1 min for Cr(VI). Because of the column length and extended retention time, a different Bio WAX nonporous 50 mm × 4.6 mm (5 μm) column was used. The Cr species were completely resolved with retention times of 0.97 min for Cr(III) and 1.98 min for Cr(VI). For both methods, good separation of standard solutions and of Cr(III) and Cr(VI) was obtained. Figure 1a,b presents the overlaid chromatograms for HPLC-ICP-MS.

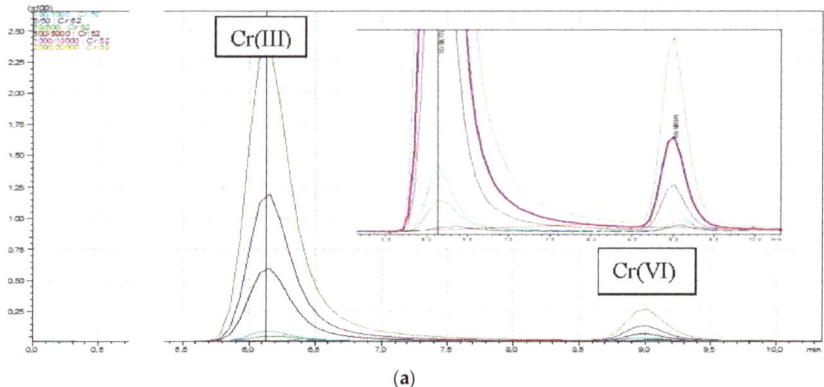

(a)

Figure 1. *Cont.*

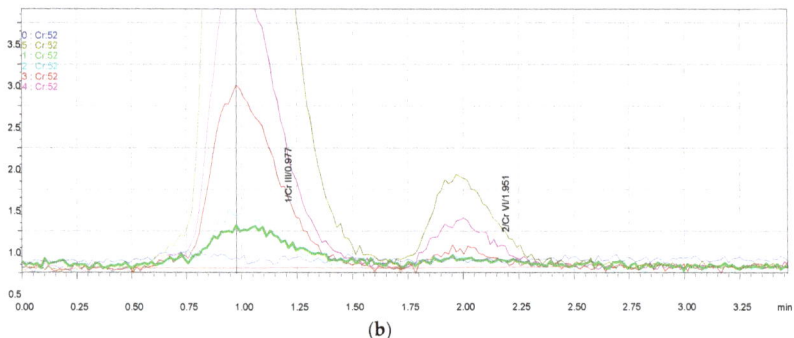

Figure 1. (a) Overlaid chromatograms for HPLC-ICP-MS with the use of Hamilton PRPX-100 analytical column. (b) Overlaid chromatograms for HPLC-ICP-MS with the use of Bio Wax analytical column.

Because of their shorter retention times for chromium, the Bio WAX column was selected for testing real samples. The LOD values for Cr(III) were equal to 1.3 ng/g in solid sample and 2.6 ng/L in solution, and for Cr(VI), 0.7 ng/g in solid sample and 1.4 ng/L in solution. However, in order to avoid tailing the peak connected with the higher concentration of Cr(III) in toys, higher concentrations of mix standard solutions containing: 10,000 ng/L Cr(III) and 1000 ng/L Cr(VI) were prepared and analyzed. In order to maintain high concentrations of Cr(III), high concentrations of Cr(VI) were also maintained, therefore peak resolution was satisfied.

2.3. Method Application for Toys' Analysis

The newly developed method was applied to determine the concentration of Cr(III and VI) in toy samples collected from several shops in Poznań city (Poland). Table 1 shows the results for samples divided into individual colors and classified to two categories: cheap and expensive.

Table 1. Concentrations values of chromium(III) for particular samples.

Sample	Black	Blue	Brown	Green	Metal	Orange	Pink	Red	Transparent	Violet	White	Yellow
						cheap toys < 5 €						
4	A	227.0 ± 3.8	A	A	A	A	A	A	A	A	A	A
7	A	A	A	357.5 ± 5.2	A	A	211.0 ± 3.1	A	145.0 ± 2.1	A	A	258.0 ± 4.4
8	A	A	A	A	A	A	A	A	A	A	A	A
9	A	A	A	315.5 ± 4.9	A	A	A	A	A	A	A	A
12	A	A	A	542.0 ± 10.6	A	261.0 ± 5.0	A	375.5 ± 8.1	A	A	A	585.0 ± 12.0
15	A	A	A	A	A	A	A	A	A	A	A	296.5 ± 7.2
16	A	A	A	510.5 ± 14.7	A	A	A	A	A	A	A	554.0 ± 13.5
17	A	A	A	A	A	A	A	A	A	A	A	84.5 ± 1.2
18	A	A	A	A	A	A	A	260.0 ± 6.8	A	A	A	A
19	A	A	A	A	A	A	A	A	A	A	291.5 ± 8.7	220.0 ± 4.1
20	A	A	A	2317 ± 60	A	A	A	A	A	A	A	A
24	A	131.0 ± 1.4	A	A	A	A	A	294.5 ± 5.5	A	A	A	584.0 ± 9.9
25	A	A	A	A	A	A	A	221.0 ± 1.9	A	108.5 ± 2.0	A	239.1 ± 5.4
26	A	A	A	A	A	285.0 ± 6.0	A	A	A	A	A	81 ± 1.1
27	A	127.5 ± 2.5	A	73.5 ± 1.3	A	A	A	56.2 ± 0.9	115.5 ± 2.0	A	A	151.5 ± d2.6
29	A	A	A	A	A	199.5 ± 2.5	140.5 ± 2.2	A	A	A	A	A
30	A	361.5 ± 7.0	A	A	A	A	A	127.5 ± 3.1	A	A	A	48.5 ± 1.0
32	A	124.5 ± 1.1	A	218.5 ± 4.7	A	A	A	A	282.3 ± 5.6	A	52.9 ± 0.9	A
1	A	A	A	A	A	A	A	A	A	A	A	A
2	A	A	A	A	A	A	A	A	A	A	A	A
5	A	109.6 ± 1.9	A	A	A	168.8 ± 2.7	A	A	A	A	A	A
7	A	A	A	A	A	A	118.5 ± 1.7	A	A	A	A	A
8	A	A	A	A	A	A	142.6 ± 2.6	A	A	A	A	A
10	A	A	A	A	A	A	A	A	102.4 ± 2.0	A	A	A
11	A	595.4 ± 10.2	A	A	A	A	A	A	A	A	A	A
13	A	A	A	A	A	A	153.9 ± 2.2	A	A	A	A	A
15	8025 ± 177	71.7 ± 1.2	65.5 ± 1.2	A	A	A	A	A	A	A	A	116.4 ± 1.8
17a	70.5 ± 1.4	145.5 ± 3.1	A	795.5 ± 15.9	A	A	A	A	A	A	A	39.1 ± 0.8
18a	A	A	A	A	312.3 ± 8.1	A	A	237.4 ± 4.4	A	A	A	80.9 ± 1.6
19	A	A	A	106.2 ± 2.4	A	A	A	A	A	A	A	130.5 ± 2.9
20	A	A	A	A	A	A	A	A	A	A	188.2 ± 3.8	A
21	A	197.6 ± 2.1	A	A	A	A	A	A	A	A	A	A
22a	A	A	A	A	A	A	87.6 ± 2.1	A	A	A	A	1096 ± 25.4

Table 1. Cont.

Sample	Cr(III) [ng/g]											
	Black	Blue	Brown	Green	Metal	Orange	Pink	Red	Transparent	Violet	White	Yellow
						expensive toys > 5 €						
1	A	245.0 ± 5.0	A	A	A	A	381.0 ± 9.0	A	A	265.5 ± 6.3	A	A
2	A	A	A	342.0 ± 6.8	A	A	A	A	A	A	A	A
3	A	209.0 ± 4.2	A	A	A	A	A	A	A	A	A	A
5	A	A	A	A	A	A	A	A	A	A	245.0 ± 4.7	A
6	A	A	A	203.5 ± 5.0	A	A	A	A	A	A	A	A
10	A	A	152.0 ± 3.1	A	A	A	A	A	A	A	A	397.0 ± 9.4
11	A	A	A	A	A	A	173.5 ± 3.5	A	A	A	A	A
13	A	A	A	A	A	A	710.0 ± 18.2	A	A	A	A	A
14	A	266.5 ± 6.8	A	A	A	-	A	A	A	A	A	A
21	A	A	A	A	A	-	A	421.0 ± 10.2	A	A	A	A
22	A	A	A	A	A	-	A	A	A	A	443.0 ± 9.4	A
23	A	A	A	349.0 ± 5.1	A	A	A	A	A	A	A	A
28	A	A	A	A	4168 ± 985	248.5 ± 5.1	A	A	154.5 ± 2.0	A	A	A
31	A	96.5 ± 1.1	A	48.5 ± 0.8	A	A	A	A	A	A	A	A
33	A	194.8 ± 1.9	A	A	A	203.7 ± 4.0	A	A	A	A	A	A
3	A	A	A	A	A	A	A	154.0 ± 2.0	A	A	A	A
6	A	A	A	A	A	A	A	A	126.0 ± 1.9	A	A	A
9	A	A	A	A	A	A	A	A	A	A	A	137.9 ± 2.4
12	59.8 ± 1.1	A	A	124.7 ± 2.9	A	A	397.2 ± 8.0	A	A	A	A	A
14	A	A	A	664.5 ± 11.3	A	A	A	51.35 ± 0.9	A	A	116.4 ± 2.0	365.5 ± 8.1
16	A	A	A	A	A	A	A	A	A	A	A	68.81 ± 1.4
Average value	310.9 ± 59.8	206.9 ± 3.7	108.8 ± 2.2	464.6 ± 10.1	2240.2 ± 494.5	227.8 ± 2.55	251.6 ± 5.26	219.8 ± 2.43	154.3 ± 2.6	187 ± 3.65	222.8 ± 4.42	276.7 ± 1.56

A - absent color in the toy.

Concentration of Cr(VI) was under LOD in each analyzed samples. This is probably because in case of toys samples, as solid samples, the extraction process was applied. The acid used in the analysis was diluted 0.07 mol/L hydrochloric acid, and this concentration was in line with the requirements of the EN-71 norm. Such a low concentration was aimed simulating natural conditions, which could occur if a child swallowed part of a toy. This low concentration of HCl was too low to extract the analyzed form of chromium, which could have been retained in the toy material. Among the collected samples, the least numbers were brown and violet—two samples each. The average concentration of chromium(III) in brown samples was 108.8 ng/g and 187.0 ng/g in violet samples. Also, a small group was made up of metallic samples in which the concentration of trivalent form of chromium was significantly higher as expected than in other samples, and simultaneously was the one which exceeded migration limits observed in the whole analysis. The average concentration of chromium(III) in metallic samples was 2240 ng/g. One group of the collected samples were blue—15 samples, green—15 samples, and yellow—20 samples. The average concentration of this form of chromium was 206.9 ng/g in blue samples, 464.6 ng/g in green samples, and 276.7 in yellow samples. The maximum concentration of chromium(III) was observed in green sample and was equal to 2317 ng/g and in yellow samples was equal 1096 ng/g. The minimum concentration of chromium(III) was noticed in yellow samples and equaled 39.1 ng/g. Another group of samples consisted of ten samples each of pink and red. The average value of concentration of the detected form of chromium was 251.6 ng/g for pink samples and 219.8 ng/g for red samples. The minimum concentration of trivalent form of chromium was 87.6 ng/g in pink samples and 51.4 ng/g in red samples. However, the maximum was 397.2 ng/g in pink samples and 375.5 in red samples. The next group were orange, transparent, and white samples—six samples each. The average concentration of chromium(III) was 227.8 ng/g in orange samples, 154.3 ng/g in transparent samples, and 222.8 ng/g in white samples. The minimum concentration of chromium(III) in orange samples was 199.5 ng/g, in transparent samples was 102.4 ng/g, and in white samples was 52.9 ng/g. The maximum was 285 ng/g in orange samples, 282.3 ng/g in transparent samples, and 443 ng/g in white samples. Higher concentrations of chromium(III) were observed in black, green, and yellow parts of the toys, which can be connected with the pigments and paints usually used in toy production processes.

2.4. Determination of Chromium, Metals, and Metalloid Concentrations in HCl Extracts by ICP-MS

In order to compare the results from speciation analysis, the concentration of chromium in the extracts was measured by ICP-MS. The obtained results between both of the methods were comparable and the differences between the results were under 5%, which indicates the correctness of the results. High concentrations of chromium were noted for black, green, and yellow samples, the same as in speciation analysis. Reviewing the data obtained by analysis of HCl extracts, which are presented in Table 2, it may be stated that the higher concentration of element in black, brown, green, red, transparent, white, yellow, and metallic samples was noted for zinc.

Table 2. Average concentration of metals and metalloids in various colors of toys in HCl extracts.

	As ng/g	Cd ng/g	Cr ng/g	Cu ng/g	Hg ng/g	Mn ng/g	Ni ng/g	Pb ng/g	Sb ng/g	Zn ng/g
Black	32.75 ± 167	1.8 ± 65	281.2 ± 163.9	44.8 ± 5161	4.133 ± 3.6	39.67 ± 182	163 ± 54.5	9.3 ± 815	46.32 ± 63.7	461.7 ± 309.5
Blue	10.8 ± 27.8	12.34 ± 51.5	213.3 ± 126.5	1163 ± 9150	0.944 ± 4.8	94.9 ± 153.5	14.5 ± 421.6	49.17 ± 699.3	43.66 ± 18.4	397.2 ± 328.4
Brown	7.6 ± 13.4	1.8 ± 70	104 ± 146	44.8 ± 538.9	3.15 ± 9.77	65.33 ± 135	14.5 ± 23.5	9.3 ± 464.1	21.48 ± 4.55	938.9 ± 385.5
Green	10.3 ± 90.5	24.74 ± 275	477.9 ± 194	864.7 ± 2900	0.838 ± 4.35	364.6 ± 1071	14.5 ± 411.7	138.1 ± 338.2	193.7 ± 583	3066 ± 8491
Orange	21 ± 103.6	22.1 ± 56	218.1 ± 115.5	1570 ± 3850	1.32 ± 2.35	337.8 ± 154.2	421.5 ± 171.1	168.7 ± 500	37.02 ± 30.05	387.2 ± 477.6
Pink	76.9 ± 1205	2.9 ± 54.5	245 ± 184	90 ± 313.9	5.115 ± 4.7	288 ± 1236	1024 ± 424.8	9.3 ± 430	28.05 ± 28.1	397.2 ± 423.5
Red	31.3 ± 321.4	14.85 ± 94	230.5 ± 209	760 ± 211.7	0.955 ± 2.75	46.73 ± 594	443.6 ± 255.5	104.7 ± 645	243.6 ± 455.5	1746 ± 885.4
Transparent	13.9 ± 41.98	29.1 ± 126	158.8 ± 185	1058 ± 2368	1.675 ± 3.23	501.8 ± 1804	402.4 ± 721.6	61.67 ± 430	35.95 ± 22.3	2548 ± 1542
Violet	26.9 ± 53.5	16.25 ± 57.5	197.5 ± 145	776 ± 65.5	2.15 ± 3.4	6.3 ± 70.5	14.5 ± 103.4	91.67 ± 440	91.03 ± 140	392.7 ± 76
White	8 ± 20.4	1.8 ± 55	233.1 ± 136	216.7 ± 606.1	0.259 ± 0.15	38.83 ± 189	14.5 ± 298	9.3 ± 435	184 ± 184.6	743.8 ± 617
Yellow	12.3 ± 26.1	1.289 ± 142.5	289.5 ± 142.5	276.3 ± 4224	0.782 ± 5.8	22.36 ± 224.5	355.8 ± 398.4	5.614 ± 460	54.23 ± 49.7	1443 ± 974
					µg/g					
Metallic	0.298 ± 0.296	0.282 ± 2.95	9.175 ± 0.194	7.35 ± 3.3	0.055 ± 0.001	119.6 ± 257.5	150.5 ± 25.39	1.622 ± 0.455	0.279 ± 0.001	902.7 ± 7.009

The higher value of concentration of zinc was observed in green samples and was equal to 3066 ng/g. For blue and violet samples, the higher concentration was noted for copper and was equal to 1163 ng/g for blue color and 776 ng/g for violet color. For the last group of samples, orange and pink, the higher concentration was observed for nickel, which was equal to 421.5 ng/g for orange samples and 1024 ng/g for pink samples.

2.5. Determination of Chromium, Metals, and Metalloids Concentrations in HCl Extracts by ICP-MS Versus Total Content after Mineralization in HNO_3/H_2O_2 Mixture

To complete the research, the determination of total content of chromium, metals (Cd, Cu, Hg, Mn, Ni, Pb, Zn), and metalloids (As, Sb) after microwave-assisted mineralization in HNO_3/H_2O_2 mixture were made. The obtained values of concentration, which are much higher than that of HCl extracts, are related to the much greater elution strength of the HNO_3/H_2O_2 mixture compared to the migration solution used in the procedure described in the EN-71 standard involving the use of HCl. This would mean that the metals and metalloids, which are contained in the toy material, are deeply bonded with this material and do not pass into the diluted HCl environment after swallowing the piece of the toy. These elements can be washed out only after using a stronger reagent such as a mixture of HNO_3/H_2O_2. Differences in efficiency of extraction of the metals and metalloids were dependent on some factors like the type of metal, color of sample, and variety of toy material. Based on this result, it may be stated that the degree of metal washing out of the toy material using dilute 0.07 mol/L HCl was the highest for As, Cd, and Cu in pink samples; Cr, Hg, and Ni in black samples; Mn and Sb in red samples; Pb in brown samples; and Zn in violet samples. While these results after mineralization process indicate that the degree of metal washing out of the toy material was the highest for As, Cd, Cr, Ni, and Pb for metallic samples; Cu in blue samples; Hg in pink and white samples; Mn in metallic and black samples; Sb in metallic and blue samples, and Zn in brown samples. Procedures using a mixture of HNO_3/H_2O_2 allowed determination of total content of chosen metals and metalloids. The obtained average content of elements in various colors of toys after ICP-MS analysis are presented in Table 3.

Table 3. Average content of metals and metalloids after mineralization in HNO_3/H_2O_2.

	As ng/g	Cd ng/g	Cr ng/g	Hg ng/g	Mn ng/g	Ni ng/g	Pb ng/g	Sb ng/g	Zn µg/g	Cu µg/g
black	67.5 ± 105	345.4 ± 65	311.1 ± 116.5	28.2 ± 3.6	541.5 ± 1261	163.0 ± 54.5	2816 ± 3025	2838 ± 846.9	6.718 ± 18.98	3.862 ± 5.092
blue	151.9 ± 427.5	115.3 ± 51.5	359.1 ± 318.5	48.2 ± 51.6	816.4 ± 875.3	394.3 ± 2087	479.2 ± 435	218.4 ± 422.2	13.45 ± 1.851	181.7 ± 18.76
brown	32.5 ± 36	56.5 ± 70	823.1 ± 1438	40.8 ± 17.2	1966 ± 3634	1806 ± 2124	449.6 ± 1193	161.9 ± 283.2	19.52 ± 2.458	0.971 ± 5.389
green	135.3 ± 134.5	127.7 ± 275	552.8 ± 1204	68.8 ± 104.7	728.5 ± 996.8	390.3 ± 618.1	724.9 ± 1455	3806 ± 981.9	32.39 ± 65.35	15.93 ± 29.25
orange	187.7 ± 154.1	125.1 ± 56	485.8 ± 696.9	47.9 ± 60.8	231 ± 557.5	421.5 ± 932.8	511.7 ± 500	198.1 ± 305.7	29.34 ± 54.37	17.89 ± 3.096
pink	105 ± 125	105.9 ± 54.5	461.2 ± 862.8	412.5 ± 26.31	2780 ± 111.1	1024 ± 734.41	690.8 ± 430	300.4 ± 1477	23.01 ± 42.66	6.767 ± 2.4
red	229.8 ± 311.5	117.9 ± 94	357.7 ± 469.2	49.2 ± 86.8	214.3 ± 17.3	443.6 ± 200	488.2 ± 645	243.6 ± 180.4	40.80 ± 48.37	1.424 ± 2.65
transparent	169.9 ± 183.5	156.5 ± 126	451.3 ± 767.5	91.9 ± 77.9	944.7 ± 382.5	402.4 ± 1175	552.9 ± 430	185.1 ± 22.3	7.185 ± 7.787	5.307 ± 2.5
violet	226 ± 340	119.3 ± 57.5	429.2 ± 64.8	57.1 ± 56.7	170.9 ± 163.1	322.9 ± 241.1	722.8 ± 440	426.9 ± 140	0.393 ± 0.01	0.340 ± 2.45
white	31.12 ± 83.5	101.8 ± 55	422.6 ± 367.9	35.3 ± 13.3	371.3 ± 601.7	508.8 ± 992.7	560.2 ± 435	184.0 ± 184.6	28.78 ± 11.36	0.615 ± 2.35
yellow	140.6 ± 591.4	104.3 ± 56.5	479.7 ± 839.3	36.7 ± 19.2	228.6 ± 465	355.8 ± 529.8	508.0 ± 460	185.7 ± 409.7	46.21 ± 66.85	1.946 ± 2.5
					mg/g					
metallic	4.729 ± 9.25	0.002 ± 0.003	0.102 ± 0.124	0.002 ± 0.002	96.79 ± 189.9	919.7 ± 1837	0.452 ± 0.0003	0.004 ± 0.04	3.725 ± 1.542	0.037 ± 0.173

The obtained results are very similar to HCl extracts, the highest content of was very much present in the parts of toys made from metallic materials. The highest obtained values relate to As, Mn, and also Ni. In the case of chromium, the higher content was observed in green and yellow parts of the toys, also similar to speciation and HCl extract analyses. The highest concentrations of zinc were noted for black, brown, green, orange, pink, red, transparent, white, and yellow samples. The highest concentration was observed in yellow samples and was equal to 46.21 ng/g (excluding metallic samples). Higher concentration of copper was noted in blue samples, similar to HCl extract analysis. In violet samples, the higher concentration was noted for lead and was equal 722.8 ng/g. Presence of metals like Cr, Cd, Mn, Pb, and Zn in toy material may be due to pigments or coloring agents, which are usually added to toy materials during the production process. In addition, Mn is usually used as main additives in paints and Pb as stabilizer to improve material properties and reduce cost on plastic. Both Cd and Hg are also used as a stabilizing factor for PVC materials. Chromium is an important dye used in PVC materials and as a heat stabilizer [32]. As mentioned, the higher content of chromium was noted in black parts of toys. Black spinel-type chromium-nickel pigment is inert with respect to alkali and acids and has good mechanical strength [33]. Higher content of chromium was found also in yellow parts of the toys, which can be associated with yellow paints containing common pigment, e.g., lead chromate [8]. Synthetically produced chrome is using in paints and as material: vinyl, rubber, and paper. Higher content of chromium was noted also in green parts of the toys. Green chromium(III) oxide is commonly used in the paint industry. In particular, it is used to color paints, plastic, construction materials, refractories enamels, etc. [34]. Results obtained are similar to previous reports employing other analytical techniques such as ICP-OES and ED-XRF; XRF was used to determine migration limits of elements from different parts of the toy. Concentration of elements in plastic parts of the toys was below the specified limits stated in the European Union Toy Safety Directive [4,10]. Similar to studies on toy jewelry, metallic parts of the toys are more problematic than other materials [12,13]. In particular, special attention should be payed to the risk for children due to possible exceedance of migration limits. Similar to research conducted by high definition X-ray fluorescence techniques, in most of the samples of this study high amounts of Zn and Cu and other elements such as As, Cr, Mn, and Ni in smaller quantities were detected [2,6]. The smallest quantity was observed for Hg in a previous study, which investigated heavy metal concentrations in toys purchased from the Palestinian Market. This can be associated with the usage of mercury as a catalyst in specific chemical reactions during plastic manufacturing in China [2]. Compared to previous legislation on potentially harmful chemicals in children's products, the migration limits of elements are significantly lower [27,35]. Possible exceedances usually refer to cadmium and lead-like factors commonly used as a stabilizer to prevent creating free chlorine radicals in materials made of PVC and also to reduce the cost of plastic [6,8,36]. The differences in metal and metalloid content in different toys and its parts are related with specificity of their compositions and differences in manufacturing processes [9]. Compared to similar speciation analysis of chromium conducted on dairy and cereal food samples, the results agree with those of this study. Trivalent chromium in yogurt and cheese samples ranges approximately from <13 to 255 ng/g. Most studies suggested the absence of hexavalent chromium in food samples like dairy and cereal products [37], chocolates, beverages, vegetables, fruits, eggs, meat and sea products [38], and flour [39], similar to the results from toy sample analyses obtained in this study.

3. Materials and Methods

3.1. Sample Collection

Toys were collected randomly from several convenience shops in urban areas in Poznań (Poland). These were shops commonly visited by people, which offer different types of toys at various prices. The samples were segregated into parts with different colors (black 3%, blue 17%, brown 2%, green 18%, metal 2%, orange 4%, pink 10%, red 10%, transparent 6%, violet 2%, white 6%, and yellow 20%).

In addition, to answer the question of whether more expensive toys are safer for the health of our children, a comparative analysis of the content of chromium in toys divided into cheap toys <5 € (34%) and expensive >5 € (66%) was made. The division is presented on Figure 2.

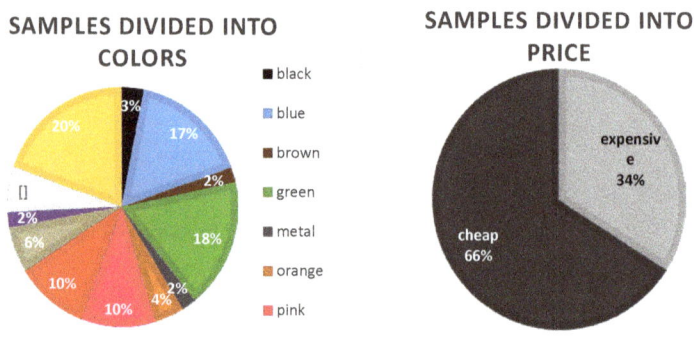

Figure 2. Samples divided into factors: colors and price.

3.2. Determination of Total Chromium Content by Energy Dispersive X-ray Fluorescence Spectrometry

In order to determine the total content of chromium in toys, energy dispersive X-ray fluorescence spectrometer (EDX) was used. Each toy categorized based on color and price was irradiated with X-rays from an X-ray tube after selecting the most appropriate irradiation diameter for the sample shape. Due to the possible heterogeneity of the toy, each one was measured several times in different parts of the toy. During analysis, a special filter for chromium was used to improve the sensitivity of detection and reduce or eliminate factors such as background, characteristic lines, and other forms of scattered radiation. The analytical conditions for EDX is presented in table (Table 4).

Table 4. Energy dispersive X-ray (EDX) analytical conditions.

Analytical Conditions	
X-ray tube	Rh target
Filter	Filter #1 (for Cr)
Voltage	Cr:30 kV
Current	5.22–6.22 keV
Atmosphere	Air
Measurement Diameter	10 mm Φ
Measurement Time	100 s
Dead Time	30%

3.3. Method Development for Speciation Analysis of Chromium(III and VI) in Toys

3.3.1. Analytical System

An ICPMS-2030 mass spectrometer (Shimadzu, Japan) directly coupled with Prominence LC 20Ai inert system was used for Cr speciation. The inert system eliminates the possibility of the metal background leaching from the components of the aperture. In addition, inert LC is the most suitable for metal speciation analysis in which the lowest possible detection limit is required. The ICP-MS operates at 1000 W with 9 L/min Ar plasma gas flow, 1 L/min nebulizer Ar gas flow, and 0.75 L/min auxiliary Ar gas flow for Hamilton PRP X100 column and 0.70 L/min auxiliary Ar gas flow for BioWAX column. The concentric (MicroMist) nebulizer with 1.0 L/min (carrier + make-up) argon gas flow was used for nebulizing the HPLC eluate. The kinetic energy discrimination (KED) mode was used for determination of chromium isotope 52.

The sampling depth was 4.5 mm for Hamilton PRP X100 column and 5.0 mm for BioWAX column. The inert LC is equipped with a binary pump LC 20Ai, a vacuum degasser (DGU 20A3R), an autosampler (SIL 20AC), a heated column compartment (CTO 20AC), and a controller (CBM 20A)(Shimadzu, Kyoto, Japan). An anion exchange column, Agilent Bio WAX 5 µm 4.6 mm × 50 mm, 5 µm, PEEK guard (Agilent, Santa Clara, CA, USA), was used for resolving of Cr species at ambient temperature. Polypropylene vials fitted with polypropylene vial caps were used. Prior to use, the vials were cleaned with dilute nitric acid and thoroughly rinsed with ultrapure deionized water (UPW) (Merck, Kenilworth, NJ, USA). Rubber, plastic, and even trace organic residues can easily cause reduction of Cr species when the sample comes into contact with them. Liquid Chromatography parameters are presented in Table 5.

Table 5. Basic Liquid Chromatogrpahy parameters for speciation analysis.

Column	Hamilton PRP X100	BioWAX Non-Porous
Mobile Phase	60 mM NH_4NO_3, pH 7.0 ± 0.1 by NH_4OH	75 mM NH_4NO_3, Ph = 7.1 ± 0.1 by NH_4OH
Mobile Phase Flow [mL/min]	1.0	0.8
Temperature	30 °C	30 °C
The Volume of the Dispensing Valve Loop [µL]	350	200

3.3.2. Reagents and Standards

Ultrapure water (<0.005 µS) obtained from a Milli-Q Direct 8 purification unit (Millipore, Burlington, MA, USA, Merck) was used to prepare all the solutions. Ammonium nitrate, potassium dichromate, standard solution of Cr(III) and Cr(VI)—1000 mg/L (Merck, USA), Na-EDTA, diluted hydrochloric acid, and ammonia (Sigma−Aldrich, St. Louis, MI, USA) to adjust the pH of the mobile phase were used for the analysis. All standard solutions used for the calibration process were prepared by volume dilution of Cr standard solution 1000 mg/L. To avoid contamination, all glassware and storage bottles were kept in 10% (v/v) nitric acid for at least 48 h, rinsed three times with ultrapure water, and preserved dried till use.

3.3.3. Sample Preparation

The procedure used HPLC-ICP-MS and followed EN71-3, which simulated gastric digestion as would occur in the case when a child swallows toy material; this is presented in Figure 3.

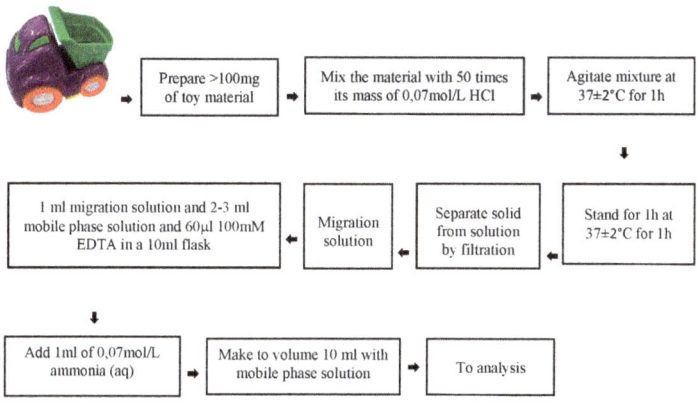

Figure 3. The sample preparation procedure for chromium speciation analysis.

The extraction (migration) solutions obtained were stabilized with EDTA and ammonia solution. The addition of ammonia to neutralize the solution preserves the chromium species extracted from toy materials for several hours with no species inter-conversion or loss by precipitation. Both Cr species were preserved for at least 24 h after the sample preparation if the solution was neutralized at pH = 7 ± 0.1. Calibration standards were also prepared by the same sample preparation method. The guidelines of the EN71-3 define conditions that may make it difficult to prepare a sample properly. The test portion of the sample should be not be less than 100 mg and shall have at least one dimension of approximately 6 mm. Therefore, in element analysis, it was impossible to use metal tools to fragment the samples. In this case, instead of a ball mill or metal scissors, a Teflon hammer and scissors were used.

3.4. Determination of Concentration of Chromium, Metals, and Metalloids in HCl Extracts by ICP-MS

In order to check the correlation between concentration of chromium and other elements: As, Cd, Cr, Cu, Hg, Mn, Ni, Pb, Sb, and Zn, ICP-MS analysis after extraction in 0.07 mol/L HCl was conducted. The sample preparation procedure was the same as in Figure 2. The results of chromium determination were compared with the data obtained from chromium speciation analysis.

3.5. Determination of Total Content of Chromium, Metals, and Metalloids after Microwave-Assisted Mineralization in HNO_3/H_2O_2

Every sample segregated based on color and price was solubilized by closed-vessel microwave-assisted acid digestion in an Anton Paar Multiwave Pro microwave oven equipped with 8NXF 100 rotor. A sample mass 100 ± 0.2 mg was directly weighted into the microwave oven polytetrafluoroethylene (PTFE) vessels. The attempt to extract a solid sample into a solution using only HNO_3 failed. Because of that, the digestion was continued further with 8 mL of high-purity concentrated nitric acid (HNO_3, 65%; Merck, USA) and 2 mL of high-purity hydrogen peroxide (H_2O_2, 30% v/v; TraceSELECT, Fluka, Seelze, Germany). This step significantly improved efficiency of this process. Each sample was analyzed in triplicates. The total content of metals and metalloids was determined using ICP-MS technique. The data obtained were compared with the results from HCl extract analysis. The parameters of ICP-MS spectrometer for analysis of both type of extracts are presented in Table 6.

Table 6. ICP-MS parameters for analysis of HCl and H_2O_2/HNO_3 extracts.

Generator Power [W]	1200
Argon flow—plasma [L/min]	8.0
Argon flow—nebulizer [L/min]	1.1
Argon flow—auxiliary gas [L/min]	0.70
Nebulizer	Concentric type, "micro"
Torch	Concentric type, "mini"
Spray chamber temperature [°C]	5.0
Collision gas—He [ml/min]	6.0
Voltage on octapole rods [V]	−21
Energy filter [V]	7.0
Sampling deep [mm]	5.0

4. Conclusions

The EDX analytical technique for detection of chromium was conducted with special filters, which allowed analysis at the level of mg/kg and did not require sample preparation. Despite using special filters for chromium, improving the sensitivity of detection, and reducing or eliminating factors such as background, characteristic lines, and other forms of scattered radiation, and measuring the toy material several times from different parts of the toy, the obtained results showed the absence of chromium in examined toy materials in the abovementioned levels. A method for speciation analysis of chromium was developed. The HPLC-ICP-MS hyphenated technique used allowed to obtain better selectivity and sensitivity. The hexavalent form of chromium was not detected in toys which were tested, which can be attributed to low elution strength of dilute HCl used in the procedure described in the standard and retaining this form of chromium in the toy material. Based on the results, the higher concentration of chromium(III) is in black, green, and yellow samples, but in none of the cases, the migration limit for this form of element was exceeded. Determination of chromium, metal (Cd, Cu, Hg, Mn, Ni, Pb, Zn), and metalloid (As, Sb) concentrations in HCl extracts by ICP-MS and of total content after microwave-assisted mineralization in HNO_3/H_2O_2 mixture were performed. The data obtained for HCl extracts were comparable with results from speciation analysis, which suggest correctness of the research. Simultaneously, it was observed that acid digestion had much higher elution strength and had significantly higher concentration values of selected metals, and thus, made it possible to determine the total content of elements. Obtained data also provides information about the potential risk of exposure by being released by saliva during chewing, sweating during skin contact, or gastric fluid after ingestion. Besides, the toy samples were bought only from Poznan city area, which may not represent the whole country; however, most of them are available in stores with the same range of products in various places in Poland or even in the whole world. Considering the division into the price of toys, no significant differences in the content of the investigated metals and metalloids were noticed. The contents of these metals were comparable with each other. Although the migration limits of certain elements from the toy's material to the environment were not detected above recommended values in these studies, toy materials may still pose a possible risk for children by creating negative health effects, particularly the metallic parts of the toys. This is because of the variety of the materials and the heterogeneity of element composition in different parts of the toy. The second argument is the possibility of bioaccumulation of heavy metals and metalloids from toys, which can happen due to ingestion, inhalation, or dermal contact, and which can last through childhood during the long times spent on playing and educating with toys.

Author Contributions: For research articles with several authors, a short paragraph specifying their individual contributions must be provided. The following statements should be used "Conceptualization, K.K. and M.F.; Methodology, K.K. and M.F.; Validation, K.K. and M.F.; Formal Analysis, K.K. and M.F.; Investigation, K.K.; Writing-Original Draft Preparation, K.K.; Writing-Review & Editing, K.K. and M.F.; Supervision, M.F.; Funding Acquisition, K.K."

Funding: The work was supported by grant no. POWR.03.02.00-00-I023/17 co-financed by the European Union through the European Social Fund under the Operational Program Knowledge Education Development.

Acknowledgments: Authors would like to thank Shim-Pol for analytical instrumentation support.

Conflicts of Interest: The authors confirm no conflict of interest. The founding sponsors had no role in the design of the study; in the collection, analyses, or interpretation of data; in the writing of the manuscript, and in the decision to publish the results.

References

1. Vareda, J.P.; Durães, L. Functionalized silica xerogels for adsorption of heavy metals from groundwater and soils. *J. Sol-Gel Sci. Technol.* **2017**, *84*, 400–408. [CrossRef]
2. Al-Qutob, M.; Asafra, A.; Nashashibi, T.; Qutob, A. Determination of Different Trace Heavy Metals in Children's Plastic Toys Imported to the West Bank/Palestine by ICP/MS-Environmental and Health Aspects. *J. Environ. Prot.* **2014**, *5*, 1104–1110. [CrossRef]
3. Guney, M.; Zagury, G.J. Contamination by Ten Harmful Elements in Toys and Children's Jewelry Bought on the North American Market. *Environ. Sci. Technol.* **2013**, *47*, 5921–5930. [CrossRef] [PubMed]
4. Guney, M.; Zagury, G. Children's exposure to harmful elements in toys and low-cost jewelry: Characterizing risks and developing a comprehensive approach. *J. Hazard. Mater.* **2014**, *271*, 321–330. [CrossRef] [PubMed]
5. Korfali, S.I.; Sabra, R.; Jurdi, M.; Taleb, R.I. Assessment of Toxic Metals and Phthalates in Children's Toys and Clays. *Arch. Environ. Contam. Toxicol.* **2013**, *65*, 368–381. [CrossRef] [PubMed]
6. Ismail, S.N.S.; Mohamad, N.S.; Karuppiah, K.; Abidin, E.Z.; Rasdi, I.; Praveena, S.M. Heavy metals content in low-priced toys. *JEAS* **2017**, *5*, 1499–1509.

7. Zhong, X.; de Cássia da Silveira e Sá, R.; Zhong, C. Mitochondrial Biogenesis in Response to Chromium (VI) Toxicity in Human Liver Cells. *Int. J. Mol. Sci.* **2017**, *18*, 1877. [CrossRef] [PubMed]
8. Turner, A.; Kearl, E.; Solman, K. Lead and other toxic metals in playground paints from South West England. *Sci. Total Environ.* **2016**, *544*, 460–466. [CrossRef] [PubMed]
9. Rebelo, A.; Pinto, E.; Almeida, A. Chemical safety of children's play paints: Focus on selected heavy metals. *Microchem. J.* **2015**, *118*, 203–210. [CrossRef]
10. Ionas, A.; Dirtu, A.; Anthonissen, T.; Neels, H.; Covaci, A. Downsides of the recycling process: Harmful organic chemicals in children's toys. *Environ. Int.* **2014**, *65*, 54–62. [CrossRef] [PubMed]
11. Xue, J.; Zartarian, V.; Moya, J.; Freeman, N.; Beamer, P.; Black, K.; Tulve, N.; Shala, S. A Meta-Analysis of Children's Hand-to-Mouth Frequency Data for Estimating Non-Dietary Ingestion Exposure. *Risk Anal.* **2007**, *27*, 411–420. [CrossRef] [PubMed]
12. Guney, M.; Zagury, G. Bioaccessibility of As, Cd, Cu, Ni, Pb, and Sb in Toys and Low-Cost Jewelry. *Environ. Sci. Technol.* **2014**, *48*, 1238–1246. [CrossRef] [PubMed]
13. Hillyer, M.; Finch, L.; Cerel, A.; Dattelbaum, J.; Leopold, M. Multi-technique quantitative analysis and socioeconomic considerations of lead, cadmium, and arsenic in children's toys and toy jewelry. *Chemosphere* **2014**, *108*, 205–213. [CrossRef] [PubMed]
14. Bruzzoniti, M.; Abollino, O.; Pazzi, M.; Rivoira, L.; Giacomino, A.; Vincenti, M. Chromium, nickel, and cobalt in cosmetic matrices: An integrated bioanalytical characterization through total content, bioaccessibility and Cr(III)/Cr(VI) speciation. *Anal. Bioanal. Chem.* **2017**, *409*, 6831–6841. [CrossRef] [PubMed]
15. Unceta, N.; Astorkia, M.; Abrego, Z.; Gómez-Caballero, A.; Goicolea, A.; Barrio, R. A novel strategy for Cr(III) and Cr(VI) analysis in dietary supplements by speciated isotope dilution mass spectrometry. *Talanta* **2016**, *154*, 255–262. [CrossRef] [PubMed]
16. Markiewicz, B.; Komorowicz, I.; Sajnóg, A.; Belter, M.; Barałkiewicz, D. Chromium and its speciation in water samples by HPLC/ICP-MS-technique establishing metrological traceability: A review since 2000. *Talanta* **2015**, *132*, 814–828. [CrossRef] [PubMed]
17. Lewicki, S.; Zdanowski, R.; Krzyżowska, M.; Lewicka, A.; Dębski, B.; Niemcewicz, M.; Goniewicz, M. The role of Chromium III in the organism and its possible use in diabetes and obesity treatment. *Ann. Agric. Environ. Med.* **2014**, *21*, 331–335. [CrossRef] [PubMed]
18. Kutscher, D.; McSheehy, S.; Wills, J.; Jensen, D. *Speciation Analysis of Cr(III) and Cr(VI) in Drinking Waters Using Anion Exchange Chromatography Coupled to the Thermo Scientific iCAP Q ICP-MS*; Application Note: 43098; Thermo Fisher Scientific: Munich, Germany, 2016.
19. Linos, A.; Petralias, A.; Christophi, C.; Christoforidou, E.; Kouroutou, P.; Stoltidis, M.; Veloudaki, A.; Tzala, E.; Makris, K.; Karagas, M. Oral ingestion of hexavalent chromium through drinking water and cancer mortality in an industrial area of Greece—An ecological study. *Environ. Health* **2011**, *10*, 50. [CrossRef] [PubMed]
20. Cui, X.Y.; Li, S.W.; Zhang, S.J.; Fan, Y.Y.; Ma, L.Q. Toxic metals in children's toys and jewelry: Coupling bioaccessibility with risk assessment. *Environ. Pollut.* **2015**, *200*, 77–84. [CrossRef] [PubMed]
21. Leist, M.; Leiser, R.; Toms, A. Low-level speciation of chromium in drinking waters using LC-ICP-MS. In *The Application Notebook. Mass Spectrom*; Varian: Palo Alto, CA, USA, 2006.
22. Misra, S.; Gupta, P. *Consumer Education Monograph Series, Toys and Safety Regulations, Consumer Education Monograph Series*; Centre for Consumer Studies, Indian Institute of Public Administration 18: New Delhi, India, 2015.
23. Sakai, K.; Song, J.; Yan, D.; Zeng, X. *LC-ICP-MS Method for the Determination of Trivalent and Hexavalent Chromium in Toy Materials to Meet European Regulation EN71-3:2012 Migration of Certain Elements*; Application Note 991-2878EN; Agilent Technologies: Santa Clara, CA, USA, 2013.
24. Krätkea, R.; Beausoleila, C.; Bartonova, A.; Schoeters, G. *Does the EU Migration Level of Chromium VI in Toys Need to Be Lowered, Chromium VI in Toys*; Scientific Committee Health and Environmental Risks SCHER Opinion on Chromium VI in Toys: Luxembourg, 2015; ISBN 978-92-79-35600-1.
25. EN 71-3:2013+A1: Safety of Toys-Part 3 Migration of Certain Elements. Available online: https://law.resource.org/pub/eu/toys/en.71.3.2015.html (accessed on 6 November 2017).
26. Vieth, B.; Pirow, R.; Luch, A. Safety limits for elements in toys: A comparison between the old and the new European toys safety directive. *Arch. Toxicol.* **2014**, *88*, 2315–2318. [CrossRef] [PubMed]

27. Dahab, A.A.; Elhag, D.E.; Ahmed, A.B.; Al-Obaid, H.A. Al-Obaid, Determination of elemental toxicity migration limits, bio accessibility and risk assessment of essential childcare products. *Environ. Sci. Pollut. Res.* **2016**, *23*, 3406–3413. [CrossRef] [PubMed]
28. Marcinkowska, M.; Komorowicz, I.; Barałkiewicz, D. New procedure for multielemental speciation analysis of five toxic species: As(III), As(V), Cr(VI), Sb(III) and Sb(V) in drinking water samples by advanced hyphenated technique HPLC/ICP-DRC-MS. *Anal. Chim. Acta* **2016**, *920*, 102–111. [CrossRef] [PubMed]
29. Séby, F.; Vacchina, V. Critical assessment of hexavalent chromium species from different solid environmental, industrial and food matrices. *Trends Anal. Chem.* **2018**, *104*, 54–68. [CrossRef]
30. Popp, M.; Hann, S.; Koellensperger, G. Environmental application of elemental speciation analysis based on liquid or gas chromatography hyphenated to inductively coupled plasma mass spectrometry—A review. *Anal. Chim. Acta* **2010**, *668*, 114–129. [CrossRef] [PubMed]
31. Barałkiewicz, D.; Pikosz, B.; Belter, M.; Marcinkowska, M. Speciation analysis of chromium in drinking water samples by ion-pair reversed-phase HPLC–ICP-MS: Validation of the analytical method and evaluation of the uncertainty budget. *Accredit. Qual. Assur.* **2013**, *18*, 391–401. [CrossRef]
32. Zeng, X.; Xu, X.; Boezen, H.M.; Huo, X. Children with health impairments by heavy metals in an e-waste recycling area. *Chemosphere* **2016**, *148*, 408–415. [CrossRef] [PubMed]
33. Vasilkov, O.O.; Barinova, O.P.; Kirsanova, S.V.; Marnautov, N.A.; Elfimov, A.B. Ceramic black pigments based on chromium-nickel spinel $NiCr_2O_4$. *Glass Ceram.* **2017**, *74*, 7–8. [CrossRef]
34. Sangeetha, S.; Basha, R.; Sreeram, K.J.; Sangilimuthu, S.N.; Nair, B.U. Functional pigments from chromium(III) oxide nanoparticles. *Dyes Pigment.* **2012**, *94*, 548–552. [CrossRef]
35. Becker, M.; Edwards, S.; Massey, R. Toxic chemicals in toys and children's products: Limitations of current response and recommendations for government and industry. *Environ. Sci. Technol.* **2010**, *44*, 7986–7991. [CrossRef] [PubMed]
36. Kumar, A.; Pastore, P. Lead and cadmium in soft plastic toys. *Curr. Sci.* **2007**, *93*, 818–822.
37. Hernandez, F.; Jitaru, P.; Cormant, F.; Noël, L.; Guérin, T. Development and application of a method for Cr(III) determination in dairy products by HPLC-ICP-MS. *Food Chem.* **2018**, *240*, 183–188. [CrossRef] [PubMed]
38. Vacchina, V. Cr(VI) speciation in foods by HPLC-ICP-MS: Investigation of Cr(VI)/food interactions by size exclusion and Cr(VI) determination and stability by ion-exchange on-line separations. *Anal. Bioanal. Chem.* **2015**, *407*, 3831–3839. [CrossRef] [PubMed]
39. Pyrzynska, K. Chromium redox speciation in food samples. *Turk. J. Chem.* **2016**, *40*, 894–905. [CrossRef]

Sample Availability: Samples of the compounds are not available from the authors.

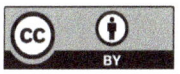

© 2018 by the authors. Licensee MDPI, Basel, Switzerland. This article is an open access article distributed under the terms and conditions of the Creative Commons Attribution (CC BY) license (http://creativecommons.org/licenses/by/4.0/).

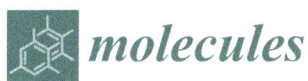

Article

Evaluation of Highly Detectable Pesticides Sprayed in *Brassica napus* L.: Degradation Behavior and Risk Assessment for Honeybees

Zhou Tong [1,2,†], Jinsheng Duan [1,2,†], Yancan Wu [3,4], Qiongqiong Liu [3], Qibao He [3], Yanhong Shi [5], Linsheng Yu [6] and Haiqun Cao [3,*]

1. Institute of Plant Protection and Agro-Product Safety, Anhui Academy of Agricultural Sciences, Hefei 230031, China; tongzhou0520@163.com (Z.T.); djszbzas@126.com (J.D.)
2. Key Laboratory of Agro-Product Safety Risk Evaluation (Hefei), Ministry of Agriculture, Hefei 230031, China
3. School of Plant Protection, Anhui Agricultural University, Hefei 230036, China; wuyancan1989@163.com (Y.W.); ahbb1104@163.com (Q.L.); heqibao0418@126.com (Q.H.)
4. Hefei Testing and Inspection Center for Agricultural Products Quality, Hefei 230601, China
5. School of Resource & Environment, Anhui Agricultural University, Hefei, 230036, China; shiyh@ahau.edu.cn
6. School of Animal Science and Technology, Anhui Agricultural University, Hefei 230036, China; yulinsheng@ahau.edu.cn
* Correspondence: haiquncao@163.com; Tel.: +86-0551-65785730
† These authors contributed equally to this work.

Academic Editor: Francesco Crea
Received: 27 August 2018; Accepted: 21 September 2018; Published: 27 September 2018

Abstract: Honeybees are major pollinators of agricultural crops and many other plants in natural ecosystems alike. In recent years, managed honeybee colonies have decreased rapidly. The application of pesticides is hypothesized to be an important route leading to colony loss. Herein, a quick, easy, cheap, effective, rugged, and safe (QuEChERS) method was used to determine eight highly detectable pesticides (carbendazim, prochloraz, pyrimethanil, fenpropathrin, chlorpyrifos, imidacloprid, thiamethoxam, and acetamiprid) in rape flowers. A field experiment was conducted at the recommended dose to evaluate the contact exposure risk posed to honeybees for 0–14 days after treatment. The initial residue deposits of neonicotinoids and fungicides among these compounds were 0.4–1.3 mg/kg and 11.7–32.3 mg/kg, respectively, and 6.4 mg/kg for fenpropathrin and 4.2 mg/kg for chlorpyrifos. The risk was quantified using the flower hazard quotient (FHQ) value. According to the data, we considered imidacloprid, thiamethoxam, chlorpyrifos, fenpropathrin, and prochloraz to pose an unacceptable risk to honeybees after spraying in fields, while fungicides (carbendazim and pyrimethanil) and acetamiprid posed moderate or acceptable risks to honeybees. Therefore, acetamiprid can be used instead of imidacloprid and thiamethoxam to protect rape from some insects in agriculture, and the application of prochloraz should be reduced.

Keywords: pesticide; honeybee; risk; field

1. Introduction

The honeybee is a social insect species. It plays a major environmental role by providing necessary ecosystem services, similar to bumblebees, solitary bees, moths, butterflies, beetles, and other insects [1]. As the most abundant pollinators globally, honeybees contribute an estimated €153 billion annually to global agriculture [2]. However, in recent decades, managed honeybee colonies have decreased in North America, Europe, and Asia-Pacific [3–9], known as colony collapse disorder (CCD). Presently, honeybees are exposed to diverse stressors, including Varroa mites (*Varroa destructor*) and viruses [10], pathogens [11], pesticides [12,13], habitats [14] and climate change [15].

Sublethal doses of pesticides have been proven to disrupt memory, learning, navigation, and foraging activities in honeybees, and affect their sensitivity to other stressors, particularly increasing pathogen vulnerability [16–19]. Concern about the risk posed to bees by pesticides not only includes the toxicity evaluation of plant protection products, but also accurate estimation of the residue exposure levels from these products in the environment. With the development of analysis technique, the quick, easy, cheap, effective, rugged, and safe (QuEChERS) approach and UPLC–MS/MS have extensive application. Some complex matrices, such as soil [20], meat product [21] et al. were extracted through the QuEChERS. The high sensitivity and selectivity have also been provided by ultra-high-performance liquid chromatography–tandem mass spectrometry (UPLC–MS/MS) [22] and gas chromatography–tandem mass spectrometry (GC–MS/MS) [23]. Meanwhile, a large number of bee product was monitored in decade. For example, pesticides have been detected in pollen, beeswax, and honeybee samples collected in Italy [24–26]. A survey conducted on apiaries in France found that honeybees are exposed to multiple miscellaneous pesticides simultaneously from other honeybees, pollen, bee bread, and beehives [27–32]. In Poland, 48 different pesticide residues have been found in honeybees [33–35]. Also, other studies on the influence of 5 different pesticides on honeybees were conducted in Poland [36]. China is a vast region with a complex climate that has a long history of honeybee management. In rapeseed crops in China, eight pesticides, namely carbendazim, prochloraz, pyrimethanil, fenpropathrin, chlorpyrifos, imidacloprid, thiamethoxam, and acetamiprid, have been detected at high residue levels in pollen samples by UPLC–MS/MS [37]. Therefore, risk assessment of these chemicals is increasingly important to protect pollinators from the adverse effects of plant protection products (PPPs).

Risk assessments for honeybees typically consider only the acute toxicity of pesticides either through topical or oral exposure for 24 or 48 h, ignoring the negative effects resulting from sustained exposure to pesticide residues over longer periods. Some evaluations have paid attention to the application rates of different chemicals to estimate a hazard quotient (HQ) [38]. In the case of environmental risk assessments for honeybees, exposure assessments have been defined in general terms. Toxicity data is combined with contact and dietary exposure, and calculated separately using two approaches that are specific to different applications. Since 2010, individual studies have used pesticide residues in a plant matrix (pollen, nectar, or the aerial part of the plant) to evaluate the toxicity exposure ratio (TER) [39] or pollen hazard quotient (PHQ) [40]. As proposed in the European and Mediterranean Plant Protection Organization (EPPO)'s document, 'Environmental risk assessment scheme for plant protection products Chapter 10: honeybees', such residues to honeybees occur through both contact with and ingestion of plant protection products. Two tiers of risk assessment are included in this document, with the primary procedure evaluating the HQ or TER in the laboratory, while field trials are proposed for a high tier risk assessment.

This study aims to assess the risk posed by some highly detectable pesticides, such as carbendazim, prochloraz, pyrimethanil, fenpropathrin, chlorpyrifos, imidacloprid, thiamethoxam, and acetamiprid [37] to honeybees following spraying in rape fields. After treatment on specific days, it is necessary to evaluate the exposure risk of these compounds, which are widely used to protect crops against aphids, *Plutella xylostella* (L.), *Sclerotinia sclerotiorum (Lib.) de Bary*, and *Peronospora parasitica (Pers.) Fr.*, to legitimately guide pesticide application and honeybee management. Pesticide residues on rape flowers were used in the exposure to calculate the flower hazard quotient (FHQ) in order to estimate the risk of contact with pollinators after pesticide spraying.

2. Materials and Methods

2.1. Chemicals and Standards

A Milli-Q ultrapure water system manufactured by Millipore (Milford, UT, USA) was used throughout experiments to provide the HPLC-grade water that was employed during analysis and to hydrate the rape flower samples. Ultragradient HPLC-grade acetonitrile and methanol were obtained from Tedia (Shanghai, China). Formic acid, acetic acid, anhydrous magnesium sulfate ($MgSO_4$), and sodium acetate (NaOAc) were supplied by Sinopharm Chemical Reagent Co., Ltd. (Shanghai, China). PSA (primary and secondary amine-bonded silica), C_{18} (octadecyl-bonded silica) and GCB (graphitized carbon black) were purchased from Agilent Technologies (Santa Clara, CA, USA).

Reference standards of imidacloprid (purity, 98%), thiamethoxam (purity, 95%), acetamiprid (purity, 95%), fenpropathrin (purity, 98.5%), chlorpyrifos (purity, 98%), carbendazim (purity, 95%), prochloraz (purity, 98%) and pyrimethanil (purity, 95%) were obtained from Dr. Ehrenstorfer GmbH (Augsburg, Germany).

Formulated pesticides of imidacloprid 10% wettable powder (WP), thiamethoxam 25% water-dispersible granules (WDG), acetamiprid 20% WP, fenpropathrin 20% emulsifiable concentrate (EC), chlorpyrifos 40% EC, carbendazim 80% WP, prochloraz 25% EC, and pyrimethanil 40% suspension concentrate (SC) were purchased from the agricultural market located in Hefei, Anhui, China.

2.2. Experimental Design and Sample Collection

Field experiments of each chemical were conducted using the same rape variety at the Experimental Station of Anhui Agriculture University, Anhui, China, in accordance with good agricultural practices (GAP). At each site, 3 m × 30 m rectangular plots spaced 1 m apart were flagged at the corners. Three replicate plots were designated for each pesticide, in addition to an untreated control plot. No mixtures were used on individual experimental plots. Spray application of the chemicals was achieved using an automatic sprayer at the recommended dose (shown in Tables 1–3) during rape flowering. The formulated compounds were dissolved in water, with 900 L/ha of water used for application. Rape flower samples were collected from five stochastically assigned subsections in each plot and combined into a plastic bag for each replicate. Flower sampling from each control was repeated 0, 1, 3, 5, 7, 10, and 14 days after spraying. The information of meteorology was listed in Table 4. All the samples were frozen immediately and stored at −20 °C until extraction for residue determination (up to 15 days). The storage stability tests were conducted before the sample analysis, and the results proved that the degradation rate of all the target compounds storing in −20 °C was lower than 5% entirely.

Table 1. Residues of neonicotinoids in rape flowers.

| Days after Treatment | Untreated Control | Residue Levels of the Neonicotinoids (ng/g) ± SD ||||||
| | | Thiamethoxam (30 g a.i./ha) ME (29%) || Imidacloprid (60 g a.i./ha) ME (75%) || Acetamiprid (60 g a.i./ha) ME (−5%) ||
		Residue	Degradation Rate (%)	Residue	Degradation Rate (%)	Residue	Degradation Rate (%)
0 day	ND	375.0 ± 35.5	-	1006.0 ± 150.3	-	1259.0 ± 108.2	-
1 day	ND	315.3 ± 45.3	15.9	390.0 ± 57.5	61.2	1099.7 ± 170.4	12.7
3 day	ND	108.7 ± 3.1	71.0	78.7 ± 1.5	92.2	394.3 ± 8.6	68.7
5 day	ND	78.7 ± 7.2	79.0	68.3 ± 3.1	93.2	337.7 ± 29.3	73.2
7 day	ND	18.7 ± 2.5	95.0	11.3 ± 1.2	98.9	87.3 ± 5.5	93.1
10 day	ND	9.3 ± 1.2	97.5	ND	-	27.3 ± 1.5	97.8
14 day	ND	8.0 ± 1.0	97.9	ND	-	10.3 ± 0.6	98.7
DT50 day	-	2.3		1.2		1.9	

Table 2. Residues of chlorpyrifos and fenpropathrin in rape flowers.

Days after Treatment	Untreated Control	Residue Levels of Insecticides (ng/g) ± SD			
		Chlorpyrifos (360 g a.i./ha) ME (22%)		Fenpropathrin (60 g a.i./ha) ME (−8%)	
		Residue	Degradation Rate (%)	Residue	Degradation Rate (%)
0 day	ND	4249 ± 821.1	-	6409 ± 656.6	-
1 day	ND	1755 ± 441.6	58.7	4824.± 778.7	24.7
3 day	ND	386.3 ± 14.3	90.9	1646 ± 129.5	74.3
5 day	ND	160.7 ± 15.6	96.2	1159 ± 246.0	81.9
7 day	ND	98.3 ± 14.0	97.7	412.0 ± 66.8	93.6
10 day	ND	57.3 ± 4.9	98.7	179.0 ± 21.1	97.2
14 day	ND	38.7 ± 5.5	99.1	58.7 ± 11.5	99.1
DT50 day	-	2.1		2.0	

Table 3. Residues of the fungicides in rape flowers.

Days after Treatment	Untreated Control	Residue Levels of the Fungicides (ng/g) ± SD					
		Carbendazim (1500 g a.i./ha) ME (50%)		Pyrimethanil (360 g a.i./ha) ME (−34%)		Prochloraz (181.5 g a.i./ha) ME (−20%)	
		Residue	Degradation Rate (%)	Residue	Degradation Rate (%)	Residue	Degradation Rate (%)
0 day	ND	32,299 ± 583.0	-	16,222 ± 573.7	-	11,684 ± 167.0	-
1 day	ND	25,316 ± 878.0	21.6	93,089 ± 724.9	42.6	4891 ± 150.3	58.1
3 day	ND	11,478 ± 814.5	64.5	1155 ± 104.4	92.9	471.7 ± 58.1	96.0
5 day	ND	8713 ± 564.2	73.0	374.3 ± 23.6	97.7	100.3 ± 4.7	99.1
7 day	ND	6196 ± 498.3	80.8	195.7 ± 2.1	98.8	57.3 ± 0.6	99.5
10 day	ND	1908 ± 477.6	94.1	50.3 ± 3.2	99.7	11.3 ± 2.9	99.9
14 day	ND	153.3 ± 17.9	99.5	9.3 ± 1.5	99.9	ND	-
DT50 day		2.0		1.3		1.0	

Table 4. The information of meteorology during the trial days.

Days after Treatment	0 Day	1 Day	3 Day	5 Day	7 Day	10 Day	14 Day
Data	27 March	28 March	30 March	1 April	3 April	6 April	10 April
Season	Spring						
Weather	Sunny	Sunny	Cloudy	Rain	Cloudy	Cloudy	Sunny
Rainfall	-	-	-	4 mm	-	-	-
Temperature	24 °C	25 °C	22 °C	22 °C	21 °C	25 °C	26 °C

2.3. Sample Preparation

Rape flower samples were grated with liquid nitrogen and 2 g of the sample were weighed into a 50 mL polypropylene centrifuge tube. Ultrapure water (3 mL) was then added and the tube was shaken for 30 s to hydrate the sample. Next, 0.1 N acetic acid in acetonitrile (10 mL) and glass beads (2 g) were added and the samples were vortexed for 2 min at room temperature, followed by freezing for 10 min at −20 °C in a freezer. $MgSO_4$ (0.5 g) and NaOAc (2 g) were then added and the tube was shaken vigorously for 60 s and centrifuged for 5 min at 3800 rpm. A 5 mL aliquot of the supernatant (acetonitrile phase) was transferred to a 15-mL centrifuge tube containing the QuEChERS (Quick, Easy, Cheap, Effective, Rugged, and Safe) salt kit (1.25 g; PSA:C18:$MgSO_4$:GCB, 1:1:3:0.15 ($w/w/w/w$)). After mixing well, the mixture was again centrifuged at 3800 rpm for 5 min, and 2.5 mL of the acetonitrile phase was transferred to a glass tube. The supernatant was then evaporated to dryness under a gentle stream of nitrogen at 30 °C. The dry residue was dissolved in methanol (0.5 mL, HPLC grade), filtered through a 0.22 μm filter membrane, and introduced into an autosampler vial for UPLC–MS/MS analysis.

2.4. Chemical Analysis

A Waters Acquity ultra-performance liquid chromatography system (Waters, Milford, MA, USA) equipped with a binary pump and Acquity EBH (ethylene bridged hybrid) C_{18} column (1.7 µm i.d., 2.1 mm × 100 mm particle size) was used for liquid chromatography. Components were separated using Milli-Q water/methanol (98:2) + 0.05 N formic acid (solvent A) and methanol + 0.05 N formic acid (solvent B) at 40 °C. Separation was performed with a flow rate of 0.45 mL/min starting with a mobile phase of 5% B in A at the injection time, which was then rapidly increased to 100% B over 0.25 min and then held at 100% mobile phase B until 8.5 min. Finally, the mobile phase was switched to 5% B in A at 8.51 min and held until 10 min to re-equilibrate the column. The injection volume was 3 µL and the total analytical time was 10 min.

A Waters Xevo TQ triple quadrupole mass spectrometer (Waters, Milford, MA, USA) equipped with an electrospray ionization (ESI) source and conducted in positive electrospray ionization mode was used for mass spectrometry detection. The ESI source temperature was 150 °C. The gas flow rates of the cone and desolvation gases were 50 and 900 L/h. The desolvation temperature was 500 °C. Helium was used as the collision gas with a flow rate of 0.15 mL/min. The mass spectrometer was operated in multiple reaction monitoring (MRM) mode to monitor two precursor ion transitions for each pesticide. The target ion transition with the highest response (primary ion transition) was used for quantification and the second target ion transition was used for confirmation [41]. Confirmation was provided through a product ion scan (PIC) of each peak, which adapted to a reference spectrum for each analysis. The quantification and confirmation calculations were calculated using Target Lynx 4.1 software (Waters Corp., Milford, MA, USA) implemented by the apparatus. Other MS settings used in this experiment, including ion transitions, cone voltages, collision energies, and dwell times, are shown in Table S1.

2.5. Preparation of Standard Solutions

All standard stock solutions (1000 ng/mL) were prepared in acetonitrile, and further diluted to prepare working standards. Calibration standards (1–100 ng/mL) were prepared by diluting the working standards. Standards with concentrations in the range 1–100 ng/mL were prepared for spiking blank rape flowers. Matrix-matched standards were prepared by adding the pesticides to the blank sample. Blank sample (1 mL) extract was evaporated to dryness under nitrogen, and the required calibration standard (1 mL) was added to prepare matrix-matched standards of the required concentrations (1–100 ng/mL).

2.6. Data Analysis

The limit of detection (LOD) was determined as the minimum concentration detectable for all target chemicals based on a signal-to-noise (S/N) ratio of 3, while the limit of quantification (LOQ) was set as a S/N ratio of 10 [42].

Matrix effects (ME) were calculated from the slopes of calibration curves in the matrix and solvent for each determination using Equation (1).

$$ME(\%) = \left(\left(\frac{Slope\ of\ calibration\ on\ curve\ in\ matrix}{Slope\ of\ calibration\ on\ curve\ in\ solvent}\right) - 1\right) \times 100 \quad (1)$$

To evaluate the risk posed to honeybees by highly detectable pesticides, we used distinct new approaches to assess oral exposure. For exposure through the uptake of pollen or honey from the flower, the oral LD50s shown in Table S2 were used to calculate the daily oral flower hazard quotient (FHQ_{do}) for honeybees exposed to 1 g of contaminated flowers per day [43].

$$FHQ_{do} = \frac{PEC(ng/g) \times MCL(g)}{_{oral}LD50(ng/bee)} \quad (2)$$

Using Equation (2), the FHQ$_{do}$ was calculated from the oral exposure dose (equal to the predicted exposure concentration (PEC) multiplied by the maximum contact level (MCL)) and the acute oral LD50 for adult bees. When the FHQ$_{do}$ value was lower than 0.1, the risk was considered acceptable, while values between 0.1 and 1 indicated moderate risks, and values greater than 1 indicated an unacceptable risk.

3. Results and Discussion

3.1. Method Validation

The LOD and LOQ were calculated from the regression data shown in Table S3. The LODs ranged from 0.0088 to 0.1064 ng/mL. Calibration curves, including the zero point, were constructed using the blank rape flower matrix spiked at six different concentration levels in the range 1–100 ng/mL after the extraction step. This calibration could reduce the impact of matrix effects in the electrospray source, such as ion enhancement or suppression. The linear region, observed throughout the concentration range studied depending on the chemicals, is shown in Table S3. Good linearity was observed in all cases, with correlation coefficients (R^2) better than 0.9902, which assumed the quantitative analysis of pesticide residues in rape flower.

During MS analysis, quantification was subject to strong matrix effects (ME) that could severely reduce or promote the response of the chemical. Therefore, the ME of each compound is described in Table 1. Among the eight pesticides, unacceptable matrix effects were observed in the range of −34% to 75%. To reduce matrix effects, we prepared analytical curves in the matrix.

Recovery studies of the eight pesticides were performed in rape flower samples at three spiked levels of 5, 50, and 500 ng/g. The accuracy and precision of the analytical method were evaluated using these studies. The recoveries and relative standard deviation (RSD) are listed in Table 5. Recoveries obtained for all chemicals ranged from 78.9% to 115.2%, with all pesticides within the satisfactory range of 70–120%. The RSD value was included in RSD$_r$ and RSD$_R$, which calculated using the standard deviation of the recovery on the same day and the three separate days, respectively. In this experiment, the RSD$_r$ values ranged from 1.2% to 10.6%. Meanwhile, the RSD$_R$ values ranged from 3.0% to 11.2%.

Table 5. Recoveries, relative standard deviations (RSDs), and matrix effects (MEs) of eight pesticide compounds in rape flowers.

Compound	ME	Spiked Level (ng/g)	Intra-Day (n = 5)						(Inter-Day) (n = 15) RSD$_R$ (%)
			Day 1		Day 2		Day 3		
			Recovery (%)	RSD$_r$ (%)	Recovery (%)	RSD$_r$ (%)	Recovery (%)	RSD$_r$ (%)	
Carbendazim	50	5	95.6	4.7	88.9	3.9	90.5	6.9	5.2
		50	88.4	3.6	78.9	2.2	92.6	6.5	4.1
		500	97.6	3.2	88.5	5.7	91.8	6.2	5.0
Thiamethoxam	29	5	100.5	1.2	97.6	5.0	95.3	4.6	3.6
		50	94.3	4.8	95.3	4.2	92.8	4.0	3.0
		500	97.1	2.4	93.2	2.8	115.2	6.1	3.8
Imidacloprid	75	5	95.7	4.2	88.4	9.7	90.6	6.3	4.7
		50	88.4	1.2	93.4	2.3	93.7	5.6	3.0
		500	96.5	2.9	93.2	5.2	95.6	4.9	4.3
Acetamiprid	−5	5	100.1	4.6	95.6	4.9	93.2	6.1	5.2
		50	91.2	2.1	105.2	5.6	92.9	4.8	4.2
		500	98.0	5.6	94.2	4.2	89.9	5.9	5.2
Pyrimethanil	−34	5	88.9	3.6	94.2	3.8	89.5	8.9	5.4
		50	89.7	4.2	91.3	4.9	90.8	5.4	4.8
		500	90.8	5.2	96.5	3.1	92.7	5.6	3.0

Table 5. Cont.

Compound	ME	Spiked Level (ng/g)	Intra-Day (n = 5)						(Inter-Day) (n = 15) RSD$_R$ (%)
			Day 1		Day 2		Day 3		
			Recovery (%)	RSD$_r$ (%)	Recovery (%)	RSD$_r$ (%)	Recovery (%)	RSD$_r$ (%)	
Procholraz	−20	5	95.7	4.2	88.4	3.7	90.6	6.3	4.7
		50	88.4	1.2	93.4	2.3	93.7	5.6	3.0
		500	96.5	2.9	93.2	5.2	95.6	4.9	4.3
Chlorpyrifos	22	5	100.1	4.6	95.6	4.9	93.2	6.1	11.2
		50	91.2	2.1	95.2	5.6	92.9	4.8	4.2
		500	98.0	10.6	94.2	4.2	89.9	5.9	5.2
Fenpropathrin	−8	5	92.3	4.8	99.2	4.5	91.2	6.2	5.2
		50	89.6	2.5	92.5	3.7	91.8	6.5	4.2
		500	95.2	6.6	94.6	2.5	88.3	5.4	4.8

3.2. Residues of Highly Detectable Pesticides on Rape Flowers

As shown in Table 1, the average initial residue deposits of the neonicotinoids were 370.0, 1006.0, and 1259.0 ng/g from treatments with thiamethoxam, imidacloprid, and acetamiprid at the recommended doses, respectively. On day 1 after treatment, 12.7–15.9% of the neonicotinoids residues had dissipated from the rape flower, which increased to 93.1–95.0% by day 7, with the exception of imidacloprid, which showed substantial degradation (61.2%) on day 1. Imidacloprid residues dissipated fast in the initial stages. On day 5 after application, more than 70% of the residues had dissipated from both treatments, which increased to about 95% by day 10. On day 10, the residue levels of imidacloprid were below the LOQ. The dissipation trend of the neonicotinoids is described in Figure 1.

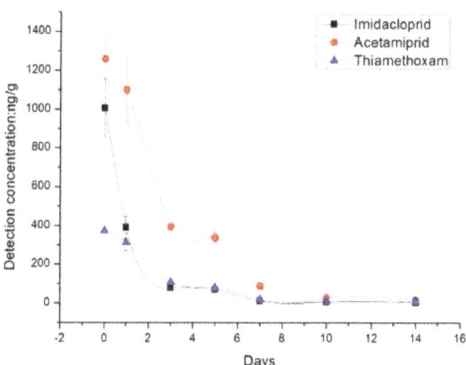

Figure 1. Residue dissipation of the Neonicotinoids on rape flower.

As shown in Table 2, the average initial residue deposits of chlorpyrifos and fenpropathrin were 4249 ng/g and 6409 ng/g, respectively, after treatment at the recommended doses. On day 1 after treatment, 24.7% of fenpropathrin residues had dissipated from the rape flower, which increased to 93.6% by day 7. In contrast, 58.7% of chlorpyrifos residues had dissipated from the rape flower by day 1, which increased to 90.9% by day 3. On day 14, the residue levels of chlorpyrifos and fenpropathrin were 38.7 ng/g and 58.7 ng/g. The dissipation trends of chlorpyrifos and fenpropathrin are described in Figure 2, showing that the degradation rate of chlorpyrifos was much faster than that of fenpropathrin.

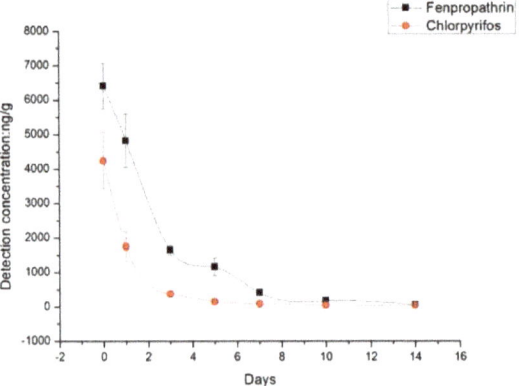

Figure 2. Residue dissipation of chlorpyrifos and fenpropathrin on rape flower.

As shown in Table 3, the average initial residue deposits of the fungicides were 32,299 ng/g, 16,222 ng/g, and 11,684 ng/g from treatments with carbendazim, pyrimethanil, and prochloraz, respectively, at the recommended doses. On day 1, 42.6–58.1% of the fungicide residues had dissipated from the rape flowers, which increased to 92.9–96.0% by day 3, with the exception of carbendazim, which showed relatively little degradation (21.8%) after day 1. Pyrimethanil and prochloraz residues dissipated rapidly during the initial stages. On day 5 after application, more than 70% of carbendazim residues had dissipated, which increased to about 90% by day 10. On day 10, the prochloraz residue level was below the LOQ. The dissipation trend of the fungicides is described in Figure 3, showing that the degradation rate of carbendazim was much slower than those of pyrimethanil and prochloraz.

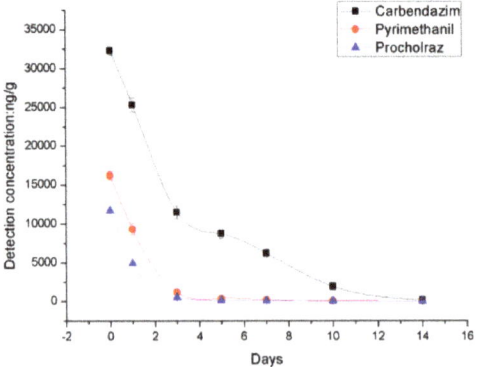

Figure 3. Residue dissipation of the Fungicides on rape flower.

3.3. Risk Assessment

To understand the risks posed to honeybees by the application of highly detectable pesticides, FHQ_{do} values (shown in Table 6) were calculated using Equation (1), as shown in the 'Data analysis' section. Risks were classed as acceptable, moderate, and unacceptable.

Among the neonicotinoids, the risk was unacceptable for all, except acetamiprid, up to day 14 after treatment. Meanwhile, imidacloprid retained the most harmful oral exposure risk. The oral risk posed by acetamiprid was much lower than those of imidacloprid and thiamethoxam, and classed as acceptable. In Jiang's research, imidacloprid and thiamethoxam have been detected and respectively ranged from 1.61 to 64.58 ng/g and ND (not detected) to 31.52 ng/g in cotton pollen after seed treatment [22]. It almost seemed that the neonicotinoids residue level of spray treatment is higher than seed treatment. Meanwhile, the risk to honeybees was unacceptable equally. Chlorpyrifos also carried an unacceptable risk level until day 3 after spraying, after which the risk decreased to moderate until day 14. Through data analysis, we considered the insecticides, comprising imidacloprid, thiamethoxam, and chlorpyrifos, to have a high oral exposure risk when used for aphid treatment, with the exception of acetamiprid. Therefore, when using plant protection products to prevent aphids on flowering rape, honeybee management could be achieved using acetamiprid instead of imidacloprid, thiamethoxam, and chlorpyrifos.

Fenpropathrin is a major chemical used to protect flowering rape against insects such as *Plutella xylostella* (L.) [44]. On the spraying day, the FHQ value reached 128.18, and remained at an unacceptable exposure risk level for honeybees until day 14 after treatment. Therefore, honeybee management will be improved at least 14 days after spraying with fenpropathrin.

Plant diseases, such as *Sclerotinia sclerotiorum* (Lib.) de Bary and *Peronospora parasitica* (Pers.) Fr, are a primary cause of oilseed rape destruction during growth. To prevent such diseases, a large number of fungicides, including carbendazim, pyrimethanil, and prochloraz, are widely used in agriculture. As shown in Table 5, the fungicides posed lower risks, with the exception of prochloraz, for which the unacceptable risk to honeybees was sustained until day 5 after treatment, and became acceptable after day 10. As the recommended dose of carbendazim was large, a moderate risk to honeybees remained until day 7 after treatment. For pyrimethanil, a moderate risk to honeybees was present on day 1 after treatment. Although the fungicides, including carbendazim and pyrimethanil, were found to pose only moderate risks to honeybees when sprayed in rape fields, recent studies have shown that fungicides have a negative effect on honeybee colonies [45]. This effect is probably due to the synergistic toxic effects that certain fungicides, specifically azoles and prochloraz, have on insects such as honeybees [46].

Table 6. Risk level of eight pesticides following spraying in a rape field.

Days after Treatment	Oral Flower Hazard Quotient (FHQ$_{do}$)							
	Thiamethoxam	Imidacloprid	Acetamiprid	Chlorpyrifos	Fenpropathrin	Carbendazim	Pyrimethanil	Prochloraz
0 day	75.02	773.78	0.09	17.71	128.18	0.65	0.32	116.80
1 day	63.15	300.21	0.08	7.31	96.48	0.51	0.19	48.91
3 day	21.76	60.76	-	1.61	32.91	0.23	0.02	4.72
5 day	15.42	52.49	-	0.67	23.19	0.17	-	1.03
7 day	3.72	8.74	-	0.41	8.24	0.12	-	0.57
10 day	1.91	3.61	-	0.24	3.58	0.04	-	0.11
14 day	1.62	2.38	-	0.16	1.17	-	-	0.02

4. Conclusions

The degradation rates of pesticide residues of eight highly detectable chemicals sprayed in an oilseed rape field were generally rapid. However, some high toxicity insecticides, including imidacloprid, thiamethoxam, chlorpyrifos, and fenpropathrin, posed unacceptable oral exposure risks to honeybees. The three fungicides assessed posed moderate risks to honeybees, with the exception of prochloraz, which produced an unacceptable risk more than five days after treatment. This showed that the logical application of pesticides is integral to honeybee management. In the future work, we have designed to determinate pesticide residues in other crop species, and risk assessment on honeybee larva would be investigated combining more toxicology data.

Supplementary Materials: The following are available online, Table S1: Ion transitions used for quantification (MRM1) and confirmation (MRM2), and dwell time, cone voltage, and collision energy for mass spectrometry settings for different pesticide compounds, Table S2: Chemical structure, and acute oral and contact LD50 values of pesticide compounds in honeybees, Table S3: Limits of determination and quantification (LOD and LOQ), and linear ranges, linear regression equations, and linearities of the method for different pesticide compounds.

Author Contributions: Conceptualization, L.Y. and H.C.; Data curation, Z.T. and J.D.; Formal analysis, Z.T., Q.L., and Q.H.; Methodology, Y.W.; Validation, J.D. and Y.S.; Writing original draft, Z.T.; Writing review & editing, Z.T.

Funding: This work was supported by the Earmarked Fund for China Agriculture Research System grant number [CARS-45-KXJ9].

Acknowledgments: We acknowledge Xingchuan Jiang and Min Liao for their assistance.

Conflicts of Interest: The authors have no conflicts of interest to declare.

References

1. Klein, A.M.; Vaissière, B.E.; Cane, J.H.; Steffan-Dewenter, I.; Cunningham, S.A.; Kremen, C.; Tscharntke, T. Importance of pollinators in changing landscapes for world crops. *Proc. Biol. Sci.* **2007**, *274*, 303–313. [CrossRef] [PubMed]
2. Gallai, N.; Salles, J.M.; Settele, J.; Vaissière, B.E. Economic valuation of the vulnerability of world agriculture confronted with pollinator decline. *Ecol. Econ.* **2009**, *68*, 810–821. [CrossRef]
3. Brodschneide, R.; Moosbeckhofer, R.; Crailsheim, K. Preliminary Results of Honey Bee Colony Losses in Austria 2010/2011. *Mellifera* **2011**, *11*, 14–15.
4. Genersch, E.; Ohe, W.V.D.; Kaatz, H.; Schroeder, A.; Otten, C.; Büchler, R.; Berg, S.; Ritter, W.; Mühlen, W.; Gisder, S. The German bee monitoring project: A long term study to understand periodically high winter losses of honey bee colonies. *Apidologie* **2010**, *41*, 332–352. [CrossRef]
5. Higes, M.; Martín-Hernández, R.; Martínez-Salvador, A.; Garrido-Bailón, E.; González-Porto, A.V.; Meana, A.; Bernal, J.L.; Del Nozal, M.J.; Bernal, J. A preliminary study of the epidemiological factors related to honey bee colony loss in Spain. *Environ. Microbiol. Rep.* **2010**, *2*, 243–250. [CrossRef] [PubMed]
6. Potts, S.G.; Biesmeijer, J.C.; Kremen, C.; Neumann, P.; Schweiger, O.; Kunin, W.E. Global pollinator declines: Trends, impacts and drivers. *Trends Ecol. Evol.* **2010**, *25*, 345. [CrossRef] [PubMed]
7. Zee, R.E.V.D.; Pisa, L.; Andonov, S.; Brodschneider, R.; Charrière, J.D.; Chlebo, R.; Coffey, M.F.; Crailsheim, K.; Dahle, B.; Gajda, A.; Gray, A.; et al. Managed honey bee colony losses in Canada, China, Europe, Israel and Turkey, for the winters of 2008-9 and 2009-10. *J. Apic. Res.* **2012**, *51*, 100–114.
8. Kulhanek, K.; Steinhauer, N.; Rennich, K. A national survey of managed honey bee 2015–2016 annual colony losses in the USA. *J. Agric. Res.* **2017**, *56*, 328–340. [CrossRef]
9. Vanengelsdorp, D.; Caron, D.; Hayes, J.; Underwood, R.; Henson, M.; Rennich, K.; Spleen, A.; Andree, M.; Snyder, R.; Lee, K.; et al. A national survey of managed honey bee 2010-11 winter colony losses in the USA: Results from the Bee Informed Partnership. *Apidologie* **2015**, *46*, 292–305. [CrossRef]
10. Wilfert, L.; Long, G.; Leggett, H.C.; Schmid-Hempel, P.; Butlin, R.; Martin, S.J.M.; Boots, M. Deformed wing virus is a recent global epidemic in honeybees driven by Varroa mites. *Science* **2016**, *351*, 594–597. [CrossRef] [PubMed]
11. Ravoet, J.; Maharramov, J.; Meeus, I.; De Smet, L.; Wenseleers, T.; Smagghe, G.; De Graaf, D.C. Comprehensive Bee Pathogen Screening in Belgium Reveals Crithidia mellificae as a New Contributory Factor to Winter Mortality. *PLoS ONE* **2013**, *8*, e72443. [CrossRef] [PubMed]
12. Goulson, D.; Nicholls, E.; Botías, C.; Rotheray, E.L. Bee declines driven by combined stress from parasites, pesticides, and lack of flowers. *Science* **2015**, *347*, 1255957. [CrossRef] [PubMed]
13. Maini, S.; Medrzycki, P.; Porrini, C. The puzzle of honey bee losses: A brief review. *Bull. Insectol.* **2010**, *63*, 153–160.
14. Naug, D. Nutritional stress due to habitat loss may explain recent honeybee colony collapses. *Biol. Conserv.* **2009**, *142*, 2369–2372. [CrossRef]
15. Memmott, J.; Craze, P.G.; Waser, N.M.; Price, M.V. Global warming and the disruption of plant-pollinator interactions. *Ecol. Lett.* **2007**, *10*, 710–717. [CrossRef] [PubMed]
16. Decourtye, A.; Armengaud, C.; Renou, M.; Devillers, J.; Cluzeau, S.; Gauthier, M.; Pham-Delègue, M.H. Imidacloprid impairs memory and brain metabolism in the honeybee (*Apis mellifera* L.). *Pestic. Biochem. Phys.* **2004**, *78*, 83–92. [CrossRef]
17. Williamson, S.M.; Wright, G.A. Exposure to multiple cholinergic pesticides impairs olfactory learning and memory in honeybees. *J. Exp. Biol.* **2013**, *216*, 1799. [CrossRef] [PubMed]
18. Sanchez-Bayo, F.; Goulson, D.; Pennacchio, F.; Nazzi, F.; Goka, K.; Desneux, N. Are bee diseases linked to pesticides?—A brief review. *Environ. Int.* **2016**, *89*, 7–11. [CrossRef] [PubMed]

19. Alburaki, M.; Boutin, S.; Mercier, P.L.; Loublier, Y.; Chagnon, M.; Derome, N. Neonicotinoid-Coated Zea mays Seeds Indirectly Affect Honeybee Performance and Pathogen Susceptibility in Field Trials. *PLoS ONE* **2015**, *10*, e0125790. [CrossRef] [PubMed]
20. Villaverde, J.; Sevilla-Morán, B.; López-Goti, C.; Alonso-Prados, J.; Sandín-España, P. Computational-Based Study of QuEChERS Extraction of Cyclohexanedione Herbicide Residues in Soil by Chemometric Modeling. *Molecules* **2018**, *23*, 2009. [CrossRef] [PubMed]
21. Chang, C.C.; Kao, T.H.; Zhang, D.; Wang, Z.; Inbaraj, B.S.; Hsu, K.Y.; Chen, B.H. Application of QuEChERS Coupled with HPLC-DAD-ESI-MS/MS for Determination of Heterocyclic Amines in Commercial Meat Products. *Food Anal. Methods* **2018**, *11*, 3243–3256. [CrossRef]
22. Jiang, J.; Ma, D.; Zou, N.; Yu, X.; Zhang, Z.; Liu, F.; Mu, W. Concentrations of imidacloprid and thiamethoxam in pollen, nectar and leaves from seed-dressed cotton crops and their potential risk to honeybees (*Apis mellifera* L.). *Chemosphere* **2018**, *201*, 159. [CrossRef] [PubMed]
23. Li, C.; Chen, J.; Chen, Y.; Wang, J.; Ping, H.; Lu, A. Graphene-Derivatized Silica Composite as Solid-Phase Extraction Sorbent Combined with GC-MS/MS for the Determination of Polycyclic Musks in Aqueous Samples. *Molecules* **2018**, *23*, 318. [CrossRef] [PubMed]
24. Martinello, M.; Baratto, C.; Manzinello, C.; Piva, E.; Borin, A.; Toson, M.; Granato, A.; Boniotti, M.B.; Gallina, A.; Franco, M. Spring mortality in honey bees in northeastern Italy: Detection of pesticides and viruses in dead honey bees and other matrices. *J. Agric. Res.* **2017**, *56*, 239–254.
25. Tosi, S.; Costa, C.; Vesco, U.; Quaglia, G.; Guido, G. A 3-year survey of Italian honey bee-collected pollen reveals widespread contamination by agricultural pesticides. *Sci. Total Environ.* **2018**, *615*, 208–218. [CrossRef] [PubMed]
26. Boi, M.; Serra, G.; Colombo, R.; Lodesani, M.; Massi, S.; Costa, C. A 10 year survey of acaricide residues in beeswax analysed in Italy. *Pest Manag. Sci.* **2016**, *72*, 1366–1372. [CrossRef] [PubMed]
27. Rortais, A.S.; Arnold, G.R.; Halm, M.-P.; Touffet-Briens, F. Modes of honeybees exposure to systemic insecticides: Estimated amounts of contaminated pollen and nectar consumed by different categories of bees. *Apidologie* **2005**, *36*, 71–83. [CrossRef]
28. Chauzat, M.P.; Faucon, J.P. Pesticide residues in beeswax samples collected from honey bee colonies (*Apis mellifera* L.) in France. *Pest. Manag. Sci.* **2007**, *63*, 11001106. [CrossRef] [PubMed]
29. Chauzat, M.P.; Martel, A.C.; Cougoule, N.; Porta, P.; Sarah Zeggane, J.L.; Aubert, M.; Carpentier, P.; Faucon, J.P. An assessment of honeybee colony matrices, *Apis mellifera* (Hymenoptera: Apidae) to monitor pesticide presence in continental France. *Environ. Toxicol. Chem.* **2011**, *30*, 103–111. [CrossRef] [PubMed]
30. Lambert, O.; Piroux, M.; Puyo, S.; Thorin, C.; Thorin, C.; L'Hostis, M.; Wiest, L.; Buleté, A.; Delbac, F.; Pouliquen, H. Widespread occurrence of chemical residues in beehive matrices from apiaries located in different landscapes of Western France. *PLoS ONE* **2013**, *8*, e67007. [CrossRef] [PubMed]
31. Giroud, B.; Vauchez, A.; Vulliet, E.; Wiest, L.; Buleté, A. Trace level determination of pyrethroid and neonicotinoid insecticides in beebread using acetonitrile-based extraction followed by analysis with ultra-high-performance liquid chromatography-tandem mass spectrometry. *J. Chromatogr. A* **2013**, *1316*, 53–61. [CrossRef] [PubMed]
32. Daniele, G.; Giroud, B.; Jabot, C.; Vulliet, E. Exposure assessment of honeybees through study of hive matrices: Analysis of selected pesticide residues in honeybees, beebread, and beeswax from French beehives by LC-MS/MS. *Environ. Sci. Pollut. Res. Int.* **2017**, *25*, 6145–6153. [CrossRef] [PubMed]
33. Lozowicka, B. The development, validation and application of a GC-dual detector (NPD-ECD) multi-pesticide residue method for monitoring bee poisoning incidents. *Ecotoxicol. Environ. Saf.* **2013**, *97*, 210–222. [CrossRef] [PubMed]
34. Barganska, Z.; Slebioda, M.; Namiesnik, J. Determination of pesticide residues in honeybees using modified QUEChERS sample work-up and liquid chromatography-tandem mass spectrometry. *Molecules* **2014**, *19*, 2911–2924. [CrossRef] [PubMed]
35. Kiljanek, T.; Niewiadowska, A.; Gawel, M.; Semeniuk, S.; Borzęcka, M.; Posyniak, A.; Pohorecka, K. Multiple pesticide residues in live and poisoned honeybees—Preliminary exposure assessment. *Chemosphere* **2017**, *175*, 36–44. [CrossRef] [PubMed]
36. Migdał, P.; Roman, A.; Popiela-Pleban, E.; Kowalska-Góralska, M.; Opaliński, S. The Impact of Selected Pesticides on Honey Bees. *Pol. J. Environ. Stud.* **2018**, *27*, 787–792. [CrossRef]

37. Tong, Z.; Wu, Y.C.; Liu, Q.Q.; Shi, Y.H.; Zhou, L.J.; Liu, Z.Y.; Yu, L.S.; Cao, H.Q. Multi-Residue Analysis of Pesticide Residues in Crude Pollens by UPLC-MS/MS. *Molecules* **2016**, *21*, 1652. [CrossRef] [PubMed]
38. Campbell, P.J.; Brown, K.C.; Harrison, E.G.; Bakker, F.; Barrett, K.L.; Candolfi, M.P.; Canez, V.; Dinter, A.; Lewis, G.; Mead-Briggs, M.; et al. A hazard quotient approach for assessing the risk to non-target arthropods from. *J. Pest Sci.* **2000**, *73*, 117.
39. Environmental Risk Assessment for Plant Protection Products. PP 3/10 (3): Chapter 10: Honeybees. *EPPO Bull.* **2010**, *40*, 323–331. [CrossRef]
40. Stoner, K.A.; Eitzer, B.D. Using a hazard quotient to evaluate pesticide residues detected in pollen trapped from honey bees (*Apis mellifera*) in Connecticut. *PLoS ONE* **2013**, *8*, e77550. [CrossRef] [PubMed]
41. Walorczyk, S.; Gnusowski, B. Development and validation of a multi-residue method for the determination of pesticides in honeybees using acetonitrile-based extraction and gas chromatography-tandem quadrupole mass spectrometry. *J. Chromatogr. A* **2009**, *1216*, 6522–6531. [CrossRef] [PubMed]
42. Kong, W.J.; Liu, Q.T.; Kong, D.D.; Liu, Q.Z.; Ma, X.P.; Yang, M.H. Trace analysis of multi-class pesticide residues in Chinese medicinal health wines using gas chromatography with electron capture detection. *Sci. Rep.* **2016**, *6*, 21558. [CrossRef] [PubMed]
43. Sanchez-Bayo, F.; Goka, K. Pesticide residues and bees—A risk assessment. *PLoS ONE* **2014**, *9*, e94482. [CrossRef] [PubMed]
44. Hermansson, J. Biology of the diamondback moth (*Plutella xylostella*) and its future impact in Swedish oilseed rape production. *Swedish Univ. Agric. Sci.* **2016**, *15*, 1–44.
45. Simondelso, N.; San, M.G.; Bruneau, E.; Minsart, L.A.; Mouret, C.; Hautier, L. Honeybee colony disorder in crop areas: The role of pesticides and viruses. *PLoS ONE* **2013**, *9*, e103073.
46. Pilling, E.D.; Bromleychallenor, K.A.C.; Walker, C.H.; Jepson, P.C. Mechanism of Synergism between the Pyrethroid Insecticide λ-Cyhalothrin and the Imidazole Fungicide Prochloraz, in the Honeybee (*Apis mellifera* L.). *Pest. Biochem. Physiol.* **1995**, *51*, 1–11. [CrossRef]

Sample Availability: Samples of the rape flowers are available from the authors.

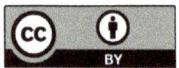

© 2018 by the authors. Licensee MDPI, Basel, Switzerland. This article is an open access article distributed under the terms and conditions of the Creative Commons Attribution (CC BY) license (http://creativecommons.org/licenses/by/4.0/).

MDPI
St. Alban-Anlage 66
4052 Basel
Switzerland
Tel. +41 61 683 77 34
Fax +41 61 302 89 18
www.mdpi.com

Molecules Editorial Office
E-mail: molecules@mdpi.com
www.mdpi.com/journal/molecules